PRAISE FOR *EATING FOR LOWER CHOLESTEROL*

"This wonderful guide artfully choreographs exp[...] reducing tactics with tasty recipes that all will enjoy."
— MEHMET OZ, MD, Coauth[...]ler
YOU: The Owner's M[...]dy
that [...]ger

"Jones and Trujillo offer a rich blend of recipes and reason: what to eat and why. I highly recommend it as a practical, healthy eating guide for the whole family."
— MALCOLM K. ROBINSON, MD, Director, Metabolic Support Service and the Program for Weight Management, Department of Surgery, Brigham and Women's Hospital, Harvard Medical School

"The sound bytes of nutritional medicine are easy-to-read, evidence-based, and up-to-date. No new scientific findings have been missed in this book! . . . A must-have for anyone interested in healthy eating for lower cholesterol and other nutrition-based disorders, such as hypertension, diabetes, and obesity . . . A big plus are the nutritional guidelines for children and adolescents, who may also suffer from cholesterol disorders and obesity. This book acknowledges the fact that preventative medicine is the best medicine for young America."
— CAROLINE M. APOVIAN, MD, FACN, Associate Professor of Medicine, Boston University School of Medicine, Director, Nutrition and Weight Management Center, Boston Medical Center

"Jones and Trujillo prove that lowering one's cholesterol does not have to require sacrifice. A bit of focus and these great recipes will do the rest. Bon appétit!"
— ERIC RIPERT, Chef and Co-owner of Le Bernardin, New York City

"An excellent resource for people who need to lower their cholesterol, as well as for people who want to keep their healthy cholesterol levels in check. This book is the perfect collaboration between a world-class chef and a talented dietitian/nutrition educator . . ."
— PENNY KRIS-ETHERTON, PHD, RD, Distinguished Professor of Nutrition, Department of Nutritional Sciences, Penn State University

"As a practicing cardiologist for twenty-five years I am always looking for tools to help my patients achieve their cardiac risk factor objectives. . . . Jones and Trujillo successfully intertwine nutritional and scientific information with a robust menu to accomplish the task. . . . I will wholeheartedly recommend this book to my patients."
— DENNIS C. FRIEDMAN, MD, FACC, Director of Cardiac Rehabilitation at Shady Grove Adventist Hospital, Medical Director of Cardiology

"In a world where childhood obesity is reaching epic proportions, parents need practical resources to create a healthy home. Whether it's cutting cholesterol or looking for creative ways to bring back the family meal, *Eating for Lower Cholesterol* serves up heart-healthy, family-friendly recipes with a side of invaluable, up-to-date nutrition information. It's a must-have for every parent's cookbook collection."

—LISA TARTAMELLA KIMMEL, MS, RD, Coauthor of
Generation Extra Large: Rescuing Our Children from the Epidemic of Obesity,
and Outpatient Nutrition Coordinator, Yale-New Haven Hospital

"*Eating for Lower Cholesterol* provides a scientifically-based, balanced approach to good nutrition and overall better health. The authors have presented a well-researched guide that provides practical nutrition information on a variety of heart-health topics. . . . This book is a wonderful resource for the entire family and brings back the joy of eating!"

—KATHY MCMANUS, MS, RD, Director, Department of Nutrition,
Brigham and Women's Hospital

"Finally, a useful resource that bridges the gap between nutrition and practice! A must-have reference for anyone working to improve their health through diet."

—CHRISTINA FERROLI, PhD, RD, Community Nutritionist,
Editor of *The Digest*, Public Health/Community Nutrition Practice Group

"*Eating for Lower Cholesterol* is so much more than just a cookbook . . . The introduction is an outstanding explanation of how our diet contributes to heart disease. The recipes are interspersed with tips, hints, and great ideas—you won't want to miss a single one. . . . Fresh herbs, enticing salsas and marinades, new ingredients and familiar ones . . . I can't wait to try them all!"

—SUSAN S. PERCIVAL, PhD, Professor, Nutritional Sciences,
University of Florida

"I recommend this book to everyone—with or without heart disease! So many delicious recipes that are heart healthy! I loved the Stocking a Heart Healthy Pantry section. I plan to use this book as a resource for our cardiac patients."

—BARBARA COURTNEY, MS, RCEP, Manager,
Cardiac Rehabilitation & EECP Center,
Shady Grove Adventist Hospital

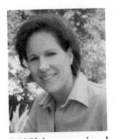

Catherine Jones, an award-winning cookbook author and food writer, graduated from La Varenne Culinary School in France and worked with the late renowned chef Jean-Louis Palladin. Her first book, *A Year of Russian Feasts* (Jellyroll Press, 2002), won *Foreword* magazine's Book of the Year Travel Essay Award and *Writer's Digest* Best Cookbook Award, and it was a finalist for the International Association of Culinary Professionals Julia Child Cookbook Award. Her cookbook *Eating for Pregnancy: An Essential Guide to Nutrition with Recipes for the Whole Family* (Marlowe and Company, 2003) has received many accolades. The daughter of a retired diplomat and wife of a foreign service officer, Jones has seen much of the world but calls Bethesda, Maryland, home. She and her family were on assignment in Vienna, Austria, when she completed this book. They currently live in Manila, the Philippines. Jones is the mother of an eight-year-old daughter and a five-year-old son.

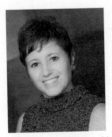

Elaine B. Trujillo, MS, RD, CNSD, is a national leader in nutrition and a certified nutrition support dietitian. She worked for ten years at the Brigham and Women's Hospital (named one of the top ten hospitals in the country by *U.S. News and World Report,* 2004), Harvard Medical School, where she was the lead dietitian responsible for patient investigation in metabolic and nutrition studies and was editor of a newsletter and a reviewer of several national nutrition journals. She has contributed to numerous publications and has lectured nationally and internationally. Currently she is at the National Cancer Institute, National Institutes of Health, and at the Cardiac Rehabilitation and EECP Center, Shady Grove Adventist Hospital in Rockville, Maryland. She is the mother of a twelve-year-old son and ten-year-old daughter. Trujillo and her family live in Rockville, Maryland.

CATHERINE JONES with
ELAINE B. TRUJILLO, MS, RD, CNSD

EATING FOR
LOWER CHOLESTEROL

*A Balanced Approach to Heart Health
with Recipes Everyone Will Love*

MARLOWE AND COMPANY
NEW YORK

EATING FOR LOWER CHOLESTEROL:
A Balanced Approach to Heart Health with Recipes Everyone Will Love

Copyright © 2005 by Catherine C. G. Jones

Marlowe & Company
An Imprint of Avalon Publishing Group Incorporated
245 West 17th Street • 11th Floor
New York, NY 10011-5300

AVALON
publishing group incorporated

Library of Congress Cataloging-in-Print data is available.

ISBN 1-56924-376-X
ISBN-13: 978-1-56924-376-3

9   8   7   6   5   4   3   2   1

Designed by Pauline Neuwirth, Neuwirth & Associates, Inc.

Printed in the United States of America

For all hearts, young and old

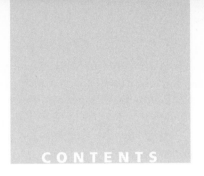

CONTENTS

EATING FOR
LOWER CHOLESTEROL

𝒯he phone rang. It was my brother Mark.

"Hi, Cathy. You're not going to believe this. Mom just had a heart attack. We're at the hospital now. She's okay. We're waiting for the test results to see if there was any heart damage."

"When did this happen? How *could* this happen?" I asked as tears welled in my eyes.

"Mom said she had chest pains at around four in the morning, but she waited until six to wake me up to drive her to the hospital," Mark said. That sounds like mom, I thought to myself.

My brother went on, "She told me she had chest pains earlier in the week but thought she just pulled a muscle wallpapering the bathroom. On Friday, they got so bad she called 911. The paramedics came and tried to take her to the hospital, but she wouldn't go. She told them that she was feeling better and signed a release form. She promised to see her doctor that afternoon, but she never did. She was too busy. Too busy! Can you believe it?!"

"Yes, I can," I said.

A week later I flew to New Hampshire to take care of my mom when she got out of the hospital. I was responsible for making sure she followed a heart-healthy diet and did her exercises. I felt like the food police and a drill sergeant rolled into one. Ironically, it was my mother who had taught me the pleasures of cooking when I was a little girl. And now here I was telling her she couldn't eat her favorite foods. In her mind, food was to enjoy, not to be measured in calories, grams of saturated fat, or milligrams of cholesterol. As for cardiovascular exercise, she considered housework and running errands exercise enough.

Soon after I returned home, I took my slender seven-year-old daughter, Allie, to her pediatrician for her annual checkup. I was shocked when he told me that her cholesterol levels were high.

"Do you have a family history of heart disease?" Dr. Balfour asked.

I couldn't believe this was happening—first my mom, then my daughter. Both of them needed cholesterol-lowering diets and I was still struggling to understand the basics of cholesterol and heart disease. What I wanted at that moment was for someone to explain LDL, HDL, triglycerides, saturated fats, omega-3 fatty acids, and partially hydrogenated oil so I could understand it all. I wanted someone to tell me what foods can raise or lower cholesterol levels and how to design heart-healthy meal plans. Plus, I wanted information on cholesterol for kids and women in particular. I found Elaine B. Trujillo, a nutritionist, who answered all of my questions and explained complicated terms in understandable words.

We decided to put our talents together to write *Eating for Lower Cholesterol.* Elaine provided the nutrition information, and, using her guidelines, I created a collection of fabulous heart-healthy recipes. I spent a summer in New Hampshire cooking with my mother, convincing her that fine cuisine can exist without butter or cream. She had some excellent ideas of her own, and together we discovered ways to cook new foods—such as buffalo, Piedmontese beef, ostrich, whole grains, egg substitutes, and tofu—and how to make old favorites heart-friendlier. We proved to ourselves, and to family and friends who dined with us, that eating can still be a pleasure if you are on a cholesterol-lowering diet.

I learned one more thing. Heart disease is the leading cause of death among American women, as well as men. It is vital to know the symptoms of a heart attack (see page 6), to listen to your body, and, if something just does not feel right, to go to the doctor, or call 911. Please don't wait, like my mother did! The earlier we begin to take care of our hearts, and those of our children, the healthier we will all be.

A FEW WORDS FROM
Elaine B. Trujillo

My parents are first-generation Americans. My Irish mother learned to cook Italian cuisine when she met my father, and food always seemed to take center stage. If we weren't eating, we were talking about eating. At lunch we discussed what we would eat for dinner, and at the Thanksgiving table we planned our Christmas feast.

When I met my husband, Roberto, who is a physician and scientist, I knew I had my work cut out for me. His idea of the perfect breakfast was cheesecake and chocolate milk, and he looked forward to a cheeseburger with fries for dinner. Although his meal choices have improved quite a bit over the years, he is stuck with his genetic predisposition for high cholesterol.

Roberto was born in Mexico, and his mother, Lupita, is the best Mexican cook I know— everyone who has tasted her lemon chicken (page 198) agrees! Not until my mother-in-law developed high blood pressure did she realize that food does not need to be highly salted to taste good. She has taught me, among other things, how Mexican food, with all of its wonderful spices and chile peppers, can easily be flavored without salt.

The need to focus on a heart-healthy diet and lifestyle was further personalized when my children, ages ten and twelve, were diagnosed with high cholesterol. A dietitian's worst nightmare! I had thought I was doing everything right with them. I certainly had more control over their diets than over my husband's, but again, genetics came into play.

I make sure my family eats a lot of vegetables and fruits, whole grains, lean meats and fish, low-fat dairy products, and (when I can sneak them in) soy products. I put into practice the same cholesterol guidelines that I am giving you. I've also taught my kids about the importance of eating healthy foods, and I've noticed that now they avoid most junk food on their own.

I began working at the Shady Grove Adventist Hospital, Cardiac Rehabilitation & EECP Center when I moved from Boston to Maryland. I knew I was going to like it when I first stepped in the door—music was blaring and everyone was exercising. My job was to walk around the room and talk nutrition in a nonthreatening manner, a very different approach from that of most hospital settings.

When Catherine Jones shared her book idea with me, I was excited at the prospect of compiling a comprehensive work that would integrate nutrition information for lowering cholesterol with healthy and, more important, tasty recipes. I often counsel my patients together with their husbands, wives, children, or other family members. As I am talking, someone inevitably jots down notes, and usually the cook in the family asks me for recipes and meal plans. Now I can give them *Eating for Lower Cholesterol*.

There is no better way to take control of your diet than to learn what foods are good for you, to shop wisely, and to cook at home. While I hope this book helps you understand the importance of lowering your cholesterol, I also hope you discover that eating and cooking for a healthy heart can be easy, delicious, and fun.

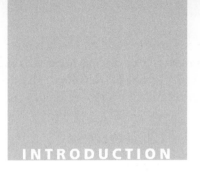

UNDERSTANDING CHOLESTEROL
AND HEART DISEASE

Welcome to the world of cholesterol! The following questions and answers are designed to help you understand what cholesterol is and how it relates to heart disease; what "your numbers" mean; factors that raise cholesterol levels and increase your risk of heart disease; treatments for high cholesterol; cholesterol in children; cholesterol in women; a condition called metabolic syndrome; and ways to control high blood pressure. These are all complex and confusing issues. Specific questions or concerns about your cholesterol levels or heart health should be addressed to your doctor or health-care provider.

How Does High Cholesterol Cause Heart Disease?

Cholesterol is a fat-like substance in your blood that builds up in the walls of your arteries. Cholesterol is normal, and cholesterol is used by your body for producing cell membranes and some hormones. Over time, however, high levels of cholesterol can cause plaque, or "hardening of the arteries." When this happens, the coronary arteries, which carry oxygen to the heart, become narrow and blood flow to the heart is slowed down or blocked. If there is not enough blood and oxygen reaching your heart, you may suffer chest pain, and if the blood supply to the heart is completely cut off, the result is a heart attack. If blood flow to the brain is blocked, this may result in a stroke.

Cholesterol and other fats do not dissolve in your blood. They are transported to and from the cells by special carriers called lipoproteins. The low-density lipoprotein (LDL) is known as the "bad" cholesterol. Too much of it can clog your arteries. High-density lipoprotein (HDL) is known as the "good" cholesterol. It carries cholesterol away from your arteries so it can be removed by your liver. High levels of HDL cholesterol may lessen your risk of a heart attack. Lowering cholesterol levels that are too high reduces the risk for developing heart disease and the chance of a heart attack. This is important for everyone, men, women, and children.

Where Does Cholesterol Come From?

Your body makes some cholesterol in the liver, and the rest comes from cholesterol in animal products that you eat, such as meats, poultry, fish, eggs, butter, cheese, and whole milk. Saturated fat from animal products and some tropical oils, such as palm kernel and coconut oil, as well as trans fats, found in stick margarines and many processed foods, are harmful because they cause your body to produce more cholesterol. *Plant foods such as fruits, vegetables, vegetable oils, and grains, do not have cholesterol.*

What Do the Numbers Mean?

Total cholesterol is the most common measurement of blood cholesterol. It is the number you normally receive as a test result, an important first step in determining your risk for heart disease. However, a critical second step is having a blood test called a "lipoprotein profile," which gives information about LDL cholesterol, HDL cholesterol, and triglycerides, as well as total cholesterol. Cholesterol levels are measured in milligrams (mg) of cholesterol per deciliter (dL) of blood. See the chart below to determine your cholesterol category.

CHOLESTEROL LEVELS AND CATEGORIES[1]

TOTAL CHOLESTEROL LEVEL	CATEGORY
Less than 200 mg/dL	Desirable
200–239 mg/dL	Borderline High
240 mg/dL and above	High

LDL CHOLESTEROL LEVEL	CATEGORY
Less than 100 mg/dL	Optimal
100–129 mg/dL	Near Optimal
130–159 mg/dL	Borderline High
160–189 mg/dL	High
190 mg/dL and above	Very high

HDL CHOLESTEROL LEVELS	CATEGORY
Less than 40 mg/dL	A major risk factor of heart disease
40-59 mg/dL	The higher these numbers, the better
60 mg/dL and above	Considered protective against heart disease

LDL, or bad cholesterol, is a better indicator of the potential risk of a heart attack than total blood cholesterol. The lower your LDL level, the lower your risk. Low HDL, or good cholesterol, can also put you at high risk for heart disease. In general, men have lower HDL levels. Most men have HDL levels in the range of 40 to 50 mg/dL, and most women in the range of 50 to 60 mg/dL. Smoking, being overweight, and being sedentary can all result in lower HDL cholesterol. You can help raise HDL levels by not smoking, by losing weight or maintaining a healthy weight, and by being physically active.

The ratio of total cholesterol to HDL cholesterol is sometimes used in place of total blood cholesterol. The ratio is obtained by dividing into the total cholesterol by the HDL cholesterol level. The goal is to keep the ratio below 5:1, and optimally at 3.5:1.

What Are Trigycerides and Acceptable Triglyceride Levels?

Triglycerides are the form in which most fat exists in food, as well as in your body. They are present in your blood and, along with cholesterol, form lipids in your blood. The calories that your body and tissues do not use immediately after eating are converted to triglycerides and transported to fat cells to be stored. Triglycerides are released from fat tissue in your body to meet the body's energy needs between meals.

High levels of triglycerides can raise your risk for heart disease. Levels that are between 150 and 199 mg/dL are borderline high. Levels that are 200 mg/dL or more are considered high and may require treatment with medication. For children two to nine years old, triglycerides should be less than or equal to 150 mg/dL. The following factors can increase triglyceride levels:

◆ Being overweight
◆ Physical inactivity
◆ Cigarette smoking
◆ Excessive alcohol use
◆ Very high carbohydrate diet
◆ Certain diseases and drugs
◆ Genetic disorders

How Often Do I Need to Have My Cholesterol and My Children's Cholesterol Checked?

Because there are no signs or symptoms of high cholesterol, most people do not know that their levels are elevated until they have a routine blood test. The cholesterol level of adults over the age of twenty should be measured at least once every five years. Cholesterol screening and the adoption of heart-healthy habits by young adults and children may be particularly valuable in delaying the development of heart disease later in life. Adults and children who especially need to have their levels checked include those with:

- ◆ Obesity
- ◆ Diabetes
- ◆ A family history of early heart disease
- ◆ At least one parent with high cholesterol

Cholesterol guidelines for children are different from those for adults (see Cholesterol Guidelines for Children). Your child's doctor or health-care provider is the best resource for concerns about your child's heart health. For more information on cholesterol in children, see Sources, page 265.

CHOLESTEROL GUIDELINES FOR CHILDREN AND ADOLESCENTS TWO TO NINETEEN YEARS OLD[2]

	DESIRABLE	BORDERLINE	HIGHER RISK
Total Cholesterol	<170	170–199	≥200
LDL Cholesterol	<110	110–129	≥130
HDL Cholesterol	Levels should be greater than or equal to 35 mg/dL		

Is a Low-Fat Diet Safe for Children?

A low-fat diet is safe for children older than two years, *but do not restrict fat and cholesterol in children less than two years of age, because fat is essential for normal growth and development.* Compelling evidence shows that the atherosclerotic process, or the buildup of fatty plaque in artery walls, begins in childhood and progresses slowly into adulthood.[3] The American Heart Association found that a low-fat diet, defined as no more than 30 percent of calories coming from fat, with 8 to 10 percent of calories from saturated fat and a cholesterol intake of less than 300 mg per day, is safe for the majority of children and will ultimately result in a lower frequency of heart disease in the general population.[4]

What Are the Risk Factors for Developing High Cholesterol?

- ◆ **Diet** A diet that is high in saturated fat, trans fats, and cholesterol can make your blood cholesterol levels go up. Conversely, reducing saturated fat and cholesterol in your diet helps lower blood cholesterol levels.
- ◆ **Weight** Being overweight can increase your blood cholesterol levels and increase your risk for heart disease. The good news is that losing weight can lower your total cholesterol, LDL cholesterol, and triglyceride levels, and it can also increase your HDL cholesterol levels.
- ◆ **Physical Activity** Being physically inactive is a risk factor for heart disease. Regular exercise can help lower LDL cholesterol and raise HDL cholesterol levels.

- ◆ **Age and Gender** As people get older, their cholesterol levels rise. Before menopause, women have lower total cholesterol levels than men of the same age. After menopause, women's LDL levels tend to rise.
- ◆ **Heredity** Your genetic background, at least in part, determines how much cholesterol your body makes.

What Factors Increase the Chances of Developing Heart Disease or Having a Heart Attack?

- ◆ High LDL cholesterol levels
- ◆ Low HDL cholesterol, of less than 40 mg/dL
- ◆ A family history of early heart disease (heart disease in a father or a brother before age fifty-five; heart disease in a mother or sister before age sixty-five)
- ◆ High blood pressure, 140/90 mmHg or higher, or being on blood pressure medication
- ◆ Age (for men, forty-five years or older; for women, fifty-five years or older)
- ◆ Cigarette smoking

How Is High Blood Cholesterol Treated?

The main goal of any cholesterol-lowering treatment, with or without medication, is to reduce LDL cholesterol levels. The usual course of treatment is to follow a cholesterol-lowering diet, to increase physical activity, and to lose weight, if necessary, or maintain a healthy weight. In addition, drug treatment may be needed to help lower LDL levels. For more information on when it is necessary to initiate diet, physical activity, and weight management and when you should consider drug therapy, see Risk Categories, LDL Cholesterol Goals, and Therapy, page 256.

What Cholesterol-Lowering Medications Are Currently Available?

Keep in mind that even if you begin drug treatment, you will still need to continue to follow a cholesterol-lowering diet, to engage in physical activity, and to manage your weight. *Drug treatment can control but does not "cure" high blood cholesterol.*

Five Major Types of Cholesterol-Lowering Medicines

- ◆ *Statins:* very effective in lowering LDL cholesterol levels, and safe for most people.
- ◆ *Bile Acid Sequestrants:* help lower LDL cholesterol levels; they are usually prescribed with another cholesterol-lowering medicine, such as statins.
- ◆ *Nicotinic Acid:* lowers LDL cholesterol and triglycerides and raises HDL cholesterol.
- ◆ *Fibrates:* lowers triglycerides and may increase HDL cholesterol levels; when used with a statin, they may increase the chances of muscle side effects.

◆ *Ezetimibe:* acts within the intestine to block cholesterol absorption, thereby lowering LDL cholesterol; it may be used with statins or alone.

Do Women Need to Worry about Their Cholesterol Levels and Heart Disease?

Yes. Heart disease is the leading cause of death in American women, and about half a million women each year die from heart disease. The increased risk of heart disease in women occurs after menopause, when levels of the female hormone estrogen are reduced. Estrogen is associated with higher levels of HDL cholesterol and lower levels of LDL cholesterol, so its protective effect is lessened after menopause. It was once thought that hormone replacement therapy (HRT) would be a promising option for women, but in recent major studies not only did HRT not prevent heart disease, it was found to result in higher rates of some cancers.

It is important to note that women and men may exhibit different symptoms when having a heart attack. Where most men may feel chest pain or discomfort on the left side or other areas of the upper body, women tend to feel a burning sensation in their upper abdomen and may also experience lightheadedness, upset stomach, and sweating. A woman may not even know she is having a heart attack, dismissing the symptoms as indigestion or an upset stomach. Heart attacks are generally more severe in women, and women are 50 percent more likely than men to die in the first year after a heart attack. *If you have any inkling that you or someone else is having a heart attack, call 911 immediately—every minute that passes without treatment means that more heart muscle dies.*

Heart Attack Signs

GENERAL WARNING SIGNS

◆ Discomfort in the center of the chest that lasts for more than a few minutes or that goes away and comes back. It can feel like uncomfortable pressure, squeezing, fullness, or pain.
◆ Discomfort in other areas of the upper body, such as one or both arms, the back, jaw, or stomach.
◆ Shortness of breath, which often accompanies chest discomfort; it can also occur before chest discomfort.
◆ Breaking out in a cold sweat, nausea, or lightheadedness.

WARNING SIGNS ESPECIALLY FOR WOMEN

◆ Pain or discomfort in the center of the chest.
◆ Pain or discomfort in other areas of the upper body, including the arms, back, neck, jaw, or stomach.
◆ Shortness of breath, breaking out in a cold sweat, nausea, severe vomiting, abnormal fatigue, or lightheadedness.

The Heart Truth Campaign and its red dress symbol is a national program to raise awareness of heart disease in women. A collection of nineteen red dresses from America's most prestigious designers symbolizes the critical nature of heart disease in women. To learn more about the program, go to www.nhlbi.nih.gov/health/hearttruth.

What Is Metabolic Syndrome, and Who Is at Risk for Developing It?

Some important risk factors for heart disease include high lipid levels, high blood pressure, high blood sugar, and obesity. When these occur simultaneously the combination is known as metabolic syndrome, or insulin resistance syndrome. Other factors may also play a role in developing insulin resistance, such as obesity in the abdominal area, physical inactivity, a family history of type 2 diabetes, heart disease, polycystic ovarian syndrome, and ethnic background (Hispanic Americans, African Americans, Asian Americans, and some Native Americans are more vulnerable).

Insulin resistance occurs when the body does not respond naturally to insulin and, therefore, not enough blood sugar is passed into cells where it can be used by the body. The result is that fats and proteins are not metabolized normally, and the process of hardening of the arteries begins, increasing the risk of cardiovascular disease. Up to 20 percent of Americans have metabolic syndrome, and about one in four of them will go on to develop type 2 diabetes. In people with type 2 diabetes, the pancreas can no longer secrete sufficient insulin to maintain normal blood sugar levels. People who develop type 2 diabetes have a two to four times greater risk of heart disease.

One reason why so many Americans are now developing metabolic syndrome and type 2 diabetes is that the number of people, both adults and children, who are overweight or obese has increased markedly in the past thirty years. It is estimated that 65 percent of adults and 16 percent of children ages twelve to nineteen years old are now overweight or obese. But with proper diet and moderate exercise, millions of overweight Americans at high risk for metabolic syndrome and type 2 diabetes can delay, and possibly prevent, their onset.

What Is High Blood Pressure and What Can I Do About It?

Blood pressure refers to the force of blood against the artery walls. It is recorded as two numbers, systolic (as the heart beats) over diastolic (as the heart relaxes between beats). When blood pressure levels are elevated over time, the resulting condition is high blood pressure, or hypertension.

CLASSIFICATION OF BLOOD PRESSURE

Category	Systolic Blood Pressure		Diastolic Blood Pressure
Normal	<120	and	<80
Prehypertension	120–139	or	80–89
Hypertension, Stage 1	140–159	or	90–99
Hypertension, Stage 2	≥160	or	≥100

High blood pressure occurs in about one out of every four American adults, and studies indicate that it is rising in children. It is especially common in African Americans. It becomes more common as people get older or when they gain weight. High blood pressure can be prevented and controlled, whether you are on medication or not, by maintaining a healthy weight, being physically active, and following a healthy eating plan. If you are at risk for heart disease, be sure to have your blood pressure checked often.

STAY BALANCED: A HEART-HEALTHY WAY OF EATING

EATING FOR LOWER cholesterol and a healthy heart is not as difficult as it may sound—and it does not require becoming a health freak or a vegetarian. Just a few simple changes can lower your cholesterol levels and, in turn, provide significant cardiac benefits.

The Stay Balanced Scale below, designed for this book by Elaine B. Trujillo, MS, RD, CNSD, is geared for people who are trying to lower their cholesterol levels; but anyone, with elevated cholesterol or not, will benefit from following a heart-healthy diet. The basic premise of the Stay Balanced Scale is that your intake of calories from healthy foods should be balanced by exercise that burns off those calories.

In 2005, the U.S. Department of Agriculture established a new personalized food pyramid, called My Pyramid, as part of the New Dietary Guidelines for Americans. My Pyramid is designed to enable you to compute the amount of food *you* need daily based on your gender, age, weight, and activity level. Customized pyramids are a huge step in the right direction, and millions of Americans can potentially benefit from this new approach.

However, for an eating plan that specifically targets lowering your cholesterol, we suggest using the Stay Balanced Scale in conjunction with the Daily Calorie Guidelines listed below. The list of Stay Balanced Food Groups that follows the scale outlines the types and amounts of food you should consume while staying within your calorie range. To help you with meal planning, a list of Food Groups and Sample Serving Sizes and Three Stay Balanced Sample Menus can be found in the Appendix, pages 257 to 260.

15 Simple Recommendations to Help You Stay Balanced

◆ Follow the guidelines in the Stay Balanced Scale while staying within your calorie allowance.

◆ Eat an abundance of vegetables and fruits.

◆ Eat whole grains instead of refined grains.

◆ Choose heart-healthy unsaturated fats from plant sources.

◆ Reduce your intake of saturated fats.

◆ Consume seafood high in omega-3 fatty acids.

◆ Eat nutrient-dense, low-fat soy protein, such as tofu or soy yogurt.

◆ Choose the leanest white and red meats, and watch portion sizes.

◆ Take a multivitamin with minerals daily.

◆ If you drink alcoholic beverages, do so in moderation—up to one drink per day for women, up to two drinks per day for men. One drink equals 12 ounces of regular beer, 5 ounces of wine, or 1½ ounces of 80-proof distilled spirits.

◆ Consume less than 2,300 mg of sodium per day. Choose and prepare foods with little salt. Individuals with hypertension, African Americans, and middle-aged and older adults should aim to consume no more than 1,500 mg of sodium per day.

◆ Avoid foods that contain trans fats or partially hydrogenated oil, such as processed foods.

◆ Limit consumption of refined carbohydrates and foods that contain high-fructose corn syrup, such as sodas, candy bars, and other junk food.

◆ Avoid fast food, especially the "value combos," which are loaded with fats and calories.

◆ Make daily exercise a priority.

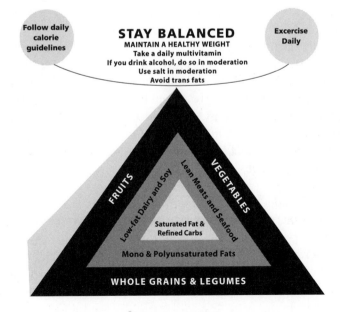

Stay Balanced Food Groups and Daily Serving Sizes

Fruits

1 TO 2¹/₂ CUPS, OR 2 TO 5 SERVINGS, *PER DAY*

Choose a variety of fruits that provide a range of vitamins and minerals. Fruits high in folic acid are particularly good for your heart. Some examples include bananas, blackberries, cantaloupe, citrus fruits, honeydew melon, papaya, raspberries, and strawberries.

Vegetables

1 TO 4 CUPS, OR 2 TO 8 SERVINGS, *PER DAY*

Choose a variety of vegetables that provide a range of vitamins and minerals. Vegetables high in folic acid are particularly good for your heart. Some examples include asparagus, beets, broccoli, brussel sprouts, corn, peas, romaine lettuce, squash, and tomato juice.

Whole Grains and Legumes

3 TO 10 SERVINGS *PER DAY*, INCLUDING AT LEAST ¹/₂ TO 3¹/₂ CUPS PER WEEK OF LEGUMES, SUCH AS BEANS, LENTILS, AND CHICKPEAS

Because whole grains have less folate than enriched refined grains (unless the whole grain has been fortified with folic acid), include some folate-fortified products, such as folate-fortified whole-grain cereals.

Low-Fat Dairy

3 SERVINGS, OR 3 CUPS LOW-FAT OR FAT-FREE PRODUCTS, *PER DAY*

Dairy products are an excellent source of calcium and heart-healthy B vitamins.

Soy

25 GRAMS OF SOY PROTEIN *PER DAY*

Soy is a low-fat, cholesterol-free source of protein that can be consumed instead of lean meat or seafood. Soy milk can also replace cow's milk and yogurt in the low-fat dairy food group. Always opt for enriched soy milk that has been fortified with calcium, vitamins A, D, and B_{12}, and riboflavin. *For children under the age of two, do not, unless under the guidance of a health-care professional, substitute soy milk for cow's milk, because infants and toddlers need more fat for development.*

Lean Meats and Seafood

2 TO 7 OUNCES (TOTAL) OF LEAN MEATS, FISH OR SHELLFISH, AND/OR EGGS OR EGG SUBSTITUTES *PER DAY*

At least twice a week, choose fatty fish and shellfish that are high in omega-3 fatty acids, such as wild salmon, albacore tuna, trout, shrimp, and scallops. Soy products, such as tofu and soy burgers, can be substituted for lean meats and seafood.

Monounsaturated and Polyunsaturated Fats
4 TO 13 SERVINGS, *PER DAY*

Keep the total fat intake between 20 to 35 percent of calories, with most fats coming in the form of monounsaturated, polyunsaturated, and omega-3 fatty acids. Sources of these heart-healthy fats include salad dressings, peanut butter, mayonnaise, avocados, olives, nuts, seeds, and vegetable oils. Some sample serving sizes include 1 tablespoon low-fat mayonnaise, 1 tablespoon peanut butter, 2 tablespoons reduced-fat salad dressing, 1 teaspoon soft margarine, and 1 teaspoon vegetable oil.

Saturated Fats
MINIMIZE CONSUMPTION

Consume less than 7 percent of calories from saturated fat and no more than 200 mg/day of cholesterol. Avoid products with trans fats or partially hydrogenated oil.

Refined Carbohydrates
MINIMIZE CONSUMPTION

Consume fewer refined carbohydrates and foods and beverages that contain added sugars and high-fructose corn syrup, such as sodas, junk food, white rice, and white bread. These products can make your blood sugar and insulin levels shoot up and then crash, which may ultimately lead to increased feelings of hunger, and weight gain. Whole-grain products have a gentler effect on your blood sugar. Avoid adding sugar to beverages.

Special Stay Balanced Recommendations for Children and Adolescents

◆ Eat lots of fruits and vegetables.
◆ Consume whole-grain products often; at least half of all grains should be whole grains.
◆ Children from two to eight years old should consume 2 cups per day of fat-free or low-fat milk or milk products. Children nine years of age and older should consume 3 cups per day of these products.
◆ Keep total fat intake at between 30 and 35 percent of daily calories for children two to three years old and between 25 and 35 percent for children and adolescents four to eighteen years old, with most fats coming in the form of polyunsaturated, monounsaturated, and omega-3 fatty acids, from sources such as fish, nuts, and vegetable oils.
◆ Limit saturated fats and avoid foods that contain trans fats or partially hydrogenated oil.
◆ Limit consumption of refined carbohydrates and foods that contain high-fructose corn syrup, such as sodas, candy bars, and other junk food.

- Avoid fast food, especially "value combos," which are loaded with fats and calories.
- Exercise daily for at least 60 minutes.

DAILY CALORIE GUIDELINES
ESTIMATED CALORIE REQUIREMENTS FOR GENDER AND AGE GROUP

			ACTIVITY LEVEL[a]	
GENDER	AGE (YEARS)	SEDENTARY[b]	MODERATELY ACTIVE[c]	ACTIVE[d]
Child	2–3	1,000	1,000–1,400[e]	1,000–1,400
Female	4–8	1,200	1,400–1,600	1,400–1,800
	9–13	1,600	1,600–2,000	1,800–2,200
	14–18	1,800	2,000	2,400
	19–30	2,000	2,000–2,200	2,400
	31–50	1,800	2,000	2,200
	51+	1,600	1,800	2,000–2,200
Male	4–8	1,400	1,400–1,600	1,600–2,000
	9–13	1,800	1,800–2,200	2,000–2,600
	14–18	2,200	2,400–2,800	2,800–3,200
	19–30	2,400	2,600–2,800	3,000
	31–50	2,200	2,400–2,600	2,800–3,000
	51+	2,000	2,200–2,400	2,400–2,800

[a] These levels are based on Estimated Energy Requirements (EER) from the Institute of Medicine (IOM) Dietary Reference Intakes Macronutrients Report, 2002, calculated by gender, age, and activity level for reference-sized individuals. "Reference size," as determined by IOM, is based on median height and weight for ages up to 18 years of age and median height and weight for that height to give a BMI of 21.5 for adult females and 22.5 for adult males.
[b] Sedentary means a lifestyle that includes only the light physical activity associated with typical daily life.
[c] Moderately active means a lifestyle that includes physical activity equivalent to walking about 1.5 to 3 miles a day at 3 to 4 miles per hour, in addition to the light physical activity associated with typical daily life.
[d] Active means a lifestyle that includes physical activity equivalent to walking more than 3 miles per day at 3 to 4 miles per hour, in addition to light physical activity associated with typical daily life.
[e] The calorie ranges shown are to accommodate needs of different ages within each group. Older children and adolescents need more calories. Older adults need fewer calories.

SOURCE: Estimated Calorie Requirements (in Kilocalories) for Each Gender and Age Group at Three Levels of Physical Activity, *Dietary Guidelines for Americans,* Sixth Edition. U.S. Department of Agriculture and the Department of Health and Human Services, U.S. Government Priority Office, January 2005.
NOTE: Estimates are rounded to the nearest 200 calories and were determined using the Institute of Medicine equation.

What Is the Body Mass Index and How Does It Work?

The Body Mass Index (BMI) is a helpful tool for determining whether or not you are at a healthy weight. It is a single number based on the ratio of your weight to your height. The basic formula for determining your BMI is to multiply your weight in pounds by 703, divide by your height in inches, then divide again by your height in inches. Alternatively, divide your weight in kilograms by your height in meters, squared (kg/m^2). To find out your BMI value, see the Body Mass Index chart in the Appendix, page 261.

An ideal BMI is less than 25. Studies have shown that a BMI above 25 increases your chances of dying early, primarily from heart disease or cancer, and that a BMI above 30 dramatically increases your chances. Because muscle and bone are denser than fat, an athletic or muscular person may have a high BMI but not be fat. It is important to lose weight if you need to. Even a 5 to 10 percent reduction in body weight will have a big effect on your health.

For children, weight status is determined by the comparison of BMI with age- and gender-specific percentile values. The goal with overweight children and adolescents is to slow the rate of weight gain while achieving normal growth and development. See Body Mass Index for Children in the Appendix, page 262.

The key to controling weight is to eat fewer calories while expending more calories through physical activity. To maintain energy balance, you need to ensure that "calories in" equals "calories out."

CALORIES IN – CALORIES OUT = ENERGY BALANCE

Keep in mind that 1 pound of body fat = 3,500 calories. So, to lose 1 pound of body fat per week, you need to eat 500 fewer calories each day. If you ate 100 fewer calories per day, you would lose 10 pounds in a year. Conversely, if you ate 100 more calories per day, you would gain 10 pounds in a year.

Is There an Ideal Diet for Losing Weight?

Making changes in your diet and level of physical activity are the best ways to lose weight. Maintaining a balanced intake while reducing calories is essential. To cut calories, consume fewer added sugars and fats, and less alcohol, and reduce your portion sizes. A balanced intake of nutrients includes the following percentages of carbohydrates, protein, and fat from total calories:

- ◆ 45 to 65 percent calories from carbohydrates
- ◆ 10 to 35 percent calories from protein
- ◆ 20 to 35 percent calories from fat

Diets that are either very low or very high in protein, carbohydrates, or fat do not provide balanced nutrition, and therefore are not advisable for long-term use. Furthermore, the long-term effects of the currently fashionable low-carbohydrate, high-protein diets are not clear. Many of these high-protein diets are loaded with saturated fat and trans fat, which can increase the risk of heart disease, regardless of the weight loss.

In a recent comparison of the Atkins, Ornish, Weight Watchers, and Zone diets for weight loss and heart-disease risk reduction, there was no correlation between weight loss and type of diet.[3] No one diet is necessarily better for weight loss than another. The study reinforces the point that reducing calories is ultimately the driving means for weight reduction.

What about Portion Sizes?

Many of us are careful about what we eat but not about how much we eat. And the food industry is not making it any easier on us with portion sizes that grow annually. As portion sizes in restaurants and for prepared foods increase, it takes a conscious effort to consume less.

Suggestions for Limiting Portion Sizes

◆ Eat breakfast every day, and try to eat three balanced meals each day, especially if you are prone to snacking on high-calorie foods between meals. Snacking can be beneficial though, if you choose low-calorie foods that then dull your appetite at mealtime.

◆ Limit your intake of high-fat and high-calorie foods. If you still feel hungry after a meal, have more salad or vegetables.

◆ Eat slowly, so that your brain gets the message that your stomach is full.

◆ Choose water or diet drinks over sugared beverages.

◆ When eating out, opt for heart-friendly menu items. Avoid all-you-can-eat buffets, fast food, and junk food, and control your portion sizes.

◆ Keep a food diary. Writing down when, what, and how much you eat will make you more aware of the amount of food you consume and the times when you may be eating too much.

◆ Avoid mindless or habitual eating in front of the TV or computer, or while busy with other activities.

What Is the Final Word on Fats and Heart Health?

Fats and oils are part of a healthful diet. They supply energy and essential fatty acids, and they help the body absorb the fat-soluble vitamins A, D, E, and K. Some fats are healthier than others. A high intake of saturated and trans fats increases LDL cholesterol levels. Trans fats also have the negative effect of lowering HDL cholesterol levels. See Limits on Saturated Fat Intake below for how to keep your saturated fat intake below 7 percent of your total calorie intake.

LIMITS ON SATURATED FAT INTAKE

Total Calorie Intake	Limit on Saturated Fat Intake
1,600	12 grams or less
2,000	16 grams or less
2,200	17 grams or less
2,500	19 grams or less
2,800	22 grams or less

It is essential to replace the saturated and trans fats in your diet with unsaturated fats. Saturated fats are found mostly in animal products, such as meat and cheese, and most are solid at room temperature. The exceptions are tropical oils such as palm oil, palm kernel, and coconut oil. Trans fats are vegetable oils that have been turned into solid fats by a process called hydrogenation. They go by the name partially hydrogenated oil on labels, and they lurk in processed foods such as crackers, cookies, chips, fast foods, and stick margarine.

Unsaturated fats, which can be either monounsaturated or polyunsaturated, are heart-healthy fats. When they replace saturated fats and carbohydrates in the diet, these fats increase HDL cholesterol. Polyunsaturated fats have the additional benefit of decreasing total and LDL cholesterol levels. Oils high in monounsaturated fat include canola, olive, and peanut. Oils high in polyunsaturated fat include corn, sunflower, safflower, and soybean.

Omega-3 fatty acids are polyunsaturated fats, and although they do not alter cholesterol levels, they can reduce triglyceride levels and the risk of heart attacks. Omega-3 fats are found in fish, such as salmon, trout, and herring, and some plant foods, including soybean oil, canola oil, walnuts, and flaxseed.

What Is the Latest on Vitamins, Minerals, Antioxidants and Heart Health?

Although a multivitamin and mineral supplement is not a substitute for a healthful balanced diet, very few of us consume all of the vitamins and minerals we need each day. (See the Daily Reference Intakes for Vitamins and Elements in the Appendix, pages 266 to 267.)

In older adults, supplementation with a multivitamin improved vitamin status to levels associated with reduced risk for chronic diseases such as heart disease and osteoporosis, or cancer.[4] In a group of adults with type 2 diabetes who were also deficient in one or more nutrients, taking a daily multivitamin and mineral supplement for one year lowered the number of infections and absenteeism.[5]

The result of supplementing your diet with antioxidants, such as vitamins A, C, and E, in terms of heart disease is not so clear. In a study that reviewed a collection of data from other studies on the relationship between heart disease and vitamins E, C, and carotenoids (precursors of vitamin A), people who took vitamin C supplements were found to have lower rates of heart disease.[6] However, a recent study found that in patients with vascular disease or diabetes, long-term vitamin E supplementation did not prevent cancer or major cardiovascular events, such as heart attack, stroke, or death from heart disease, and may even have increased the risk for heart failure.[7] Bottom line: Taking a daily multivitamin with minerals is advisable. The benefits and risks of long-term vitamin E supplementation may depend on your health status and whether you take it before or after you develop heart disease.

Why Is Physical Activity Important to Heart Health?

Physical activity is essential to overall good health, not just to heart health. Cardio-respiratory fitness in early adulthood significantly decreases the chance of developing high blood pressure and diabetes, both major risk factors for heart disease. Improving fitness in healthy young adults prevents weight gain and obesity and can cut the risk for diabetes and the metabolic syndrome by as much as 50 percent. Exercise is also a great tool for reducing stress. For more information on exercise and exercise guidelines for children, see Sources, page 266, or Dietary Guidelines for Americans, 2005, at www.healthierus.gov/dietaryguidelines.

Benefits of Regular Exercise
◆ Reduces your risk of heart disease, high blood pressure, osteoporosis, diabetes, and obesity.
◆ Helps you maintain a healthy weight.
◆ Keeps joints, tendons, and ligaments flexible so it is easier to move around.
◆ Contributes to your mental well-being and helps relieve stress and anxiety.
◆ Increases your energy and endurance.
◆ Helps you sleep better.

Ideal Levels of Physical Activity
◆ Engage in at least 30 minutes of moderate-intensity physical activity on most days.
◆ To help maintain desirable body weight and prevent gradual body weight gain in adulthood, engage in approximately 60 minutes of moderate- to vigorous-intensity activity on most days.
◆ To sustain weight loss in adulthood, engage in at least 60 to 90 minutes of daily moderate-intensity physical activity.

Physical Activity Recommendations for Children and Adolescents
◆ Engage in at least 60 minutes of physical activity daily, if possible.

▶ **Health Tip:** If you have had a heart attack, have been diagnosed with heart disease, or have any of the risk factors that may cause heart disease, consult with your doctor or health-care provider before you begin an exercise program. If you experience chest discomfort, severe or unusual fatigue, dizziness or faintness, irregular or rapid heartbeat, shortness of breath, or nausea while exercising, immediately stop exercising and get help. These could be symptoms of a heart attack.

What Effect Does Stress Have on Heart Disease?

We all feel stress for different reasons and we all deal with it differently. Stress is a part of a healthy life, but it can lead to health problems if not kept in check. As a matter of fact, stress is a contributor to 60 to 80 percent of all diseases, including heart disease, and to behaviors that can lead to heart disease, such as smoking, alcohol abuse, and overeating.

Researchers are trying to determine the exact connection between mental stress and heart disease, but it is prudent to try to reduce stress in your life now, today, particularly if you are at risk for developing heart disease. There is no perfect stress-reduction strategy that works for everyone. Listen to your mind and body to try and figure out which coping methods work best for you. Some suggestions include aerobic exercise, strength training, walking, yoga, better nutrition, meditation, keeping a journal, joining a stress management support group (sometimes offered by cardiac rehabilitation programs), or engaging in deep breathing or other mind and body therapies with professional therapists. (For more information on stress management, see Sources, page 267.)

SOME COMMON STRESSORS

Loss of a loved one or divorce
Bad relationship
Separation from a loved one
Job-related problems or overwork
Raising children
Financial difficulties

Excessive driving and traffic jams
Excessive noise levels or stimulation
Crowded situations or new situations
Schedule changes
Competition

COMMON STRESS-INDUCED SIGNS AND SYMPTOMS

Physical
Fatigue
Headache
Indigestion
Muscle tension or back pain
Heart palpitations
Insomnia
Constipation or diarrhea
High blood pressure
Mental/Emotional
Irritability
Anger

Depression
Anxiety
Confusion
Loneliness
Difficulty concentrating
Behavioral
Overeating
Smoking
Alcohol abuse
Substance abuse and illegal drug use

For a list of web sites, organizations, and publications offering more information on cholesterol, weight loss, exercise, how to quit smoking, or stress management, see Sources, pages 265–67.

Recipes

$\mathcal{W}$**e have made** every effort to ensure that you will have success with the recipes in *Eating for Lower Cholesterol*. Each recipe is designed to be as tasty and easy to prepare as possible, using the healthiest ingredients for your heart. The recipes in each chapter are arranged sequentially according to degree of difficulty; the recipes at the beginning of each chapter are the easiest. For best results, follow the recipes exactly; or, if necessary, modify them to accommodate dietary restrictions, such as sodium or calorie limitations, prescribed by your doctor or health-care provider.

We have also tried to make the nutritional information as straightforward and as easy to understand as possible. To this end, each recipe is headed by the phrase Heart-Health Benefits. The nutrients that follow are those that the recipe provides 20 percent or more of the Daily Value per serving, based on a 2,000-calorie diet. A Daily Value of 5 percent or less of a nutrient is considered low, and a Daily Value of 20 percent or more is considered high. A recipe may also be heart-healthy because it is fat free, cholesterol free, or sodium free.

All of the nutritional values in the recipes and text were calculated using Nutritionist Pro software from First DataBank (2004 First DataBank, Inc.). Unless otherwise stated, all of the ingredients in each recipe were included in the calculations for the Approximate Nutritional Information that follows each recipe.

Every recipe in *Eating for Lower Cholesterol* lists the following breakdowns and the percentages of their Daily Values based on a 2,000-calorie diet: calories (cals), protein (grams), total fat (grams), saturated fat (grams), cholesterol (milligrams), carbohydrates (grams), fiber (grams), sodium (milligrams), and diabetic exchanges (based on the American Diabetic Association ADA exchange system). The vitamin K content is also listed for each recipe because if you are taking blood thinners (anticoagulant medicines), it is important to maintain a consistent intake of vitamin K (the amount of vitamin K in your diet may affect how well these medicines work). Your doctor or health-care professional will give you the correct dose of medicine based on your blood levels. Vitamins and minerals are also listed when a recipe provides 20 percent or more of the Daily Value per serving. None of the recipes contain trans fats, also referred to as partially hydrogenated oil. The two terms are used interchangeably throughout the text.

The "percentage of calories from fat" is listed after the Approximate Nutritional Information. The ideal percentage should be 20 to 35 percent or less. Recipes that have a higher percentage are followed by a note that explains why their value is greater than 35 percent. Usually the reason is that the recipe is low in calories and includes heart-healthy oils or nuts, which drive up the percentage figures. For instance, in the recipe for Brussels Sprouts with Walnuts and Walnut Oil (page 122), calories from fat are 67 percent, but there are only 98 calories per serving. Most of the calories from fat come from the heart-healthy omega-3 walnut oil and walnuts.

As a final word, *Eating for Lower Cholesterol* does not endorse any specific products, food or other, even though they may be mentioned occasionally in the recipes or the text.

STOCKING A
HEART-HEALTHY PANTRY

TURNING YOUR KITCHEN, pantry, and refrigerator into cardiac-friendly zones is easier than you think. Most important, you need to be willing to throw out food—yes, as awful as it may seem, you need to get rid of the bad stuff, without feeling guilty. Once you've done the initial sweep, be vigilant about keeping undesirable foods out of your house and out of your mouth.

When shopping, look for products with 3 grams or less total fat per serving and no trans fats, also called partially hydrogenated oil in the ingredient list.

IN	OUT
Dairy	
Egg substitutes, egg whites (see page 46)	Whole eggs, egg yolks
Fat-free buttermilk	Full-fat buttermilk
Fat-free and 1% cottage cheese	Full-fat cottage cheese
Fat-free and low-fat cream cheese	Regular cream cheese
	Full-fat frozen yogurt
Fat-free half-and-half	Half-and-half and nondairy creamers with
Fat-free ice cream, frozen ice milk,	trans fats
frozen yogurt (see page 236)	Full-fat ice cream
Fat-free or 1% milk, soy milk	Whole milk and 2% milk
Fat-free ricotta cheese	Full-fat ricotta cheese
Fat-free and low-fat sour cream,	Sour cream and crème fraîche
soy sour cream, and silken tofu	
Frozen soy desserts (see page 235)	Full-fat ice cream and frozen desserts
Fruit sorbets or fruit ices	Full-fat ice cream
Heart-healthy margarine	Butter and margarines with trans fats
without trans fats (page 193)	
Nonfat and low-fat yogurt, soy yogurt, and kefir	Full-fat yogurt
Reduced-fat cheeses (all kinds; see page 85)	Full-fat cheeses
Soy-based cheeses (see page 89)	Full-fat cheeses
Whipped light cream (in a spray can)	Whipped cream, heavy cream
Dry, Canned, Bottled, and Jarred Goods	
Breakfast cereals	Breakfast cereals with trans fat
without trans fats (see page 32)	
Brown rice and brown basmati rice	White rice and white basmati rice
Dark chocolate (see page 254)	Milk chocolate, white chocolate
Fat-free reduced-sodium chicken stock	Regular chicken stock
Low-fat, low-sodium condiments	High-fat, high-sodium condiments

IN	OUT
Low-calorie, high-fiber breakfast cereals (see page 32)	Low-calorie, low-fiber breakfast cereals
Low-fat mayonnaise, light mayonnaise, and soy mayonnaise (see page 82)	Full-fat mayonnaise and mayonnaise-based spreads and dressings
Low-fat salad dressings (see page 77)	Creamy high-fat salad dressings
Low-fat, low-sodium canned soups	High-fat, high-sodium canned soups
Low-sodium or lite soy sauce	Regular soy sauce
Nonfat sweetened condensed milk	Regular sweetened condensed milk
No-yolk egg noodles and rice noodles	Egg noodles and refrigerated pasta
Trans fat–free boxed meals or meal starters (see page 201)	Boxed meals or meal starters with trans fat
Trans fat–free bread crumbs	Bread crumbs with trans fats
Trans fat–free canned soups (see page 56)	Soups with trans fats
Trans fat–free croutons (see page 65)	Croutons with trans fats
Trans fat–free graham crackers	Graham crackers with trans fats
Trans fat–free peanut butter and nut butters (soy and almond butter; see page 98)	Peanut butter with trans fats
Trans fat–free whole wheat tortillas, wraps, flat breads, and pita bread	Tortillas and breads with trans fats
Trans fat–free low-fat all-natural cereal bars (see page 244)	High-fat cereal bars with trans fats
Trans fat-free low-fat all-natural cookies (see page 237)	High-fat cookies with trans fats
Trans fat–free low-fat whole wheat crackers (see page 240)	High-fat crackers with trans fats
Reduced-sodium teriyaki sauce	Regular teriyaki sauce
Reduced-sodium V-8 juice or tomato juice	Regular V-8 juice or tomato juice
Reduced-sodium Worcestershire sauce	Regular Worcestershire sauce
Whole-grain bagels and English muffins	Plain bagels and English muffins
Whole-grain bread (see page 58)	White bread
Whole grains (see page 106)	Refined grains
Whole wheat couscous	Regular couscous
Whole-grain flours (see page 250)	Refined, bleached white flour
Whole wheat pasta	Regular pasta

Meats (white and red)

IN	OUT
Ground turkey, chicken, at least 95% lean ground beef	Ground beef that is less than 95% lean
Low-fat breakfast meats (turkey or soy bacon); (see page 41)	Bacon, sausages, pork patties, bacon bits
Low-fat cuts of red meat (see page 207)	High-fat cuts of red meat

IN	OUT
Low-fat cuts of white meat	High-fat cuts of white meat
Low-fat reduced-sodium cold cuts (see page 62)	High-fat, high-sodium lunch meats

Fish and Shellfish

IN	OUT
All fresh or frozen plain fish and shellfish, especially those high in omega-3 fatty acids (see page 158)	Fish or shellfish cooked with saturated fats (such as butter)

Soy Products

IN	OUT
All kinds (see page 131)	Full-fat dairy products

Vegetables and Fruits

IN	OUT
All types fresh, frozen, or dried (see page 113)	Potato chips, corn chips, and other fried snack foods
Canned fruits packed in natural juices or light syrup	Canned fruits packed in heavy syrup

Frozen Foods

IN	OUT
Baked frozen foods	Deep-fried frozen foods
Low-fat, reduced-sodium frozen foods	High-fat, high-sodium frozen foods
Trans fat–free frozen waffles (see page 43)	Frozen breakfasts with trans fats
Trans fat–free frozen dinners (see page 176)	Frozen dinners with trans fats
Plain frozen vegetables	Frozen vegetables cooked with butter or trans fats
Plain frozen fruits and berries	Frozen fruits with added sugar

Prepared Foods

IN	OUT
Low-fat, low-sodium prepared foods	High-fat, high-sodium prepared foods
Homemade salads with heart-healthy oils	Store-bought salads with creamy dressings

Beverages

IN	OUT
Green and black tea (see page 50)	Instant ice tea and instant green tea
Natural fruit juices	Sweetened fruit juice
Red wine or red grape juice (see page 217)	High-calorie mixed drinks (such as piña coladas)
Water (see page 71)	High-sugar, high-calorie soft drinks

OTHER GOOD FOODS USED IN THE RECIPES

High-quality all-natural store-bought, tomato sauce
Buffalo (see page 215)
Candied ginger
Canned and dried beans and legumes (all kinds; see page 89)
Canned artichoke hearts in brine
Canned chickpeas
Canned diced tomatoes
Canned Mandarin oranges in light syrup
Canned or jarred hearts of palm
Canola oil cooking spray
Capers
Cocktail sauce
Dijon mustard
Dried fruit (all kinds)
Dried herbs: bay leaves, herbes de Provence, Italian seasoning, marjoram, mint, oregano, tarragon, thyme
Fish sauce
Fresh ginger and garlic
Fresh herbs (all kinds)
Fruit sauces, unsweetened (all kinds)
Grass-fed beef (see page 211)
Ground flaxseed (not whole seeds; see page 127)
Heart-healthy oils: canola, olive, soybean, walnut, etc. (see page 116)
Hoisin sauce
Lemons and limes
Light canned tuna
Near East Taboule Mix (or similar)

Nuts: cashews, peanuts, pecans, pine nuts, walnuts, etc. (see page 93)
Oat flour
Old Bay Seasoning
Ostrich (see page 219)
Peanut sauce
Piedmontese beef (see page 210)
Pitted olives (black and green)
Prepared basil pesto
Pure vanilla extract
Rolled oats and oat meal (see page 39)
Salsa
Salt substitutes (see page 181)
Seeds (all kinds) (see page 97)
Sesame seeds (toasted or not)
Solid-pack pumpkin
Soy nuts (see page 131)
Spices: caraway seeds, cardamom, chili powder, cumin seeds, curry powder, garlic powder (not garlic salt), ginger, ground cumin, nutmeg, paprika, red pepper flakes
Splenda sugar substitute or other artificial sweetener (see page 247)
Sun-dried tomatoes in oil
Tabasco or other hot sauce
Tahini
Toasted sesame oil
Vinegars: balsamic, red wine, seasoned rice, sherry
Wasabi
Wheat germ

FOODS THAT SHOULD NOT BE IN YOUR KITCHEN

Any item that contains high amounts of saturated fat (such as butter or lard)
Crisco and other solid vegetable shortenings containing trans fats
Deep-fried anything
Hard margarines that contain trans fats (see page 193)
High-calorie foods with little or no nutritional value
High-sodium foods

ONE

GREAT
BEGINNINGS

HEART-HEALTH TIPS AT A GLANCE

▶ Make breakfast a healthy habit, a nutritious breakfast provides energy, protein, vitamins, calcium, and fiber. What Is the Ideal Breakfast?, page 26, and Sample Breakfast Menus . . . for Kids Too!, page 28, will help get you started.

▶ Good protein sources include egg substitutes, egg whites, reduced-fat cheese, fat-free and low-fat dairy products, smoothies (made with nonfat yogurt or silken tofu), peanut butter or other nut butters, and homemade pancakes (Oat Flour Buttermilk Pancakes, page 44), French toast (Calcium-Rich Whole Wheat French Toast, page 38), and cholesterol-free popovers (Cholesterol-Free Popovers, page 48).

▶ Get vitamins and folic acid into your meal plan with fresh fruit or juice.

▶ If you are taking medications for high cholesterol, high blood pressure, angina, or arrhythmia, avoid grapefruit or any foods that contain grapefruit products. See The Dangers of Grapefruit, page 30.

▶ Get calcium into your diet with fat-free and low-fat dairy products such as milk, yogurt, and cottage cheese. Select calcium-fortified products (orange juice, bread, cereal, etc.) to help meet your daily calcium requirements.

▶ Try to eat a serving of cholesterol-busting soluble fiber every morning in the form of whole-grain breakfast cereals, oatmeal, whole-grain frozen waffles, whole-grain breakfast bars, ground flaxseed, wheat germ, or psyllium.

▶ Avoid fatty, high-cholesterol breakfast meats, such as bacon and sausages (see Fake Bacon and Sausages, page 41).

▶ Avoid high-fat frozen breakfast items; see Frozen Waffles: The Best Buys, page 43, and Pancakes and French Toast: Homemade Wins for Health and Taste, page 41.

> ▶ Avoid fast-food breakfast items such as egg sandwiches, doughnuts, and pastries. (See Breakfasts on the Go . . . Maybe Not!, page 45, if you need convincing.)

> ▶ Use weekends to make breakfasts you can freeze and enjoy on weekday mornings.

What Is the Ideal Breakfast?

MEN, ACTIVE WOMEN, older children, and teenage girls need about 2,200 calories per day. Depending on your eating habits, breakfast usually consumes about 550 calories, or 25 percent of this daily allowance.

The 550-Calorie Breakfast
▶ 165 calories from fat, or 18 grams of total fat, with no more than 36 calories, or 4 grams from saturated fat
▶ 110 calories from protein, or 28 grams of protein
▶ 275 calories from carbohydrates, or 69 milligrams of carbohydrates
▶ 600 milligrams of sodium
▶ 50 milligrams of cholesterol
▶ 9 grams of fiber

Young children (ages two to six), women, and some older adults need about 1,600 calories per day. Breakfast usually consumes 400 calories, or 25 percent, of this daily allowance.

The 400-Calorie Breakfast
▶ 120 calories from fat, or 13 grams of total fat, with no more than 30 calories, or 3 grams, coming from saturated fat
▶ 80 calories from protein, or 20 grams of protein
▶ 200 calories from carbohydrates, or 50 milligrams of carbohydrates
▶ 600 milligrams of sodium
▶ 50 milligrams of cholesterol
▶ 8 grams of fiber

Fresh Fruit
with Yogurt and Honey

Heart-Health Benefits: Protein, vitamin C, B vitamins, folic acid, and calcium

This breakfast staple is a winning combination. If you like thick and creamy yogurt but without the fat, Fage Total 0% Fat Authentic Greek Yogurt is an excellent choice. Choose fruits in season for maximum flavor. Artificial sweetener can be used in place of the honey, if desired. If you don't have wheat germ, top with low-fat granola, muesli, or nuts for added fiber and crunch.

■ *Serves 1* ■

1 cup whole or cut-up fresh fruit of your choice
   (washed and hulled or peeled as needed)
$1/2$ cup nonfat plain or vanilla yogurt

1 tablespoon honey
1 to 2 tablespoons wheat germ (such as
   Kretschmer Honey Crunch Wheat Germ)

Arrange the fruit in a serving bowl and top with the remaining ingredients.

Approximate Nutritional Information: Serving size: 1 serving fresh fruit with yogurt made with $1/2$ cup blueberries and $1/2$ cup strawberries; Calories: 247 cals, 12%; Protein: 12 g, 24%; Total fat: 1.6 g, 3%; Saturated fat: 0.2 g, 1%; Cholesterol: 2.4 mg, 1%; Carbohydrates: 51 g, 17%; Fiber: 4 g, 17%; Sodium: 97 mg, 4%; Vitamin C: 51 mg, 84%; Thiamin: 0.3 mg, 20%; Riboflavin: 0.4 mg, 26%; Folic acid: 83 mcg, 21%; Calcium: 268 mg, 27%; Vitamin K: 16 mcg, 20%; Diabetic Exchange Values: 1 Milk, 1 Starch, $1^{1}/2$ Fruit

Percentage of calories from fat: 6%

Sample Breakfast Menus
. . . for Kids Too!

Two Homemade Breakfast Menus

Fresh Fruit with Yogurt and Honey (page 27)

Bran Muffin with Pineapple and Dried Cranberries (page 51)

1 tablespoon peanut butter

Raspberry-Banana Yogurt Smoothie (page 35) or Strawberry-Banana Silken Soy Smoothie, (page 36)

Calcium-Rich Whole Wheat French Toast (page 38)

Lynn Rudolf's Rhubarb-Banana Topping (page 30)

Two Hot Breakfast Menus

1^1/$_2$ cups oatmeal cooked with water

^{1}/$_2$ cup fat-free milk

8 ounces nonfat plain or light fruit yogurt

8 ounces fruit juice or 1 medium fresh fruit

Scrambled eggs made with ^{1}/$_2$ cup liquid egg substitute (see Lynn Rudolf's Southwestern-Style Breakfast Burrito, page 40)

2 slices whole wheat toast with 2 teaspoons jam

8 ounces fruit juice or 1 medium fresh fruit

Two Cold Breakfast Menus

1^1/$_2$ cups whole-grain cereal (see Choose the Right Breakfast Cereal, page 32)

1 cup fat-free milk

1 banana or ^{1}/$_2$ cup berries

8 ounces nonfat plain or light fruit yogurt

8 ounces fruit juice or 1 medium fresh fruit

1 whole-grain bagel (see Healthy Bagels and Bagel Toppings, page 33)

2 tablespoons peanut butter

8 ounces nonfat plain or light fruit yogurt

8 ounces fruit juice or 1 medium fresh fruit

Note: An 8-ounce cup of coffee or tea with fat-free milk or fat-free half-and-half and a sugar substitute can be added to any of these menus.

Two Kids' Breakfast Menus

$3/4$ cup whole-grain cereal or General Mills Cheerios mixed with a higher-fiber cereal (such as Barbara's Bakery Puffins)

1 slice whole wheat bread with 1 tablespoon peanut butter plus jam

4 ounces fat-free or 1% milk

4 ounces fat-free or low-fat fruit yogurt

4 ounces fruit juice or 1 small fresh fruit or $1/2$ cup berries

2 frozen whole wheat waffles (see Frozen Waffles: The Best Buys, page 43), with 3 tablespoons maple syrup, peanut butter, or jam

4 ounces fat-free or low-fat fruit yogurt

4 ounces fruit juice or 1 small fresh fruit or $1/2$ cup berries

Lynn Rudolf's
Rhubarb-Banana Topping

Heart-Health Benefits: Fat free and cholesterol free

An **easy-to-cook** topping that makes everything taste great. You'll find yourself eating it straight out of the saucepan.

■ *Makes about 1¹/₂ cups* ■

6 ounces fresh rhubarb, trimmed and cut into
  ¹/₂-inch slices (about 1¹/₂ cups)
1 large banana, thinly sliced

¹/₂ cup water
5 tablespoons sugar, or to taste

In a small saucepan, combine all of the ingredients and bring to a boil. Reduce the heat and simmer, uncovered, stirring occasionally, for 15 to 20 minutes, or until the mixture thickens slightly. Remove from heat and let cool. Refrigerate leftovers.

Approximate Nutritional Information: Serving size: A little less than ¹/₂ cup Lynn Rudolf's rhubarb-banana topping; Calories: 94 cals, 5%; Protein: 0.7 g, 1%; Total fat: 0 g, 0%; Saturated fat: 0 g, 0%; Cholesterol: 0 mg, 0%; Carbohydrates: 24 g, 8%; Fiber: 2 g, 6%; Sodium: 2 mg, 0%; Vitamin K: 19 mcg, 24%; Diabetic Exchange Values: 1¹/₂ Fruit

Percentage of calories from fat: 2%

THE DANGERS OF GRAPEFRUIT

CHECK WITH YOUR doctor or pharmacist before eating fresh grapefruit or any foods containing grapefruit products if you are taking medications for high cholesterol (such as Lipitor or Zocor), high blood pressure, angina, or arrhythmia. Compounds found in grapefruit called furanocoumarins, and possibly some of the flavonoids it contains, are responsible for elevating the levels of these drugs in your blood, thereby increasing the risk of adverse reactions or side effects. Grapefruit also inhibits metabolism in some of the antiarrhythmics.

Simple Strawberry-Raspberry Syrup

Heart-Health Benefits: Vitamin C; fat free and cholesterol free

---

This syrup livens up pancakes, French toast, waffles, yogurt, oatmeal, and desserts.

■ *Makes about 2¹/₂ cups* ■

²/₃ cup sugar

3 tablespoons water

2 cups (scant 1 pound) fresh strawberries,
   washed, hulled, and quartered

(see Cooking Tip below for frozen berries)

2 cups fresh raspberries

¹/₂ teaspoon pure vanilla extract (optional)

1. Combine the sugar and water in a large nonstick skillet, stir, and bring to a boil. Reduce the heat slightly and cook for 2 minutes.
2. Add the berries, stir, and return to a boil. Reduce the heat slightly and cook, uncovered, for 7 to 10 minutes, or until the consistency of a thin syrup. Remove from the heat and stir in the vanilla extract, if using. Serve warm or at room temperature. Refrigerate any leftovers.

▶ **Cooking Tip:** Four cups frozen unsweetened berries can be substituted for the fresh berries. Defrost (at room temperature or in a microwave) and drain, then proceed with the recipe. Frozen berries may take slightly longer to reach the thin syrup consistency.

Approximate Nutritional Information: Serving size: ¹/₄ cup simple strawberry-raspberry syrup; Calories: 71 cals, 4%; Protein: 0.4 g, 1%; Total fat: 0.2 g, 0%; Saturated fat: 0 g, 0%; Cholesterol: 0 mg, 0%; Carbohydrates: 18 g, 6%; Fiber: 2.1 g, 9%; Sodium: 0 mg, 0%; Vitamin C: 23mg, 39%; Vitamin K: 3 mcg, 3%; Diabetic Exchange Values: 1 Fruit

Percentage of calories from fat: 3%

Choose the Right Breakfast Cereal

THE BEST, AND perhaps easiest, way to choose the right breakfast cereal is through the process of elimination. Whole foods stores tend to carry a wider variety of healthy, high-fiber cereals than grocery stores, although more and more grocery stores are carrying whole food products. If none of the following healthy choices excite you, try mixing these cereals with your slightly less healthy favorites.

- ▶ Avoid all cereals with trans fats. Yes, even those high in fiber and vitamins.
- ▶ Choose cereals high in fiber, about 7 grams per serving. You need 25 grams of fiber per day, so 7 grams at breakfast is a good start.
- ▶ Choose whole-grain cereals. Look for the word "whole" at the beginning of the ingredient list, as in whole wheat, whole grain, whole oats or rolled oats, whole barley, etc. This ensures that the grains have not been subjected to fiber-refining processing.
- ▶ Check the calorie content, especially if you are trying to lose weight. Dried fruits (such as raisins) add extra calories.
- ▶ Choose cereals with no more than 2 grams of fat.

Cereals that contain at least 7 grams of fiber per serving and no trans fats (grams of fiber)

General Mills Fiber One (14 grams of fiber)
Kashi Good Friends (12 g)
Kashi Go Lean (10 g)
Kellogg's All Bran Original (10 g)
Nature's Path Optimum Power Breakfast Cereal Flax, Soy, and Blueberry (10 g)
Peace Cereal Organic Essential 10 (10 g)
Kashi Go Lean Crunch! (8 g)
Kashi Good Friends Cinna-Raisin Crunch (8 g)
Post Shredded Wheat 'n Bran (8g)
Back to Nature High Fiber Multi-Bran Cereal (8 g)
General Mills Multi Bran Chex (7 g)
Kellogg's Raisin Bran (7 g)
Post Raisin Bran (7 g)

Cereals that contain 2 to 6 grams of fiber per serving and no trans fats

Health Valley Organic Golden Flax Cereal (6 g)
Post Grape Nuts (6 g)
Post Shredded Wheat (6 g)
Barbara's Bakery Puffins (6 g)
Quaker Squares Crunchy Oatmeal Cereal (5 g)
Post Bran Flakes (5 g)
Kashi Heart to Heart Honey Toasted Oat Cereal (5 g)
Kellogg's Smart Start Soy Protein (4 g)

Breadshop's Granola Strawberry 'n Cream (4g)
Original Alpen (4 g)
Health Valley Organic Amaranth Flakes (4 g)
Health Valley Banana Gone Nuts (4 g)
Organic Weetabix Whole Grain Wheat Cereal (4 g)
Familia Swiss Muesli (4 g)
General Mills Multi Grain Cheerios (3 g)
General Mills Wheaties (3 g)
General Mills Cheerios (3 g)
Quaker Life (2 g)

Attention Parents: The gimmicks that go with kids' cereals make them tough competition for the healthier brands. When shopping, look for cereals that have the most fiber and the highest percentage of nutrients per serving. If necessary, mix healthier cereals with less-nutritious brands. Also, try to encourage your kids to drink the milk in the bottom of their cereal bowls. Aside from the calcium benefits, many of the vitamins added to fortify cereals end up in the milk.

HEALTHY BAGELS AND BAGEL TOPPINGS

THE AVERAGE LARGE plain bagel contains about 200 calories (sometimes up to 400 calories) and has very little nutritional value. In order to enjoy a guilt-free bagel, opt for whole wheat or multi-grain bagels that provide some fiber. Thomas' Whole Wheat Bagels, with 8 grams of fiber per bagel, are a good choice. Be wise about your bagel toppings, which can turn a healthy breakfast into a high-fat nightmare. Following are some suggestions for healthy toppings.

▶ Low-fat or fat-free cream cheese
▶ Spreadable processed cheese wedges, such as Laughing Cow Original or Light, Creamy Swiss, and Swiss Knight by Gerber
▶ Tub margarine that does not contain partially hydrogenated oil or margarine spray (see Tips for Choosing Healthy Margarines, page 193)
▶ Fat-free ricotta cheese
▶ Reduced-fat (50 to 75 percent reduced-fat) cheddar cheese or other hard cheese (see You Can Have Your Cheese and Eat It, Too, page 85)
▶ Healthy Choice or other brand-name low-fat (97 to 98 percent fat-free) lunch meats (see Smart Choice Cold Cuts, page 62)
▶ Peanut butter or other nut butter that does not contain partially hydrogenated oil
▶ Hummus (see Four Hummus Variations, page 90)
▶ Store-bought bean dips without partially hydrogenated oil
▶ Marmite (a yeast-based, vitamin-rich savory spread)
▶ Low-sugar or no-sugar jams

Two Smoothies

Simple and tasty, smoothies are the perfect way to get calcium, protein, vitamins, and fiber into your diet. Prepared smoothies are available in the dairy section of grocery stores, and frozen smoothie mixes can be found in the frozen food section. Look for nonfat, zero-cholesterol varieties, and, for fewer calories, the word "light."

The Raspberry-Banana Yogurt Smoothie recipe can be modified to suit your taste and texture preferences. Adding the banana produces a thick smoothie; if you prefer a thinner version, simply omit the banana and double the amount of other fruit. Just about any fresh, frozen, or canned fruit (packed in light syrup or natural juices) can be used. Tasty options include raspberries, blueberries, strawberries, pineapple, or peaches, or a mixture of these. Unless you like thin smoothies, avoid fruit with a high water content, such as melon, apples, oranges, and grapes.

▶ **Attention Parents:** Smoothies are a great breakfast or snack for kids, especially those who don't get enough calcium from milk. Let your kids help prepare them, and go wild with smoothies!

Raspberry-Banana Yogurt Smoothie

Heart-Health Benefits: Protein, vitamin C, riboflavin, calcium, and fiber

---

■ *Serves 1 (makes about 1¹/₂ cups)* ■

6 ounces (³/₄ cup) nonfat plain or vanilla yogurt or soy yogurt

¹/₃ large ripe banana or ¹/₂ medium banana

¹/₂ cup fresh raspberries

1 teaspoon artificial sweetener or sugar, or to taste

A drop of pure vanilla extract (optional)

1 to 2 ice cubes (optional)

Place all of the ingredients in a blender and process until smooth. Serve immediately.

▶ **Calcium Boost:** Add ¹/₃ cup pasteurized fat-free dry milk (or to taste) before blending.

▶ **Diabetic Tip:** Use artificial sweetener, not sugar.

Approximate Nutritional Information: Serving size: 1¹/₂ cups raspberry-banana yogurt smoothie (without added sugar); Calories: 180 cals, 9%; Protein: 11 g, 22%; Total fat: 0.9 g, 1%; Saturated fat: 0.2 g, 1%; Cholesterol: 3.4 mg, 1%; Carbohydrates: 34 g, 11%; Fiber: 6 g, 22%; Sodium: 132 mg, 6%; Vitamin C: 23 mg, 38%; Riboflavin: 0.5 mg, 28%; Calcium: 357 mg, 36%; Vitamin K: 5 mcg, 7%; Diabetic Exchange Values: 1 Milk, 1 Starch, ¹/₂ Fruit

Percentage of calories from fat: 4%

Strawberry-Banana Silken Soy Smoothie

Heart-Health Benefits: Vitamins A, C, D, E, and B$_{12}$, calcium, and fiber; cholesterol free

Don't hesitate about using silken soy instead of yogurt—it's a powerhouse of nutrients, and it tastes good, too.

■ *Serves 1 (makes about 1^1/$_3$ cups)* ■

^{1}/$_2$ cup silken tofu

1 cup washed and quartered fresh strawberries

^{1}/$_3$ large ripe banana or ^{1}/$_2$ medium ripe banana

1 teaspoon artificial sweetener or sugar, or to taste

A drop of pure vanilla extract (optional)

1 to 2 ice cubes (optional)

Place all of the ingredients in a blender and process until smooth. Serve immediately.

Approximate Nutritional Information: Serving size: 1^1/$_3$ cups strawberry-banana silken soy smoothie (without added sugar); Calories: 129 cals, 6%; Protein: 8 g, 15%; Total fat: 2 g, 3%; Saturated fat: 0.6 g, 3%; Cholesterol: 0 mg, 0%; Carbohydrates: 25 g, 8%; Fiber: 5 g, 20%; Sodium: 67 mg, 3%; Calcium: 326 mg, 33%; Vitamin A: 1,555 IU, 31%; Vitamin C: 90 mg, 150%; Vitamin D: 120 IU, 30%; Vitamin E: 10 IU, 32%; Vitamin B$_{12}$: 2 mcg; 30%; Vitamin K: 3 mcg, 4%; Diabetic Exchange Values: 1 Milk, 1 Fruit

Percentage of calories from fat: 10%

Yogurt: Easy-to-Digest Calcium

THE DAILY CALCIUM requirement can be hard to meet, especially for people who are lactose intolerant. Some good news is that yogurt is more easily digested than other dairy products. Why? The short answer is because yogurt contains active cultures that break down lactose, a milk sugar that can be difficult to digest.

Try to eat 6 ounces of fat-free yogurt a day, which will satisfy 30 percent of the daily calcium requirement. Creamy cultured soy yogurt, such as Silk cultured soy, is an excellent alternative to dairy yogurt, and it is surprisingly good. If you like the creaminess of higher-fat yogurt without the fat, try Fage Total 0% Fat Authentic Greek Yogurt. If you are trying to lose weight, choose plain fat-free yogurt or light fruit-flavored brands that are sweetened with artificial sugar.

Five Ways to Eat Fat-Free Yogurt

▶ For breakfast, eat yogurt with fresh fruit and granola, wheat bran, or ground faxseeds, on top of pancakes or waffles, or in a smoothie.

▶ For lunch, use yogurt in place of some or all of the mayonnaise in dressings for chicken or tuna salad, add a dollop to soup, or use it to top vegetarian dishes such as stuffed grape leaves or vegetable curry.

▶ For a snack, make a dip using yogurt and a packaged dip mix to eat with fresh vegetables. Or make a sweet dip using yogurt, honey, and a drop of vanilla extract to eat with fruit slices or berries.

▶ For dessert, try fat-free frozen yogurt—but watch the calories! Flavors like chocolate brownie are loaded with calories.

▶ For baking, try substituting yogurt for sour cream, heavy cream, or full-fat buttermilk.

Attention Parents: As with kids' cereals, sales of kids' yogurt are driven by the superhero packaging and by the flavor and color of the month, such as lime-green citrus, hot pink watermelon, and neon-blue cotton candy. Try to choose low-fat or fat-free varieties. Also, switch to nonfat frozen yogurt instead of ice cream—it contains more calcium and tastes great.

Calcium-Rich
Whole Wheat French Toast

Heart-Health Benefits: Protein, B vitamins, folic acid, and calcium

---

For a fantastic breakfast, try this French toast with Lynn Rudolf's Rhubarb-Banana Topping (page 30) or the Simple Strawberry-Raspberry Syrup (page 31). Use calcium-rich whole wheat bread, such as Calcium Rich Roman Meal, to get the maximum nutritional bang for your buck!

■ *Makes 3 slices* ■

¹⁄₄ cup liquid egg substitute

2 large egg whites

¹⁄₄ cup fat-free milk

¹⁄₂ teaspoon pure vanilla extract (optional)

Dash of ground cinnamon (optional)

Canola oil cooking spray

3 slices calcium-enriched whole wheat bread

Maple syrup, jam, or your favorite topping

1. In a shallow bowl, mix the egg substitute, whites, milk, and vanilla extract and cinnamon, if using.
2. Spray a nonstick skillet with cooking spray and heat over medium-high heat.
3. Place a slice of bread in the egg mixture and turn to coat both sides, then add the slice to the skillet and cook for 2 minutes on each side, or until thoroughly cooked and golden brown on both sides. Repeat with the remaining bread. Serve warm, topped with maple syrup.

Approximate Nutritional Information: Serving size: 3 slices calcium-rich whole wheat French toast without topping: Calories: 318 cals, 16%; Protein: 23 g, 46%; Total fat: 5.2 g, 8%; Saturated fat: 0.4 g, 2%; Cholesterol: 1.8 mg, 1%; Carbohydrates: 46 g, 15%; Fiber: 1.5 g, 6%; Sodium: 699 mg, 29%; Thiamin: 0.5 mg, 31%; Riboflavin: 0.8 mg, 47%; Niacin: 4 mg, 19%; Folic acid: 87 mcg, 22%; Calcium: 394 mg, 39%; Vitamin K: 3 mcg, 4%; Diabetic Exchange Values: 2 Starch, 2 Lean Meat, 1 Fruit

Percentage of calories from fat: 15%

Cholesterol-Busting Oats

OATS ARE A POWERHOUSE of soluble fiber, particularly beta glucan, which has been proven to reduce levels of LDL, or bad, cholesterol.[1] Because of this, labels on oat products are allowed to make a heart-health claim. Eat oatmeal for breakfast as often as possible, and experiment with adding rolled oats to muffins, breads, pancake mixes, and casseroles. For people on the go, packages of instant oatmeal or instant oatmeal in a cup are easy to transport and heat up.

Ten Ways to Jazz Up a Bowl of Oatmeal
- Fresh fruit.
- Dried fruit such as raisins, apricots, dates, or prunes.
- Other dried fruit that has no moisture, such as raspberries, peaches, strawberries, apricots, apples, and blueberries. One excellent brand available at whole foods stores is Just Raspberries (and other "Just" fruits), which has "absolutely nothing added." To order this product by phone, call Just Tomatoes at 209-894-5371 or 800-537-1985.
- Apple, pear, apricot, or other fruit sauce (see Lynn Rudolf's Rhubarb-Banana Topping, page 30).
- Low-sugar or sugar-free jam or fruit compote.
- Molasses, maple syrup, fruit syrup, or honey (see Simple Strawberry-Raspberry Syrup, page 31).
- Fat-free plain or fruit-flavored light yogurt.
- Ground (not whole) flaxseed.
- Ground spices such as cinnamon, allspice, or ginger.
- Nuts such as toasted sliced almonds or chopped walnuts.

Lynn Rudolf's
Southwestern-Style Breakfast Burrito

Heart-Health Benefits: Protein, calcium, B vitamins, and folic acid

ot just for breakfast, this burrito also makes a nutritious lunch or dinner. Add your favorite fillings, from avocado and cilantro to jalapeño peppers and part-skim mozzarella cheese.

■ *Serves 1* ■

1 large (burrito-size) whole wheat tortilla or flavored wrap (such as spinach or sun-dried tomato)

2 tablespoons canned black beans, rinsed and drained, or 2 tablespoons vegetarian refried beans

2 tablespoons grated low-fat cheddar cheese or feta cheese, or to taste

Canola oil cooking spray

1/4 cup Southwestern Egg Beaters or your favorite liquid egg substitute

1 tablespoon salsa, or to taste

1. Place a slightly damp paper towel on the microwave turntable. Lay the tortilla on the counter and place the black beans and cheese in the center. Transfer the tortilla to the paper towel.
2. Heat a small nonstick skillet over medium heat. Spray with cooking spray and heat again for a few seconds, then add the egg substitute. Cook, stirring occasionally, just until the eggs are set. Remove the skillet from the heat.
3. Heat the tortilla, uncovered, in the microwave for about 30 seconds, or until the cheese is melted. Carefully transfer the tortilla to a serving plate, and top with the salsa and the eggs. Fold the sides of the tortilla over to form a pocket and serve immediately.

Approximate Nutritional Information: Serving size: 1 Southwestern-style breakfast burrito; Calories: 245 cals, 12%; Protein: 19 g, 38%; Total fat: 7 g, 11%; Saturated fat: 4 g, 18%; Cholesterol: 20 mg, 7%; Carbohydrates: 25 g, 8%; Fiber: 3 g, 12%; Sodium: 443 mg, 18%; Calcium: 268 mg, 27%; Thiamin: 0.4 mg, 25%; Riboflavin: 0.9 mg, 57%; Vitamin B_{12}: 1.4 mcg, 24%; Folic Acid: 132 mcg, 33%; Vitamin K: 2 mcg, 2%; Diabetic Exchange Values: 2 Starch, 2 Lean Meat

Percentage of calories from fat: 27%

FAKE BACON AND SAUSAGES

IF YOU ARE a member of the Bacon-of-the-Month Club, now is the time to cancel your membership. This is heart-wrenching news for some, but there are alternatives. *(Health Note: If you are on a sodium-restricted diet, be aware that these options are high in sodium.)* Turkey bacon contains about 65 percent less fat than pork bacon; it weighs in at about 165 calories and 14 grams of fat per ounce (4 slices). One thick slice of Canadian bacon, which looks and tastes more like ham than bacon, has about 50 calories and 2 grams of fat per ounce. Vegetarian bacons made from soy are another low-fat, cholesterol-free healthy choice. Admittedly, for bacon lovers, none of these options comes close to the real thing, but they can make a decent substitute.

Like bacon, pork sausages and patties contain high levels of saturated fat and cholesterol and they should be avoided. Instead try vegetarian breakfast links or patties made with soy protein. Some brands include Boca Meatless Breakfast Links and Morningstar Farms Veggie Breakfast Sausage Links and Patties. Or look in the frozen section of the grocery stores for Shelton's Turkey Sausage Patties, Turkey Italian Sausages, Turkey Breakfast Sausages, and Hans' All Natural Skinless Chicken Breakfast Links.

Pancakes and French Toast: Homemade Wins for Health and Taste

ALMOST ALL BRANDS of store-bought frozen pancakes and French toast contain partially hydrogenated oil. Whole foods stores are your best bet for finding healthy brands that are cholesterol- and saturated fat–free. You might also have some luck finding ready-made pancakes that do not contain any partially hydrogenated oil in the refrigerated dairy section of grocery stores, usually near the eggs.

When buying boxed pancake or waffle mixes, be sure to read labels carefully, because many of them contain partially hydrogenated oil—you'd be surprised! Once again, a whole foods store is probably the best place to find an all-natural brand. Some healthy choice mixes include Arrowhead Mills, Up Country Organics, and Maple Grove Farms of Vermont.

Bottom line: Homemade pancakes and French toast are the way to go. The easy and delicious recipes here include High-Calcium Yogurt-Vanilla Pancakes (page 42), Oat Flour Buttermilk Pancakes (page 44), Hearty Mixed-Grain Pancakes (page 47), and Calcium-Rich Whole Wheat French Toast (page 38).

Attention Parents: In addition to pancakes and French toast, turnovers, toaster strudels, cinnamon toast, and other frozen breakfast items that contain partially hydrogenated oil should be avoided. Most of them have zero nutritional benefit.

High-Calcium Yogurt-Vanilla Pancakes

Heart-Health Benefits: Protein, calcium, and B vitamins

*P*acked with protein and calcium, these thin crêpe-like pancakes are fabulous topped with fresh fruit and a dusting of powdered sugar, Lynn Rudolf's Rhubarb-Banana Topping (page 30), or the Simple Strawberry-Raspberry Syrup (page 31). Or keep it simple and spread them with jam, marmalade, or honey.

■ *Makes about twelve 6-inch pancakes* ■

8 ounces nonfat plain yogurt

1 cup fat-free milk

½ cup liquid egg substitute

2 tablespoons canola oil

1 teaspoon pure vanilla extract

1 tablespoon sugar

Pinch of salt

¼ teaspoon baking soda

1 cup all-purpose flour

Canola oil cooking spray

1. Combine the yogurt, milk, egg substitute, canola oil, and vanilla extract in a large bowl and whisk together. Add the remaining ingredients (except the cooking spray) and whisk until smooth.
2. Spray a large nonstick skillet with cooking spray and heat over medium to medium-high heat until hot. Add slightly less than ⅓ cup batter to the skillet and immediately swirl the batter to form a thin pancake about 6 inches in diameter. Cook the pancake until the surface bubbles and then sets and the underside is golden brown, about 1 minute. Flip the pancake with a wide spatula and cook for 1 more minute. Serve warm. Repeat with the remaining batter.

▶ **Storage Tip:** Cover leftover pancakes with plastic wrap and refrigerate. Reheat in a microwave oven before serving.

Approximate Nutritional Information: Serving size: 4 high-calcium yogurt-vanilla pancakes; Calories: 267 cals, 13%; Protein: 13 g, 25%; Total fat: 8.3 g, 13%; Saturated fat: 0.8 g, 4%; Cholesterol: 2.7 mg, 1%; Carbohydrates: 35 g, 12%; Fiber: 0.8 g, 3%; Sodium: 209 mg, 9%; Thiamin: 0.3 mg, 22%; Riboflavin: 0.5 mg, 30%; Calcium: 199 mg, 20%; Vitamin K: 9 mcg, 11%; Diabetic Exchange Values: 1½ Milk, 1 Starch, 2 Fat

Percentage of calories from fat: 28%

Frozen Waffles: The Best Buys

FROZEN WAFFLE CHOICES are endless . . . and endlessly confusing! First, scan ingredient lists to rule out brands that contain trans fats. Next, look for brands with ingredient lists that start with whole wheat flour, followed by enriched calcium, vitamins, flax, and other nutrients. Also look for waffles that are cholesterol free (egg and dairy free) and that have the least amount of saturated fat. Dietary fiber is important, too, so choose a brand with a high value, over 5 grams of fiber.

Two brands particularly high in fiber are Kashi Go Lean Original All Natural Frozen Waffles and Van's All Natural Organic Soy Flax Gourmet Waffles. Both have 6 grams of fiber per two waffles, or 22 to 24 percent of the Daily Value. Van's 97% Fat-Free Gourmet Waffles with 5 grams of fiber, or 20 percent comes in second. Some other excellent choices include any of the waffles by Life Stream made with organic grains (such as Soy Plus and 8 Grain Sesame), and Kellogg's Eggo Nutri-Grain Low-Fat Whole Wheat Waffles.

For a fiber and vitamin boost, add fresh berries, such as raspberries, blueberries, or strawberries to your waffles—or to pancakes, oatmeal, dry cereal, or other breakfast items. Half a cup of raspberries contains about 4 grams of fiber.

Attention Parents: Many of the frozen waffles that cater to children (such as Pillsbury Waffle Sticks with Dippin' Cups) contain trans fats and very few nutritional benefits. Opt for the healthy waffle brands mentioned above and lure your kids into trying them by topping them with a bit of chocolate syrup, by making your own dipping cup filled with maple syrup, or by adding sugar sprinkles. They'll be hooked before you know it, and breakfast will become a simple, healthy meal.

Oat Flour Buttermilk Pancakes

Heart-Health Benefits: Protein and calcium

The taste of oats, cinnamon, and buttermilk makes these surprisingly light pancakes irresistible. Serve them on Saturday morning topped with maple syrup, molasses, honey, Lynn Rudolf's Rhubarb-Banana Topping (page 30), Simple Strawberry-Raspberry Syrup (31), or fresh fruit, and ease into the weekend.

■ *Makes about twelve 6-inch pancakes* ■

1 cup oat flour

$^1/_2$ cup all-purpose flour

3 tablespoons sugar

1$^1/_2$ teaspoons baking powder

$^1/_2$ teaspoon baking soda

Pinch of salt

1$^1/_2$ cups fat-free buttermilk

3 tablespoons canola oil

$^1/_2$ cup liquid egg substitute

2 large egg whites

Canola oil cooking spray

1. Combine the dry ingredients in a medium bowl and mix with a whisk.
2. Combine the remaining ingredients (except the cooking spray) in another medium bowl and whisk to blend. Add the wet ingredients to the dry ingredients and mix just until combined.
3. Spray a large nonstick skillet with cooking spray and heat over medium heat until hot. Add slightly less than $^1/_3$ cup batter to the skillet and immediately swirl the batter to form a 6-inch pancake. Cook the pancake until the surface bubbles and then sets and the underside is golden brown, about 1 minute. Flip the pancake with a wide spatula and cook for 1 minute more. Stir the batter between pancakes to release some of the air bubbles. Serve warm. Repeat with the remaining batter.

▶ **Storage Tip:** Cover leftover pancakes with plastic wrap and refrigerate. Reheat in a microwave oven before serving.

▶ **Substitutions:** Whole wheat flour can be substituted for the oat flour.

Approximate Nutritional Information: Serving size; 3 oat flour buttermilk pancakes; Calories: 341 cals, 17%; Protein: 14 g, 27%; Total fat: 14 g, 21%; Saturated fat: 1.3 g, 7%; Cholesterol: 2.1 mg, 1%; Carbohydrates: 42 g, 14%; Fiber: 3 g, 11%; Sodium: 447 mg, 19%; Calcium: 197 mg, 20%; Vitamin K: 13 mcg, 16%; Diabetic Exchange Values: 1 Milk, 2 Starch, 3 Fat

Percentage of calories from fat: 36%. **Note:** This percentage is a bit high because oat flour contains a surprisingly high amount of healthy fat (about 9 grams per cup).

Breakfasts on the Go . . . Maybe Not!

BEFORE YOU PULL into the fast food drive-through lane to pick up breakfast, remember these sobering nutritional breakdowns and percentages of RDAs based on a 2,000-calorie-per-day diet.

MCDONALD'S EGG MCMUFFIN	PERCENTAGE OF DAILY VALUE
300 calories	15%
12 g total fat	18%
5 g saturated fat	25%
235 mg cholesterol	78%
18 g protein	36%
29 g carbohydrates	10%

MCDONALD'S BACON, EGG, AND CHEESE BISCUIT	
460 calories	23%
28 g total fat	42%
9 g saturated fat	45%
245 mg cholesterol	82%
21 g protein	42%
32 g carbohydrates	11%

MCDONALD'S BACON, EGG, AND CHEESE MCGRIDDLES	
440 calories	22%
21 g total fat	32%
7 g saturated fat	5%
240 mg cholesterol	80%
19 g protein	38%
43 g carbohydrates	14%

MCDONALD'S SAUSAGE BREAKFAST BURRITO	
290 calories	15%
16 g total fat	25%
6 g saturated fat	30%
170 mg cholesterol	57%
13 g protein	26%
24 g carbohydrates	8%

MCDONALD'S HAM, EGG, AND CHEESE BAGEL	
550 calories	28%
23 g total fat	35%
8 g saturated fat	40%
255 mg cholesterol	85%
26 g protein	52%
58 g carbohydrates	19%

continued on next page

BURGER KING SOURDOUGH BREAKFAST SANDWICH WITH BACON, EGG, AND CHEESE	PERCENTAGE OF DAILY VALUE
380 calories	19%
22 g total fat	32%
8 g saturated fat	40%
190 mg cholesterol	63%
16 g protein	32%
30 g carbohydrates	10%

DUNKIN' DONUTS BAGEL, EGG, BACON, AND CHEESE SANDWICH

500 calories	25%
13 g total fat	20%
6 g saturated fat	30%
135 mg cholesterol	35%
26 g protein	52%
71 g carbohydrates	24%

SUBWAY WESTERN EGG BREAKFAST SANDWICH

285 calories	14%
12 g total fat	18%
2.5 g saturated fat	13%
182 g cholesterol	61%
13 g protein	26%
31 g carbohydrates	10%

THE SKINNY ON EGG SUBSTITUTES

MOST EGG SUBSTITUTES are basically egg whites that have been colored yellow with beta carotene and thickened with vegetable gums in an attempt to make them resemble real eggs. Naturally high in protein and low in calories, many brands are fortified with vitamins and minerals to give you the same nutritional benefits as real eggs, without the cholesterol and fat; see the comparison below.

A few egg substitutes, such as Ener G Egg Replacer, contain no egg at all but are made from starches, tapioca flour, and similar ingredients. These types of egg substitutes are not good for baking, but if you are allergic to eggs, or if you are a vegan, they might be worth a try. Experiment with different brands to find the one that works best for you.

1 Large Egg	**¼ cup Liquid Egg Substitute**
74 calories	30 calories
212 g cholesterol	0 g cholesterol
5 g fat	0 g fat
1.5 saturated fat	0 saturated fat
70 mg sodium	115 mg sodium
6.3 g protein	6 g protein
27 mg calcium	33 mg calcium

Hearty Mixed-Grain Pancakes

Heart-Health Benefit: Protein

f you prefer traditional pancakes, this is the recipe for you. Maple syrup is all you need!

■ *Makes about ten 5-inch pancakes* ■

1 cup whole wheat flour

³/₄ cup all-purpose flour

¹/₃ cup cornmeal

¹/₄ cup rolled oats (quick-cooking or old fashioned)

2 tablespoons brown sugar

2 teaspoons baking powder

¹/₂ teaspoon baking soda

¹/₂ teaspoon salt

¹/₂ teaspoon ground cinnamon

1³/₄ cups fat-free buttermilk

3 tablespoons canola oil

¹/₄ cup maple syrup

3 large egg whites

Canola oil cooking spray

1. In a large bowl, whisk together the whole wheat flour, all-purpose flour, cornmeal, oats, brown sugar, baking powder, baking soda, salt, and cinnamon.
2. In a medium bowl, whisk together the buttermilk, canola oil, maple syrup, and egg whites. Pour the wet ingredients over the dry ingredients and whisk together until combined.
3. Spray a large nonstick skillet with cooking spray and heat over medium heat until hot. Add ¼ cup batter to the skillet and gently spread the batter with back of a spoon to form a round pancake. Cook the pancake until the surface bubbles and then sets and the underside is golden brown, about 1 minute. Flip the pancake with a wide spatula and cook for 1 more minute. Stir the batter between pancakes to release some of the air bubbles. Serve warm. Repeat with the remaining pancakes.

▶ **Storage Tip:** Cover leftover pancakes with plastic wrap and refrigerate. Reheat in a microwave oven before serving.

Approximate Nutritional Information: Serving size: 2 hearty mixed grain pancakes; Calories: 369 cals, 18%; Protein: 12 g, 24%; Total fat: 9 g, 14%; Saturated fat: 0.7 g, 4%; Cholesterol: 1.7 mg, 1%; Carbohydrates: 63 g, 21%; Fiber: 4 g, 16%; Sodium: 484 mg, 20%; Vitamin K: 11 mcg, 13%; Diabetic Exchange Values: 4 Starch, 2 Fat

Percentage of calories from fat: 22%

Cholesterol-Free Popovers

Heart-Health Benefits: Protein, B vitamins, and folic acid; cholesterol free

f you're looking for a heart-friendly popover, you've found one. Light and airy, these are delicious hot straight from the oven with a spoonful of jam.

■ *Makes 6 large popovers* ■

1 cup all-purpose flour

1 cup fat-free milk

¼ cup liquid egg substitute

3 large egg whites

2 tablespoons canola oil

Pinch of salt

Canola oil cooking spray

1. Preheat the oven to 450 degrees F. Have ready a six-cup nonstick popover pan.
2. In a large bowl, combine all of the ingredients (except the cooking spray) and beat with an electric mixer on high speed for 30 seconds. Scrape down the sides of the bowl and beat on high speed for 15 seconds more. (Note: Don't be concerned if you see tiny lumps of flour, but mash any big lumps against the side of the bowl with the back of a spatula.)
3. Preheat the popover pan in the oven for 2 minutes, then remove it and spray with cooking spray. Divide the batter evenly among the popover cups.
4. Bake for 20 minutes, then reduce the heat to 350 degrees F and bake for 20 more minutes, or until the popovers are golden brown and puffed. Remove from the oven and serve immediately.

▶ **Cooking Tip:** The ¼ cup egg substitute is necessary to give the popovers some color and to prevent them from immediately collapsing when removed from the oven. Store-bought "all whites" egg products do not have enough rising power for popovers; use the fresh egg whites called for in the recipe.

▶ **Storage Tip:** To freeze the popovers, cool completely, then place in a zip-top bag and freeze. To reheat, place the popovers on a piece of foil in a preheated 350 degrees F oven for about 10 minutes. Do not microwave, or they will become soggy.

Approximate Nutritional Information: Serving size: 2 cholesterol-free popovers; Calories: 295 cals, 15%; Protein: 13 g, 26%; Total fat: 10 g, 16%; Saturated fat: 0.9 g, 5%; Cholesterol: 0 mg, 0%; Carbohydrates: 36 g, 12%; Fiber: 1 g, 5%; Sodium: 129 mg, 5%; Thiamin: 0.4 mg, 26%; Riboflavin: 0.6 mg, 33%; Folic acid: 85 mcg, 21%; Vitamin K: 11 mcg, 14%; Diabetic Exchange Values: 2 Starch, ½ Milk, 1 Medium-Fat Meat, 1 Fruit

Percentage of calories from fat: 32%

How Much Caffeine Is Okay?

THE CONSENSUS OF scientific opinion is that for most people, consumption of caffeine in moderation is safe. Moderation means 300 mg, or about 3 cups of brewed coffee per day. More than a hundred studies have focused on whether any association exists between caffeine consumption and high blood pressure, cardiac arrhythmia, or coronary heart disease. Most of the research has concluded that moderate amounts of caffeine are not associated with any increased risk for cardiovascular disease, but individuals who are sensitive to caffeine should consult their health-care providers about caffeine consumption.[2]

Beverage	Caffeine Content (mg)
Coffee	
Coffee, drip (8 ounces)	115–175
Coffee, brewed (8 ounces)	80–135
Espresso/cappuccino (2 ounces)	100
Instant coffee (8 ounces)	65–100
Decaffeinated coffee, brewed (8 ounces)	3–4
Decaffeinated coffee, instant (8 ounces)	2–3
Tea	
Tea, brewed (8 ounces)	40–60
Iced tea (8 ounces)	47
Green tea (8 ounces)	15
"Energy Drinks" (8.2 ounces)*	70–80
Selected caffeinated soft drinks (8 ounces)	10–55
Hot cocoa (8 ounces)	14
Baker's chocolate (1 ounce)	26
Dark chocolate (1 ounce)	20
Milk chocolate (1 ounce)	6
Chocolate-flavored syrup (1 ounce)	4
Caffeinated water (12 ounces)	60–125
Anacin or Midol (2 pills)	64
Excedrin (2 pills)	130
NoDoz (2 pills)	200
Over-the-counter diet pills, various brands (1 dose)	80–200

* Examples of energy drinks include Red Bull, SoBe Adrenaline Rush, and Starbucks Double Shot.

Beware of Non-Dairy Creamers, Flavored Instant Coffees, and Hot Cocoa Mixes

MOST NON-DAIRY creamers (liquid and powder form), flavored instant coffees, and instant hot cocoa mixes contain partially hydrogenated oil. Regular instant coffees do not. Also, unsweetened cocoa powder, used for baking, does not contain partially hydrogenated oil.

Attention Parents: Choose cocoa mixes free of partially hydrogenated oil, such as Swiss Miss Diet with Calcium Hot Cocoa Mix or Nestlé Fat-Free with Calcium Hot Cocoa Mix. Or make hot chocolate the old-fashioned way by heating 2% or fat-free milk with a hot chocolate mix that is fortified with nutrients, such as Ovaltine.

FROTH AU LAIT: A FAT-FREE WAY TO ENJOY YOUR COFFEE

IF YOU THINK you can't live without half-and-half in your morning coffee, invest in an amazing gadget called Froth au Lait. This machine froths up fat-free milk to a wonderfully thick consistency comparable to the foam whipped up by the best baristas at Starbucks. In fact, the froth is so thick it can be sweetened with a sugar substitute and used on fresh fruit and other desserts instead of whipped cream. To order a Froth au Lait (which also comes with a Froth 'n Sauce attachment), see Sources, page 267.

THE BENEFITS OF GREEN AND BLACK TEAS

ANIMAL STUDIES SUGGEST that the antioxidants contained in green and black teas may reduce cholesterol levels, especially LDL cholesterol. Green and black teas are produced from the leaves of *Camellia sinensis*. The leaves are picked, rolled, dried, and heated. For black tea, the leaves are allowed to ferment and oxidize. Green tea forgoes the fermentation process, and as a result it contains higher levels of antioxidants than black tea. One study showed that steeping either green or black tea for about five minutes released more than 80 percent of its catechins, or antioxidants. Instant iced tea, on the other hand, contains negligible amounts of catechins.[3]

Bran Muffins with Pineapple and Dried Cranberries

Heart-Health Benefits: Fiber, B vitamins and folic acid; cholesterol free

These muffins are so good you can't believe they're healthy. For extra protein, spread a little all-natural peanut or other nut butter on your muffin. The batter can be made the night before and the muffins baked in the morning.

◾ *Makes about 15 regular muffins* ◾

Canola oil cooking spray or muffin cup liners

$3^1/2$ cups All Bran Original cereal

1 cup boiling water

$^1/4$ cup canola oil

$^3/4$ cup sugar

1 cup fat-free buttermilk

3 large egg whites

$1^1/4$ cups all-purpose flour

$1^1/2$ teaspoons baking soda

$^1/4$ teaspoon salt

$^1/2$ cup crushed pineapple (from one 8-ounce can crushed pineapple in its own juices; do not drain)

$^1/2$ cup dried cranberries or chopped dried apricots

$^1/2$ cup chopped walnuts or pecans

1. Preheat the oven to 400 degrees F. Spray 15 muffin cups with cooking spray or line with muffin liners.
2. Place the cereal in a small bowl and pour the boiling water over it; do not stir. Set aside.
3. Combine the canola oil and sugar in a large bowl and whisk together. Add the buttermilk and whites and whisk again. Add the flour, baking soda, and salt and whisk just until well combined. Add the All Bran mixture and mix with a spoon, then add the pineapple, cranberries, and walnuts and mix just until combined. (The batter will be quite thick.) Let the batter sit at room temperature for 10 minutes (or cover and refrigerate overnight).
4. Gently stir the batter, then divide evenly among the muffin cups. Bake until a tester inserted in the center of a muffin comes out clean: about 20 minutes. Transfer the muffins to a rack and let cool slightly.

▶ **Storage Tip:** These muffins retain their moisture when covered and left at room temperature for up to 2 days. They keep well tightly wrapped and refrigerated for up to 4 days. They can also be frozen for up to one month and reheated for a few seconds in a microwave oven.

Approximate Nutritional Information: Serving size: 1 bran muffin with pineapple and dried cranberries; Calories: 201 cals, 10%; Protein: 5 g, 11%; Total fat: 6.6 g, 10%; Saturated fat: 0.4 g, 2%; Cholesterol: 0 mg, 0%; Carbohydrates: 35 g, 12%; Fiber: 6 g, 22%; Sodium: 235 mg, 10%; Vitamin B_6: 0.9 mg, 48%; Vitamin B_{12}: 2.8 mcg, 47%; Folic acid: 207 mcg, 52%; Vitamin K: 5 mcg, 6%; Diabetic Exchange Values: 2 Starch, 1 Fat

Percentage of calories from fat: 27%

TWO
SOUPS

HEART-HEALTH TIPS AT A GLANCE

▶ Soups can be a great source of protein, vitamins, minerals, and calcium. They are a terrific way to get vegetables into your diet. Eat soup for lunch or dinner, or as a snack.

▶ Homemade soups are the best, mainly because you control what goes into them. But store-bought soups can also be nutritious—if you choose low-fat, low-sodium, and low-cholesterol varieties.

▶ If you are worried that a soup will not be hearty enough for a meal, try adding canned beans, tofu, or cooked chicken for extra protein.

▶ Eat soup with a sandwich or a salad. Get inspired by the recipes for salads in Chapter Three, and check out Smart Choice Cold Cuts, page 62, and Choosing the Healthiest Breads, page 58, for sandwich ideas.

▶ To save time when preparing soups, make use of canned beans; precut and ready-to-use vegetables from a salad bar; prepackaged washed and cut vegetables; canned or jarred vegetables; and canned fat-free low-sodium stock or bouillon cubes. The recipes in this chapter and throughout the book call for fat-free low-sodium stock. Vegetable and chicken stocks are preferred because they have a mild flavor; both are cholesterol free.

▶ Instead of heavy cream or regular half-and-half, use fat-free half-and half, fat-free sour cream, fat-free buttermilk or fat-free milk, nonfat plain yogurt, or silken tofu to make a soup creamy.

▶ A hand-held blender is an excellent way to puree soups. (It is also a useful gadget for making salad dressings and smoothies.)

- ▶ Choose healthy soup garnishes, such as low-fat cheese, nuts, seeds, wheat germ, tofu cubes, fresh herbs, heart-healthy oils (see Understanding Heart-Healthy Oils, page 116), and thinly sliced fresh vegetables.

- ▶ Make a big batch of soup and freeze to have on hand. As a rule, freeze a soup before adding any pasta or rice, tofu, or dairy products. Freeze in small portions in zip-top freezer bags or plastic containers to make reheating for one or two people easy.

- ▶ A slow-cooker can be used for soups with a long cooking time.

- ▶ Introduce children to soups at a young age, and they will return to them as comfort food later in life.

Two Miso Soups

If you're unfamiliar with miso, see page 132 for a full description of miso and its different uses. Basically, miso is a fermented soybean paste that is added to water to make a broth. You can add whatever you like to this broth—simple Western ingredients, such as chicken and tomatoes, or traditional Asian additions, such as tofu and bonito flakes or fish flakes (see Cooking Tip on page 54).

▶ **Health Tip:** Because miso has a high sodium content, if you are on a sodium-restricted diet, you should avoid it.

Miso Soup
with Tofu and Rice Noodles

Heart-Health Benefits: Protein and calcium; cholesterol free

■ *Serves 2 (makes about 4 cups)* ■

3 cups water

Handful of rice noodles (about 1 ounce)

1/2 cup diced tomato

2 tablespoons thinly sliced scallions

2 slices fresh ginger

7 1/2 ounces extra-firm tofu, cut into 1/2-inch dice
   (about 1 cup)

3 tablespoons miso (any kind)

2 tablespoons chopped fresh basil or cilantro

Pinch of bonito flakes (optional)

A couple of drops of lite soy sauce, or to taste

1. Bring 2½ cups of the water to a boil in a medium saucepan. Add the noodles and return to a boil. Add the tomatoes, scallions, ginger, and tofu and simmer for 5 minutes.
2. Meanwhile, combine the remaining ½ cup water with the miso in a small bowl and stir until blended.
3. Add the miso mixture to the soup and heat until hot; remove from the heat. *Do not boil the soup after you add the miso.* Stir in the basil, soy sauce, and bonito flakes, if using, adjust the seasoning, and serve immediately.

▶ **Cooking Tip:** Bonito flakes are a traditional component of Japanese miso soup and dashi broth. Bonito is a type of mackerel. For the flakes, it is steamed, then dried until hard and shaved into flakes. The soluble flakes are used as a seasoning for soups, salads, vegetables, stews, and other dishes. Bonito is often included in the miso soup that one gets at a Japanese restaurant, so if you like that, add a pinch of bonito flakes to your homemade soup.

Approximate Nutritional Information: Serving size: 2 cups miso soup with tofu and rice noodles; 194 cals, 10%; Protein: 12 g, 24%; Total fat: 6.4 g, 10%; Saturated fat: 0.9 g, 5%; Cholesterol: 0 mg, 0%; Carbohydrates: 25 g, 8%; Fiber: 2 g, 10%; Sodium: 953 mg, 40%; Calcium: 203 mg, 20%; Vitamin K: 24 mcg, 30%; Diabetic Exchange Values: 1 Starch, 2 Vegetable, 1 Medium-Fat Meat

Percentage of calories from fat: 28%

Miso Soup with Chicken and Bok Choy

Heart-Health Benefits: Protein, vitamins A, C, and K, and B vitamins

A more traditional miso recipe that uses bok choy instead of rice noodles. If you want a cholesterol-free soup, omit the chicken.

■ *Serves 2 (makes about 4 cups)* ■

3 cups water

3 ounces boneless, skinless chicken breast or
  tenders, finely diced

2 cups thinly sliced baby bok choy

3 tablespoons miso (any kind)

A couple of drops of lite soy sauce, or to taste

Pinch of bonito flakes (optional)

1. Bring 2½ cups of the water to a boil in a medium saucepan. Add the chicken breasts and the bok choy, return to a boil, then reduce the heat and simmer for 5 minutes.
2. Meanwhile, combine the remaining ½ cup water with the miso in a small bowl and stir until blended.
3. Add the miso mixture to the soup and heat until hot; remove from the heat. *Do not boil the soup after you add the miso.* Stir in the lite soy sauce and bonito flakes, if using, and serve immediately.

Approximate Nutritional Information: Serving size: 2 cups miso soup with chicken and bok choy; Calories: 132 cals, 7%; Protein: 17 g, 35%; Total fat: 3.2 g, 5%; Saturated fat: 0.6 g, 3%; Cholesterol: 36 mg, 12%; Carbohydrates: 9 g, 3%; Fiber: 2 g, 8%; Sodium: 1,017 mg, 42%; Vitamin A: 3,159 IU, 63%; Vitamin C: 32 mg, 53%; Niacin: 6 mg, 32%; Vitamin B_6: 0.4mg, 22%; Vitamin K: 33 mcg, 41%; Diabetic Exchange Values: 2 Vegetable, 2 Very-Lean Meat

Percentage of calories from fat: 22%

Soups:
Cans, Boxes, Mixes, and Styrofoam Cups

WHEN NAVIGATING THE soup aisles of grocery stores, choose store-bought soups that are:

- ▶ Low-fat or fat-free
- ▶ Low-sodium
- ▶ Free of trans fats
- ▶ Free of palm oil (this is contained in some brands of ramen noodles)
- ▶ All natural if possible

Opt for broth-based soups over cream soups, as cream soups tend to have a higher fat content. Most soup mixes in a pouch or "cup" contain partially hydrogenated oil and should be avoided. Soups mixes that contain dried beans, rice, and seasonings, such as Bean Cuisine brand, are an excellent source of fiber.

SMART CHOICE BOXED AND CANNED SOUPS

Amy's Organic Low-Fat

Campbell's Healthy Request "30% less sodium than our regular product, 98% fat-free, no msg, low cholesterol"

Hain Pure Foods

Healthy Choice "all the flavor 40% less sodium"

Health Valley Regular and Fat-Free and No Salt Added

Imagine Organic

Shelton's All Natural

Walnut Acres

Westbrae Natural

Quick Chicken Soup with No-Yolk Noodles

Heart-Health Benefits: Protein, vitamin A, and niacin

This **quick-cooking** chicken soup may not compete with your grandmother's, but it is undoubtedly lower in fat and cholesterol, and therefore healthier. Add your favorite vegetables or whole grain to the soup, if you like.

■ *Serves 4 (makes about 6 cups)* ■

5¹⁄₂ cups fat-free low-sodium chicken stock

6 ounces boneless, skinless chicken breasts or
    tenders, cut into bite-size pieces

2 carrots, peeled and sliced, or 1 cup sliced peeled
    baby carrots

1 celery stalk, thinly sliced

¹⁄₂ cup thinly sliced leeks (optional)

1 cup very thin no-yolk noodles

2 tablespoons chopped fresh parsley

Freshly squeezed lemon juice (optional)

Salt and freshly ground pepper, to taste

1. Place the stock in a large saucepan and bring to a boil. Add the chicken, carrots, celery, and leeks and return to a boil, then reduce the heat and simmer, uncovered, for 15 minutes, or until the carrots are tender.
2. Stir in the noodles and continue to simmer until they are soft (cooking time will depend on the thickness of the noodles). Add the parsley and lemon juice, if using, adjust the seasoning, and serve immediately. Refrigerate leftovers.

Approximate Nutritional Information: Serving size: 1¹⁄₂ cups quick chicken soup with no-yolk noodles; Calories: 161 cals, 8%; Protein: 19 g, 37%; Total fat: 1.7 g, 3%; Saturated fat: 0.4 g, 2%; Cholesterol: 36 mg, 12%; Carbohydrates: 17 g, 6%; Fiber: 2 g, 6%; Sodium: 849 mg, 35%; Vitamin A: 4,052 IU, 81%; Niacin: 9 mg, 43%; Vitamin K: 43 mcg, 54%; Diabetic Exchange Values: 1 Starch, 2 Very-Lean Meat

Percentage of calories from fat: 10%

Choosing the Healthiest Breads

WHAT MAKES BREAD healthy? Look for whole wheat or whole-grain breads that are high in fiber and low in added sugars, fats, and cholesterol (usually from butter). Many healthy brands bear the American Heart Association endorsement logo on their packaging. If wheat flour, not whole wheat flour, is listed as the first ingredient, it means that the bread is made from refined white flour. Also, color is not a good indicator of a whole-grain product—just because a loaf is brown, not white, doesn't mean that it is made from whole grains.

Smart Choice Breads
Alvarado Street Bakery
Food for Life
Mestemacher All Natural Famous German
Milton's whole-grain
Pepperidge Farm Natural Whole Grain
Roman Meal Sandwich Bread Calcium Rich "as much calcium in 2 slices as a glass of milk"
Shiloh Farms
The Baker
Vermont Bread Company

Attention Parents: Start your children with whole wheat bread at a young age, and they may never ask for white bread. For kids who do not like the coarseness or density of whole wheat bread, try a soft whole wheat bread variety. A rule of thumb is to make sure that the first ingredient has the word "whole" in it. Also, bread is naturally low in fat, so don't go crazy looking for a low-fat bread or be deceived by labels claiming to be low in fat, and free of trans fats—unless, or course, you are choosing croissants or other prepared breads that normally contain added fats and sugars.

Easy Black Bean Soup
with Fresh Cilantro

Heart-Health Benefits: Protein, vitamins A and C, folic acid, and fiber; cholesterol free

Canned beans make preparing this soup a cinch. The spices add great flavor, and pureeing a portion of the soup gives it a wonderful creamy consistency without adding any cream. Garnish with fat-free sour cream and low-fat cheddar cheese, if desired.

■ *Serves 6 (makes about 8 cups)* ■

2 tablespoons canola oil

1 onion, finely chopped

4 carrots, peeled and sliced, or 2 cups sliced
   peeled baby carrots

1/4 cup diced red bell pepper

3 garlic cloves, minced

2 teaspoons ground cumin

2 teaspoons dried oregano (ground or whole
   leaves) or dried basil

1/2 teaspoon chili powder

Two 19-ounce cans black beans, rinsed and
   drained

5 cups fat-free low-sodium stock or water

1 cup low-sodium V-8 juice or tomato juice

Salt and freshly ground pepper, to taste

Chopped fresh cilantro, for garnish

1. Heat the canola oil in a 6-quart saucepan over medium-high heat until hot. Add the onion and sauté for 3 minutes. Add the carrots, red bell pepper, garlic, cumin, oregano, and chili powder and sauté for 3 minutes. Add the beans, stock, and V-8 juice and bring to a boil, then reduce the heat and simmer, uncovered, for 20 minutes, or until the carrots are tender.
2. Allow the soup to cool slightly, then puree 3 cups of it in a blender or food processor. Return the pureed soup to the saucepan, stir, and adjust the seasoning. Add the cilantro and serve immediately.

▶ **Cooking Tip:** Additional stock or water can be substituted for the V-8 juice.
▶ **Storage Tip:** This soup keeps refrigerated for about 1 week and it can be frozen for up to 1 month.

Approximate Nutritional Information: Serving size: 1 1/3 cups easy black bean soup with fresh cilantro; Calories: 208 cals, 10%; Protein: 11 g, 22%; Total fat: 5.3 g, 8%; Saturated fat: 0.4 g, 2%; Cholesterol: 0 mg, 0%; Carbohydrates: 30 g, 10%; Fiber: 10g, 40%; Sodium: 599 mg, 25%; Vitamin A: 5,527 IU, 111%; Vitamin C: 18 mg, 30%; Folic acid: 144 mcg, 36%; Vitamin K: 14 mcg, 18%; Diabetic Exchange Values: 2 Starch, 1 Medium-Fat Meat

Percentage of calories from fat: 23%

Lentil Soup with Brown Rice

Heart-Health Benefits: Protein, iron, vitamin A, B vitamins, folic acid, and fiber; cholesterol free

*Y*ou can't beat lentils for protein, iron, folic acid, and fiber. The balsamic vinegar added to the soup just before serving gives it a wonderful tang, and the heart-healthy olive oil adds richness to the broth. Slow-Cooker Instructions follow.

■ *Serves 6 (makes about 8 cups)* ■

2 tablespoons olive oil

1 onion, finely chopped

2 garlic cloves, minced

4 carrots, peeled and finely diced, or 2 cups sliced
   peeled baby carrots

1/2 cup uncooked brown rice (or any rice except
   instant)

1 tablespoon dried thyme

2 bay leaves

10 cups fat-free low-sodium stock or water, or
   more as needed

1 cup green lentils, picked over and rinsed

Salt and freshly ground pepper, to taste

A couple of drops of balsamic or red wine vinegar,
   for garnish (optional)

A couple of drops of olive oil, for garnish (optional)

1. Heat the olive oil in a 6-quart saucepan over medium-high heat until hot. Add the onion and sauté for 3 minutes. Add the garlic, carrots, brown rice, thyme, and bay leaves and sauté for 2 minutes. Add the stock and lentils, stir, and bring to a boil. Skim off the foam with a spoon, then reduce the heat and simmer, uncovered, for about 40 minutes, or until the lentils are tender.
2. Thin the soup with additional stock or water, if desired. Remove the bay leaves, adjust the seasoning, and serve immediately. Drizzle vinegar and oil over each serving to taste.

▶ **Storage Tip:** This soup keeps refrigerated for about 1 week, and it can be frozen for up to 1 month.

Slow-Cooker Instructions
Use only 9 cups stock or water, or as needed.

1. In a large nonstick skillet, sauté the onion in the oil as directed in Step 1, then add the garlic, carrots, thyme, and bay leaves and sauté for 3 minutes more.
2. Transfer the contents of the skillet to the slow-cooker. Add the lentils and stock. Cover and cook on high for 6 hours, or until the carrots and lentils are soft. Add the brown rice and cook 30 minutes longer. (Note: Do not leave the slow cooker unattended while cooking the brown rice.) Thin the soup with additional stock or water if desired, and finish it as directed in Step 2.

Approximate Nutritional Information: Serving size: $1^1/_3$ cups lentil soup with brown rice (balsamic vinegar and olive oil are not included); Calories: 265 cals, 13%; Protein: 16 g, 33%; Total fat: 5.4 g, 8%; Saturated fat: 0.7 g, 4%; Cholesterol: 0 mg, 0%; Carbohydrates: 39 g, 13%; Fiber: 12 g, 49%; Sodium: 958 mg, 40%; Iron: 5 mg, 29%; Vitamin A: 4,916 IU, 98%; Niacin: 4.8 mg, 24%; Folic acid: 160 mcg, 40%; Vitamin K: 22 mcg, 28%; Diabetic Exchange Values: 2 Starch, 1 Medium-Fat Meat, 2 Vegetable

Percentage of calories from fat: 18%

Smart Choice Cold Cuts

COLD CUTS CAN be a fat and sodium dietary nightmare. Choose brands that are reduced in fat—some brands are 98 percent fat-free—and low in sodium.

Smart Choices

- ▶ Applegate Farms Certified Organic Roasted Turkey Breast 0% Fat, and other products
- ▶ Healthy Choice 97% fat-free chicken breast, turkey breast and white turkey, pastrami, and ham
- ▶ Jennie-O-Turkey Store Extra Lean Turkey Breast 97% Fat-Free (does not contain nitrites or nitrates)
- ▶ Original Field Roast Vegetarian Grain Meat (such as Sliced Wild Mushroom, Smoked Tomato, and Lentil Sage)
- ▶ Oscar Mayer Louis Rich Fat-Free Variety-Pak
- ▶ Tyson 98% Fat-Free rotisserie-flavor chicken breast, honey-roasted turkey breast, and oven-roasted chicken breast
- ▶ Wellshire Farms All Natural Uncured 98% Fat-Free Extra Lean Virginia Baked Deli Ham (and other products)

When Making a Sandwich

- ▶ Choose whole-grain or whole wheat bread (see Choosing the Healthiest Breads, page 58).
- ▶ Go easy on the light mayonnaise and/or light or reduced-fat cheese spreads.
- ▶ Add vegetables, such as lettuce, sprouts, avocado, and tomatoes, for fiber and vitamins.
- ▶ Choose a low-fat cheese (see You Can have Your Cheese and Eat It, Too, page 85).

Conjugated Linoleic Acid:
A Natural Trans Fatty Acid

THE MAJORITY (80 to 90 percent) of dietary trans fatty acids (also known as trans fats) found in the average American diet comes from harmful manmade partially hydrogenated vegetable oils that are used in cooking and preparation of processed foods. The remaining small percentage of trans fatty acids occur naturally, coming from food products derived from ruminants, such as cows. One of these naturally occurring trans fatty acids is conjugated linoleic acid (CLA), which is found in beef and some other meats, as well as in dairy products.

In animal studies, CLA has been shown to stimulate animals' immune systems, reduce body fat, protect against certain kinds of cancer, and improve cardiovascular health. For human beings, the evidence is not yet there.[2] Bottom line: Avoid unhealthy manmade trans fats, and stay tuned for more information on CLA as the research results unfold.

WHAT IS PARTIALLY HYDROGENATED OIL AND WHY IS IT BAD FOR YOU?

HYDROGENATION IS THE process of passing hydrogen bubbles through heated oil. The fatty acids in the oil then acquire some of the hydrogenation, which makes them denser. If you fully hydrogenate an oil, you create a solid out of it, or a solid fat. If you stop partway, you create a semi-solid, or partially hydrogenated, oil that has the rich consistency of butter. Partially hydrogenated oil is cheaper than natural fats such as butter, which is why it is so commonly used in processed foods.[1]

Both hydrogenated and partially hydrogenated oils can be harmful because they contain high levels of trans fats. Trans fats have been shown to raise LDL (bad cholesterol) levels and to lower HDL (good cholesterol) levels, and to increase levels of lipoprotein and triglycerides. Trans fat information can be found in the nutrition information of food labels and in the ingredient lists as partially hydrogenated oil.

Turkish-Style Red Lentil Soup with Mint

Heart-Health Benefits: Protein, iron, vitamin A, folic acid, and fiber; cholesterol free

---

*R*ed lentils, also called pink lentils, are a nutrition powerhouse. For a finer, creamier consistency, puree all of the soup, or a portion, of it. Slow-Cooker Instructions follow.

■ *Serves 7 (makes about 9 cups)* ■

2 tablespoons canola oil or olive oil

1 onion, finely chopped

2 garlic cloves, minced

1 teaspoon dried mint

Dash of paprika or cayene pepper

3 carrots, peeled and sliced, or 1½ cups sliced peeled baby carrots

1½ cups red lentils, picked over and rinsed

7 cups fat-free low-sodium stock or water, or as needed

Salt and freshly ground pepper, to taste

1. Heat the oil in a 6-quart saucepan over medium-high heat. Add the onion and sauté for 3 minutes. Add the garlic, mint, paprika, carrots, red lentils, and stock and bring to a boil. Reduce the heat and simmer, uncovered, for 30 minutes, or until the carrots are soft and the lentils are mushy.
2. Thin the soup with additional stock or water, if desired. Adjust the seasoning and serve immediately.

▶ **Cooking Tip:** The red lentils (which really are orange) will lose their color during cooking and the finished soup will be a golden yellow color.

▶ **Storage Tip:** This soup keeps refrigerated for about 1 week, and it can be frozen for up to 1 month.

Slow-Cooker Instructions

Use only 6½ cups of stock of water, or as needed.

1. In a large nonstick skillet, sauté onion in the oil as directed in step 1, then add the garlic, mint, paprika, and carrots and sauté for 2 minutes more.
2. Transfer the contents of the skillet to the slow-cooker. Add the lentils and stock, cover, and cook on high for 4 hours, or until the carrots are tender. Finish the soup as directed in Step 2.

Approximate Nutritional Information: Serving size: 1¼ cups Turkish-style red lentil soup with mint; Calories: 215 cals, 11%; Protein: 14 g, 28%; Total fat: 4.8 g, 7%; Saturated fat: 0.4 g, 2%; Cholesterol: 0 mg, 0%; Carbohydrates: 30 g, 10%; Fiber: 6 g, 22%; Sodium: 576 mg, 24%; Iron: 4 mg, 22%; Vitamin A: 3,163 IU, 63%; Folic acid: 96 mcg, 24%; Vitamin K: 8 mcg, 10%; Diabetic Exchange Values: 1 Starch, 1 Medium-Fat Meat, 3 Vegetable

Percentage of calories from fat: 20%

High Calcium Intake from Dairy Products —or Following the DASH Diet— May Lower Blood Pressure

FINDINGS INDICATE THAT adding low-fat dairy products to a diet rich in fruits, vegetables, and nuts, with reduced saturated and total fats, may lower blood pressure.

The DASH study (Dietary Approaches to Stop Hypertension) by the National Heart, Lung, and Blood Institute of the National Institutes of Health (NIH) looked at the effects of various eating patterns on lowering blood pressure in more than 450 adults in different parts of the country. Three diets were studied: a typical American diet (including 450 mg of calcium from dairy products); a diet high in fruits and vegetables (including 450 mg of calcium from dairy products); and the DASH diet, which is a diet high in fruits and vegetables *and* in low-fat dairy products (including 1,240 mg of calcium from dairy products). Of the three, the DASH diet resulted in the greatest decrease in blood pressure.

A second study, called DASH-Sodium, looked at the effect on blood pressure of reduced-dietary sodium intake while participants followed one of two diets: the DASH diet (outlined above) or a typical American diet. Participants were randomly assigned to one of the two diets, which they then followed for a month each at three different sodium levels: a high intake, of about 3,300 mg per day (the level consumed by most Americans); an intermediate intake, of about 2,400 mg per day; and a low intake, of about 1,500 mg per day.

Results showed that reducing dietary sodium lowered blood pressure with both the DASH diet and the typical American diet, but at each of the three levels, blood pressure was lower on the DASH diet than on the typical American diet. The biggest blood pressure reductions were for the DASH diet on the low-sodium intake of 1,500 mg per day.

Bottom line: The DASH diet plus low sodium intake equals lower blood pressure, and lower blood pressure equals a healthier heart.[3]

MAKE YOUR OWN FAT-FREE CROUTONS

ALMOST ALL BRANDS of store-bought croutons contain partially hydrogenated oil. A couple that do not are Rothbury Farms Fat-Free Seasoned Croutons, Olivia's Crouton Company, and Chatham Village Croutons. The good news is that making your own fat-free croutons is super-easy. Any type of bread (fresh or stale) can be used. French baguettes make light, delicate croutons, hearty country, sourdough, rosemary, olive, and whole wheat breads make more robust and flavorful croutons.

Preheat the oven to 350 degrees F. Cut the bread into small cubes. Distribute the cubes evenly on a baking sheet lined with foil (for easier cleanup) and bake for 20 minutes. Turn the croutons, and continue baking for 5 to 10 minutes, or until they are hard and light golden brown. Cool completely, then store them in an airtight container or zip-top bag.

Red Beet Soup
with Horseradish Cream

Heart-Health Benefits: Vitamin C and folic acid; fat free

If **you like** beets, this gorgeous pink soup is for you. The tangy horseradish is the perfect foil to the sweetness of the beets. To avoid beet-stained hands, wear powder-free rubber gloves while handling the beets.

■ *Serves 6 (makes about 7 cups)* ■

2 pounds beets (about 4 to 5 medium beets), peeled and diced

6½ cups fat-free low-sodium stock

2 tablespoons prepared horseradish, or to taste

1 cup fat-free sour cream

1 tablespoon freshly squeezed lemon juice, or to taste

Salt and freshly ground pepper, to taste

1. Combine the beets and stock in a large saucepan and bring to a boil. Reduce the heat and simmer, uncovered, for about 45 minutes, or until the beets are soft. (Note: Beets require a long cooking time. The smaller you dice the beets, the shorter the cooking time will be.)
2. Remove the saucepan from the heat and allow the soup to cool slightly. Then puree the soup in batches in a regular blender, or using a handheld blender, until as smooth and silky as possible. Return the pureed soup to the saucepan (if necessary).
3. In a small bowl, whisk together the horseradish and sour cream. Add it to the soup, whisking until well incorporated. Thin the soup with extra stock, if desired. Add the lemon juice and adjust the seasoning. Reheat, and serve immediately.

▶ **Storage Tip:** The pureed soup (without the sour cream and lemon juice) can be frozen up to 3 months.

Approximate Nutritional Information: Serving size: 1 heaping cup red beet soup with horseradish cream; Calories; 128 cals, 6%; Protein: 7 g, 15%; Total fat: 0.3 g, 0%; Saturated fat: 0 g, 0%; Cholesterol: 3.3 mg, 1%; Carbohydrates: 24 g, 8%; Fiber: 5 g, 19%; Sodium: 788 mg, 33%; Vitamin C: 17 mg, 28%; Folic acid: 170 mcg, 43%; Diabetic Exchange Values: 1 Starch, 2 Vegetable

Percentage of calories from fat: 2%

Pumpkin Soup with Pumpkin Oil and Pumpkin Seeds

Heart-Health Benefits: Vitamins A and C

This slightly sweet, earthy soup is best made with Hokaido or Asian pumpkin (which have an intense pumpkin flavor and give the soup a creamy texture), though any small orange-fleshed pumpkin will work. Pumpkin oil and seeds, available in whole foods or gourmet stores, are rich in heart-healthy omega-3 fatty acids.

■ *Serves 6 (makes about 7 cups)* ■

2 tablespoons canola oil

1 onion, chopped

2¹/₂ pounds pumpkin, peeled, seeds and strings
   removed, and flesh cut into medium dice (about
   2 pounds, or about 6 cups diced pumpkin)

4 cups fat-free low-sodium stock, or as needed

¹/₂ cup fat-free sour cream

A couple of drops of pumpkin seed oil

1/3 cup unsalted roasted pumpkin seeds

1. Heat the canola oil in a large nonstick skillet over medium-high heat. Add the onion and sauté for 3 minutes. Then add the pumpkin and sauté for 5 minutes. Add the stock and bring to a boil, then reduce the heat and simmer, uncovered, for 15 to 20 minutes, or until the pumpkin is tender.
2. Remove the saucepan from the heat and allow the soup to cool slightly. Puree the soup in batches in a regular blender, or using a handheld blender, until smooth and silky. Return the pureed soup to the saucepan (if necessary).
3. Add the sour cream to the soup, whisking until well incorporated. Thin with extra stock, if desired. Adjust the seasoning and ladle into bowls. Garnish each with a few drops of pumpkin oil and some pumpkin seeds, and serve immediately.

▶ **Cooking Tip:** Use a sharp knife to remove the skin from the pumpkin; it makes the job a lot easier.

▶ **Storage Tip:** The pureed soup (without the sour cream) can be frozen for up to 3 months.

Approximate Nutritional Information: Serving size: 1¹/₃ cups pumpkin soup with pumpkin oil and pumpkin seeds (without pumpkin oil); Calories: 136 cals, 7%; Protein: 6 g, 11%; Total fat: 5.3 g, 8%; Saturated fat: 0.5 g, 3%; Cholesterol: 2 mg, 1%; Carbohydrates: 17 g, 6%; Fiber: 1 g, 4%; Sodium: 491 mg, 20%; Vitamin A: 9,972 IU, 199%; Vitamin C: 14 mg, 24%; Vitamin K: 7 mcg, 9%; Diabetic Exchange Values: 1 Starch, 1 Vegetable, 1 Fat

Percentage of calories from fat: 35%

How Much Calcium Do You Need?

AGE (FOR MALES AND FEMALES)	DAILY CALCIUM REQUIREMENT (MG)[4]
0 to 6 months	210
7 to 12 months	270
1 to 3 years	500
4 to 8 years	800
9 to 13 years	1,300
14 to 18 years	1,300
19 to 50 years	1,000
51 plus years	1,200

High-Calcium Dairy Products
with Less than 5 Grams of Fat per Serving

FOOD	SERVING SIZE	CALCIUM (MG)
Fat-free plain yogurt	1 cup	488
Low-fat plain yogurt	1 cup	448
Fat-free milk	8 ounces	301
Reduced-fat 1% milk	8 ounces	300
Nonfat dry milk	⅓ cup	283
Part-skim mozzarella cheese	1 ounce	222
Fat-free ricotta cheese	¼ cup	200
Weight Watchers Fat-Free Swiss Cheese	2 slices	150
Fat-free American cheese	1 slice	150
Reduced-fat buttermilk	½ cup	142
Fat-Free frozen yogurt (avoid chocolate)	½ cup	138
Parmesan cheese, grated	2 tablespoons	138
Reduced-fat crumbled feta cheese	¼ cup	80
Low-fat 2% cottage cheese	½ cup	78
Fat-free cottage cheese	½ cup	60
Laughing Cow Light Swiss Cheese	¾ ounce wedge	60
Fat-free sour cream	2 tablespoons	40

Note: There are two other popular cheeses that contain slightly more than 5 grams of fat per serving. Reduced-Fat Alpine Lace Swiss Cheese: one slice contains 7 grams of fat and 350 mg of calcium. Cracker Barrel 2% Milk Cheddar Cheese: one ounce contains 6 grams of fat and 200 mg of calcium.

Curried Cauliflower-Broccoli Soup with Silken Tofu

Heart-Health Benefits: Vitamins C; cholesterol free

$\mathcal{A}$ **smooth and creamy** bright green soup with flavors of ginger and curry. The silken tofu gives the soup a rich creaminess without adding fat.

■ *Serves 5 (makes about 6 cups)* ■

2 tablespoons canola oil

1 small onion, chopped

1 tablespoon minced fresh ginger

$1/2$ teaspoon curry powder, or to taste

5 cups mixed broccoli and cauliflower florets

1 medium potato, peeled and diced

4 cups fat-free low-sodium stock

$1/2$ cup silken tofu or $1/3$ cup fat-free sour cream

2 tablespoons chopped fresh cilantro

Salt and freshly ground pepper, to taste

1. Heat the canola oil in a 6-quart saucepan over medium heat. Add the onion and sauté for 1 minute. Add the ginger and curry powder and sauté for 30 seconds.
2. Add the broccoli and cauliflower florets and potato and sauté for 30 seconds. Add the stock and bring to a boil, then reduce the heat and simmer, uncovered, for 10 minutes, or until the potatoes are soft.
3. Remove from the heat and allow the soup to cool slightly. Add the silken tofu and cilantro to the soup, then puree it in batches in a regular blender, or using a handheld blender. Return the pureed soup to the saucepan (if necessary).
4. Reheat the soup. Add the cilantro, adjust the seasoning, and serve immediately.

Approximate Nutritional Information: Serving size: 1 heaping cup curried cauliflower-broccoli soup with silken tofu; 104 cals, 5%; Protein: 6 g, 12%; Total fat: 5 g, 8%; Saturated fat: 0.5 g, 2%; Cholesterol: 0 mg, 0%; Carbohydrates: 10 g, 3%; Fiber: 3 g, 11%; Sodium: 413 mg, 17%; Vitamin C: 55 mg, 92%; Vitamin K: 50 mcg, 62%; Diabetic Exchange Values: 2 Vegetable, 1 Fat

Percentage of calories from fat: 41%. **Note:** It is more important to focus on the total fat value of this recipe, which is 5 grams, or 8% Daily Value per serving, than on the percentage of calories from fat.

Classic Minestrone

Heart-Health Benefits: Protein, iron, vitamins A and C, B vitamins, folic acid, and fiber; cholesterol free

No one will be able to turn down a bowl of this hearty, soul-warming minestrone. A tiny bit of pesto or sliced fresh basil leaves and a dash of grated Parmesan cheese are the perfect garnishes. Serve with a good whole-grain bread.

■ *Serves 6 (makes about 8 cups)* ■

3 tablespoons olive oil or canola oil

1 onion, finely chopped

2 garlic cloves, crushed

2 carrots, peeled, cut lengthwise in half, and sliced, or 1 cup sliced peeled baby carrots

1 cup thinly sliced leeks (optional)

1 medium potato, peeled and cut into small dice

2 celery stalks, thinly sliced

2 teaspoons dried oregano, or to taste

1 medium zucchini, washed, quartered lengthwise, and cut into small dice

1 cup frozen green peas

1 cup canned great northern beans (or any other small canned beans), rinsed and drained

8 cups fat-free low-sodium stock, or as needed

3/4 cup ditalini pasta or other small pasta

One 14.5-ounce can diced tomatoes (do not drain) or 2 cups diced fresh tomatoes

Salt and freshly ground pepper, to taste

A spoonful of pesto or sliced fresh basil leaves, for garnish (optional)

Grated Parmesan cheese, for garnish (optional)

1. Heat the olive oil in a 6-quart saucepan over medium-high heat. Add the onion and sauté for 2 minutes. Add the garlic, carrots, leeks, if using, potato, celery, and oregano and sauté for 3 minutes, stirring constantly. Add the zucchini, peas, beans, and stock and bring to a boil. Reduce the heat and simmer, uncovered, for 5 minutes.
2. Add the pasta and tomatoes and simmer for 10 minutes, or until the pasta is cooked.
3. Adjust the seasoning, and thin the soup with additional stock or water, if desired. Garnish with the pesto (or basil leaves) and Parmesan cheese, if using, and serve immediately.

▶ **Cooking Tip:** Feel free to substitute your favorite vegetables for the ones called for in this recipe.
▶ **Storage Tip:** This soup keeps refrigerated for about 1 week. It does not freeze well.

Approximate Nutritional Information: Serving size: 1¹/₃ cups classic minestrone (without pesto and Parmesan cheese); 244 cals, 12%; Protein: 11 g, 22%; Total fat: 5.7 g, 9%; Saturated fat: 0.7 g, 4%; Cholesterol: 0 mg, 0%; Carbohydrates: 37 g, 12%; Fiber: 5 g, 20%; Sodium: 598 mg, 25%; Vitamin A: 2,787 IU, 56%; Vitamin C: 18 mg, 31%; Thiamin: 0.4 mg, 24%; Niacin: 4 mg, 21%; Folic Acid: 119 mcg, 30%; Vitamin K: 22 mcg, 27%; Diabetic Exchange Values: 2 Starch, 2 Vegetable, 1 Fat

Percentage of calories from fat: 21%

REASONS TO STAY HYDRATED WITH WATER

WATER IS ESSENTIAL to life; every cell depends on it. Try to drink 4 cups, or 32 ounces, of water per day. People exercising strenuously, doing hard physical work, or flying on a long flight need even more water.

> ► To aid with digestion.
> ► To avoid constipation, especially if you are increasing your fiber intake.
> ► To reduce the risk of urinary tract infections and kidney stones.
> ► To avoid headaches from dehydration.
> ► To eliminate toxins and to flush medications out of your system.
> ► To help regulate body temperature.

THREE

SALADS, WHOLE GRAINS, AND LEGUMES

HEART-HEALTH TIPS AT A GLANCE

▶ Get as many heart-healthy greens, whole grains, and legumes into your diet as possible. They are excellent sources of fiber, antioxidants, vitamins (folic acid and vitamins A, C, and E), minerals, and plant protein. The text boxes in this chapter will help get you started; then branch out and use your imagination to create your own favorite combinations.

▶ Use heart-healthy oils, such as olive oil and canola oil, in salads and salad dressing (see Understanding Heart-Healthy Oils, page 116, and Heart-Health Claim for Olive Oil, page 74).

▶ Use salad dressings in moderation. Avoid creamy ones, and make your own whenever possible. See How to Choose Store-Bought Salad Dressings, page 77.

▶ Keep your salad ingredients healthy, and you can't go wrong. Some top choices include: romaine lettuce, spinach, colorful vegetables (see The Top 15 High Antioxidant Fruits and Vegetables, page 113), whole grains, legumes, nuts, seeds, low-fat or reduced-fat cheeses (see You Can Have Your Cheese and Eat It, Too, page 85), and dried or fresh fruit.

▶ Add a lean protein to turn a salad into a meal. Some good choices include cooked fish or shellfish, poultry, tofu, lean cold cuts, reduced-fat cheeses, and legumes.

▶ Toss legumes into salads and soups, or puree them to make dips or spreads. In case you are wondering what legumes are, *The Food Lover's Companion* defines legumes as "any thousands of plant species that have seed pods that split along both sides when ripe." Some common examples include beans, chickpeas, lentils, peanuts, peas, and soybeans. If you come across the word "pulses," it simply means the dried seeds of a legume, such as dried lentils or soybeans.

- Whole grains, such as tabbouleh, whole wheat couscous, and quinoa, are excellent sources of cholesterol-lowering soluble fiber, B vitamins, and minerals. Try to replace refined grains, such as white rice, regular pasta, and regular couscous, with whole grains.

- Make nuts and seeds part of your diet. See Go Nuts for Nuts, page 93, and Healthy Seeds, page 97. Keep in mind, though, that nuts are high in calories and heart-healthy oils—so when you eat nuts, cut back on calories and fats from less healthy foods.

- Eat your salad before you eat the rest of your meal. This will fill you up, causing you to eat less of your main course.

THREE SALAD DRESSINGS

Lizzie Abernethy's Reduced-Fat Vinaigrette

Heart-Health Benefits: Reduced fat and cholesterol free

This light dressing is lovely on all greens.

Makes about ²/₃ cup

3 tablespoons red wine vinegar	Pinch of minced garlic (optional)
¹/₄ cup fat-free milk	3 tablespoons canola oil
1 teaspoon Dijon mustard	Salt and freshly ground pepper, to taste

Combine all of the ingredients except the canola oil in a small bowl and whisk until well blended. Add the oil and mix until emulsified, then adjust the seasoning. Refrigerate any leftovers.

Approximate Nutritional Information: Serving size: 1 tablespoon reduced-fat vinaigrette; Calories: 39 cals, 2%; Protein: 0.3 g, 1%; Total fat: 4 g, 6%; Saturated fat: 0.2 g, 1%; Cholesterol: 0 mg, 0%; Carbohydrates: 0.4 g, 0%; Fiber: 0 g, 0%; Sodium: 15 mg, 1%; Vitamin K: 5 mcg, 6%; Diabetic Exchange Values: 1 Fat

Percentage of calories from fat: 93%. **Note:** It is more important to focus on the total fat value of this vinaigrette recipe, which is 4 grams, or 6% Daily Value, per serving, than on the percentage of calories from fat.

Omega-3 Power Dressing

Heart-Health Benefit: Cholesterol free

$\mathcal{S}$oybean and walnut oil are good sources of heart-healthy omega-3 fatty acids (see Understanding Heart-Healthy Oils, page 116).

■ *Makes about ¹/₄ cup* ■

1 tablespoon red wine vinegar

1 teaspoon Dijon mustard

2 tablespoons soybean oil

1 tablespoon walnut oil

Salt and freshly ground pepper, to taste

Combine the vinegar and mustard in a small bowl and whisk until well blended. Add the soybean oil and walnut oil and mix until emulsified. Adjust the seasoning. Refrigerate any leftovers.

▶ **Storage Tip:** Always refrigerate soybean and walnut oil, as they are susceptible to damage from heat, light, and oxygen when overexposed to the elements, and the fatty acids in these oils become oxidized or rancid. See Storing and Cooking Heart-Healthy Oils, page 118.

Approximate Nutritional Information: Serving size: 1 tablespoon omega-3 power dressing; Calories: 91 cals, 5%; Protein: 0.2 g, 1%; Total fat: 10.2 g, 16%; Saturated fat: 1.2 g, 6%; Cholesterol: 0 mg, 0%; Carbohydrates: 0 g, 0%; Fiber: 0 g, 0%; Sodium: 30 mg, 1%; Vitamin K: 14 mcg, 17%; Diabetic Exchange Values: 2 Fat

Percentage of calories from fat: 98%. **Note:** It is more important to focus on the total fat value of this dressing recipe, which is 10 grams, or 16% Daily Value, per serving, than on the percentage of calories from fat.

HEART-HEALTH CLAIM FOR OLIVE OIL

OLIVE OIL IS IN! Add olive oil to your diet by using it in salad dressings, for cooking (over moderate heat), or in baking as a substitute for butter.

The U.S. Food and Drug Administration has issued a qualified health claim for a correlation between monounsaturated fat from olive oil and reduced risk for heart disease. There is limited, but not conclusive, evidence that suggests that consumers may reduce their risk of coronary heart disease if they substitute about 2 tablespoons (23 grams) of monounsaturated fat from olive oil and olive oil–containing foods in place of foods high in saturated fat, while keeping the total number of calories consumed daily at the same level.[1]

Caesar Salad Dressing with Silken Tofu

Heart-Health Benefits: Low fat and cholesterol free

S **erve this delicious** salad dressing with romaine lettuce, fat-free croutons (see Make Your Own Fat-Free Croutons, page 65), and a dusting of grated Parmesan cheese. The dressing can also be used as a dip for raw vegetables.

■ *Makes ⅔ cup* ■

4 ounces silken tofu

½ garlic clove

2 tablespoons grated Parmesan cheese

1 teaspoon Dijon mustard

1 teaspoon red wine vinegar

1½ tablespoons freshly squeezed lemon juice, or
   to taste

1½ teaspoons olive oil or canola oil

½ teaspoon capers

1 anchovy fillet or a squirt of anchovy paste
   (optional)

Salt and freshly ground pepper, to taste

Combine all of the ingredients in a blender or food processor and process until smooth, scraping down the sides of the bowl as needed. Adjust the seasoning (go easy on the salt if using the anchovy). Refrigerate any leftovers.

Approximate Nutritional Information: Serving size: 1 tablespoon Caesar salad dressing with silken tofu; Calories: 17 cals, 1%; Protein: 1.5 g, 3%; Total fat: 1.1 g, 2%; Saturated fat: 0.3 g, 2%; Cholesterol: 0 mg, 0%; Carbohydrates: 0 g, 0%; Fiber: 0 g, 0%; Sodium: 56 mg, 2%; Diabetic Exchange Values: FREE

Percentage of calories from fat: 58%. **Note:** It is more important to focus on the total fat value of this dressing recipe, which is 1 gram, or 2% Daily Value, per serving, than on the percentage of calories from fat.

Simple Tuna Salad

Heart-Health Benefits: Protein and B vitamins

This tuna salad makes a great sandwich or main course. If you are concerned about mercury levels in tuna, use light tuna instead of albacore tuna—it contains less methylmercury (see Mercury Levels and Fish Consumption: Warnings for Women and Children, page 159). Light tuna tends to be darker in color and flakier than albacore tuna, but the flavor is the same. If you want to eliminate all of the fat from this salad, use a thick plain fat-free yogurt instead of the mayonnaise.

■ *Serves 2* ■

One 6- to 6¹/₂-ounce can or 7-ounce pack light tuna in water, drained, rinsed, and drained again

1 tablespoon thinly sliced scallion greens or fresh chives

2 tablespoons finely diced celery

1 tablespoon light mayonnaise

1¹/₂ teaspoons freshly squeezed lemon juice, or to taste

Salt and freshly ground pepper, to taste

Combine all of the ingredients in a bowl and mix until well blended. Adjust the seasoning and serve.

▶ **Cooking Tip:** Add chopped fresh dill, parsley, or your favorite fresh herbs; a few drained capers or finely diced dill pickles; a little dill relish (such as Mt. Olive Dill Relish); or a dash of mustard.

Approximate Nutritional Information: Serving size: ¹/₂ cup simple tuna salad; Calories: 136 cals, 7%; Protein: 24 g, 47%; Total fat: 3.2 g, 5%; Saturated fat: 0.7 g, 4%; Cholesterol: 30 mg, 10%; Carbohydrates: 2.2 g, 1%; Fiber: 0.5 g, 1%; Sodium: 365 mg, 15%; Niacin: 12 mg, 61%; Vitamin B$_{12}$: 2.7 mcg 46%; Vitamin K: 14 mcg, 18%; Diabetic Exchange Values: 4 Very Lean Meat

Percentage of calories from fat: 22%

Salad Bar Tips

▶ Scan the salad bar to check for cleanliness and a well-maintained general appearance.

▶ Avoid prepared salads made with mayonnaise (such as macaroni or potato salads).

▶ For the best nutritional values, choose romaine, Boston, Bibb, loose-leaf, or iceberg lettuce, in that order.

▶ Try to include a grain (such as brown rice, tabbouleh, whole wheat couscous, or wheat berries) and a legume (such as chickpeas, kidney beans, lentils, or black beans) in your salad. Avoid the croutons, as most brands contain partially hydrogenated oil and have a high fat content.

▶ Opt for a low-fat salad dressing, especially if you're craving something in the creamy dressing category. Even better, make your own olive oil–and–vinegar dressing. Often dressings are not clearly labeled and you don't know what you're getting.

▶ Top your salad with seeds (such as sesame, sunflower, or pumpkin) or nuts (any kind).

▶ Avoid or go easy on the cheese unless it is low-fat, such as low-fat cottage cheese or low-fat or fat-free feta cheese (see You Can Have Your Cheese and Eat It, Too, page 85).

▶ Add dried or fresh fruit to your salad.

▶ Avoid bacon bits, whether real or artificial.

▶ Avoid tofu unless it is stored in clean water and kept well chilled.

▶ Compose a healthy fruit salad for breakfast, dessert, or snack.

HOW TO CHOOSE STORE-BOUGHT SALAD DRESSINGS

THERE IS NO shortage of store-bought salad dressings on the market today. In general, bottled vinaigrettes are a better choice than creamy fat-filled salad dressings. If you do opt for a creamy ranch-style or French dressing, it is best to buy a "light" or fat-free version. A vinaigrette-type dressing does not have to be fat-free unless you are trying to lose weight. Some healthy favorites include Newman's Own Lighten Up low-fat dressings, Annie's Naturals low-fat dressings, and Spectrum Naturals fat-free, low-fat dressings. Whatever your taste, look for the following when choosing a salad dressing:

▶ No partially hydrogenated oil

▶ A low-calorie value

▶ No high-fructose corn syrup

▶ Olive oil or canola oil base

▶ A short ingredient list (meaning fewer additives)

Coleslaw
with Lemon–Olive Oil Dressing

Heart-Health Benefits: Vitamins A and C; cholesterol free

To save time, buy a packaged coleslaw mix, or pick up both the shredded cabbage and carrots from a salad bar.

■ *Serves 4* ■

8 ounces (about 4 cups) thinly sliced cabbage, white or red or a mixture of both, or 8 ounces packaged coleslaw mix

¹/₄ cup grated carrots

¹/₄ cup thinly sliced celery

1 tablespoon chopped fresh parsley (optional)

Lemon–Olive Oil Dressing

1 tablespoon olive oil or canola oil

1¹/₂ tablespoons freshly squeezed lemon juice, or to taste

1 tablespoon light mayonnaise

Salt and freshly ground pepper, to taste

1. Combine the cabbage, carrots, celery, and parsley, if using, in a large bowl and toss gently.
2. Add the olive oil and toss, then add the lemon juice, mayonnaise, and salt and pepper and toss again. Adjust the seasoning and serve. Refrigerate leftovers.

Approximate Nutritional Information: Serving size: 1 cup coleslaw (no dressing): Calories: 21 cals, 1%; Protein: 1 g, 2%; Total fat: 0 g, 0%; Saturated fat: 0 g, 0%; Cholesterol: 0 mg, 0%; Carbohydrates: 5 g, 2%; Fiber: 2 g, 8%; Sodium: 171 mg, 7%; Vitamin A: 1,072 IU, 21%; Vitamin C: 25 mg, 41%; Vitamin K: 61 mcg, 77%; Diabetic Exchange Values: 1 Vegetable

Percentage of calories from fat: 4%

Approximate Nutritional Information: Serving size: one-quarter lemon-olive oil dressing; Calories: 44 cals, 2%; Protein: 0g, 0%; Total fat: 5g, 7%; Saturated fat: 0 g, 0%; Cholesterol: 0 mg, 0%; Carbohydrates: 0g, 0%; Fiber: 0g, 0%; Sodium: 23 g, 1%; Vitamin K: 7 mcg, 9%; Diabetic Exchange Values: 1 Fat

Percentage of calories from fat: 91%. **Note:** It is more important to focus on the total fat value of this dressing recipe, which is 5 grams, or 7% Daily Value, per serving, than on the percentage of calories from fat.

Healthy Lentil Salad
with Tomatoes and Radishes

Heart-Health Benefits: Folic acid and fiber; cholesterol free

This easy, tasty, and extremely healthy salad is a fantastic accompaniment to fish, meat, or poultry. Sherry vinegar adds a nice touch, but any vinegar can be used.

■ *Serves 4* ■

One 15-ounce can lentils, rinsed and drained, or
   1¹/₂ cups cooked lentils

¹/₄ cup finely diced celery

¹/₄ cup quartered and sliced red radishes

1 small vine-ripened tomato, cut into small dice,
   or 12 cherry tomatoes, quartered

¹/₄ teaspoon minced garlic

¹/₂ teaspoon dried thyme

1 tablespoon olive oil or canola oil

2 teaspoons sherry vinegar or other vinegar, or to
   taste

Salt and freshly ground pepper, to taste

Combine all of the ingredients in a bowl and mix gently. Adjust the seasoning and serve.

Approximate Nutritional Information: Serving size: ¹/₂ cup healthy lentil salad with tomatoes and radishes; Calories: 126 cals, 6%; Protein: 7 g, 14%; Total fat: 3.7 g, 6%; Saturated fat: 0.3 g, 1%; Cholesterol: 0 mg, 0%; Carbohydrates: 17 g, 6%; Fiber: 6 g, 26%; Sodium: 154 mg, 6%; Folic acid: 142 mcg 35%; Vitamin K: 9 mcg, 12%; Diabetic Exchange Values: 1 Starch, 1 Lean Meat

Percentage of calories from fat: 26%

The Healthiest Salad Greens

ROMAINE WINS ON almost all fronts (spinach takes the prize for vitamin A)—and iceberg lettuce comes in last. A rule of thumb for choosing greens is the darker, the better. Why? Because darker vegetables contain more antioxidants, which are good for your heart and for preventing cancer. The following common salad greens are listed in order of nutrients contained in a 1-cup serving (a cup of lettuce ranges from 5 to 10 calories).

	VITAMIN A	VITAMIN C	FOLIC ACID
Romaine	1,456 IU	13 mg	76 mcg
Spinach	2,813 IU	8 mg	58 mcg
Boston, Bibb, or Butterhead	534 IU	4 mg	40 mcg
Loose Leaf	1,064 IU	10 mg	28 mcg
Iceberg	182 IU	2 mg	30 mcg

Tomato and Great Northern Bean Salad with Fresh Basil

Heart-Health Benefits: Vitamins A and C; cholesterol free

Use the best vine-ripened tomatoes you can get—such as those from your garden or from a local farm stand. Make a pretty border around the tomatoes with watercress or baby arugula, if desired.

■ *Serves 4* ■

2 teaspoons red wine vinegar

$^1/_2$ teaspoon Dijon mustard

$1^1/_2$ tablespoons olive oil or canola oil

3 vine-ripened tomatoes, thinly sliced

1 cup canned great northern beans or cannellini beans, rinsed and drained

Squeeze of fresh lemon juice, or to taste

Salt and freshly ground pepper, or to taste

$^1/_3$ cup sliced fresh basil leaves

1. Combine the red wine vinegar and mustard in a small bowl and mix. Add the olive oil and mix until emulsified; set aside.
2. Arrange the tomato slices in a circle on a large rimmed plate or platter, leaving space in the middle for the beans; set aside.
3. Place the beans in a small bowl and toss with 1 tablespoon of the dressing. Add the lemon juice and season to taste with salt and pepper. Arrange the beans in the middle of the tomatoes. Drizzle the remaining dressing over the tomatoes, season lightly with salt and pepper, and garnish with the basil leaves. Let the salad sit at room temperature for 15 minutes before serving to allow the flavors to develop.

Approximate Nutritional Information: Serving size: one-quarter tomato and great northern bean salad with fresh basil; Calories: 138 cals, 7%; Protein: 6 g, 12%; Total fat: 5.5 g, 9%; Saturated fat: 0.8 g, 4%; Cholesterol: 0 mg, 0%; Carbohydrates: 18 g, 6%; Fiber: 4 g, 18%; Sodium: 160 mg, 7%; Vitamin A: 955 IU, 19%; Vitamin C: 14 mg, 23%; Vitamin K: 25 mcg, 31%; Diabetic Exchange Values: 1 Starch, 1 Vegetable, 1 Fat

Percentage of calories from fat: 35%

The Best Mayonnaise

MAYONNAISE IS NOT as bad for you as you may think, but don't overindulge, and always choose "light" or fat-free varieties. For a healthy twist, try replacing some of the usual amount of mayonnaise called for in salad recipes (such as tuna, chicken, or noodle salads) with plain fat-free yogurt, and use more mustard than mayonnaise on your sandwiches. Soy-based sandwich spreads are another good option. Following are some nutritional breakdowns for a 1-tablespoon serving size, starting with the highest calorie and fat content, Hellman's Real Mayonnaise, and ending with fat-free soy-based Nayonaise.

	CALORIES	TOTAL FAT	SATURATED FAT	CHOLESTEROL	SODIUM
Hellman's Real Mayonnaise	90	10 g	1.5 g	5 mg	75 mg
Hellman's Light Mayonnaise	45	4.5 g	0.5 g	<5 mg	120 mg
Fat-Free Mayonnaise Dressing (such as Smart Beat)	10	0	0	0	120 mg
Nasoya Fat-Free Nayonaise (soy-based)	10	0		0	100 mg

Super-Easy Bean Salad

Heart-Health Benefits: Folic acid and fiber; cholesterol free

Customize this basic bean salad recipe by adding your favorite beans and vegetables, such as cucumbers, tomatoes, red or yellow bell peppers, serrano chiles, tomatillos, or corn.

■ *Serves 6* ■

1 cup canned black-eyed peas, rinsed and drained

1 cup canned black beans, rinsed and drained

1 cup canned chickpeas, rinsed and drained

$^1/_4$ cup finely chopped red onion

$^1/_2$ cup diced celery

1 teaspoon minced garlic

2 tablespoons freshly squeezed lime juice, or to taste

2 tablespoons chopped fresh cilantro or parsley

2 teaspoons seasoned rice vinegar

1 tablespoon canola oil

Dash of chili powder, or to taste

Dash of ground cumin, or to taste

Salt, to taste

Combine all of the ingredients in a bowl and mix gently. Adjust the seasoning and serve.

Approximate Nutritional Information: Serving size: $^1/_2$ cup super easy bean salad; Calories: 142 cals, 7%; Protein: 7 g, 15%; Total fat: 3.3 g, 5%; Saturated fat: 0.3 g, 2%; Cholesterol: 0 mg, 0%; Carbohydrates: 22 g, 7%; Fiber: 7 g, 27%; Sodium: 210 mg, 9%; Folic Acid: 154 mcg 38%; Vitamin K: 6 mcg, 8%; Diabetic Exchange Values: 1 Starch, 1 Vegetable, 1 Fat

Percentage of calories from fat: 21%

Terrific Tabbouleh

Heart-Health Benefits: Vitamins A and C, magnesium, and fiber; cholesterol free

*A*dding healthy ingredients, like tomatoes, red bell peppers, chickpeas, and pine nuts, to an already good thing, like tabbouleh salad, makes it that much tastier and healthier! For a light lunch, serve this salad with hummus (see Four Hummus Variations, page 90), or serve as a side dish with grilled fish or chicken. Chopped fresh mint would add a welcome summery flavor. (Note: For instructions on preparing bulgur grains that are not part of a boxed tabbouleh mix, see A Guide to Cooking Healthy Grains, page 106.)

■ *Serves 4* ■

One 6-ounce package Near East Tabbouleh Mix (or any other brand of wheat salad mix)

2 tablespoons freshly squeezed lemon juice, or to taste

1 tablespoon olive oil or canola oil

2 vine-ripened tomatoes, cut into small dice

$^2/_3$ cup finely diced red bell pepper

$^1/_2$ cup canned chickpeas or your favorite canned beans, rinsed and drained

$^1/_2$ cup pine nuts, toasted

Salt and freshly ground pepper, to taste

1. Place the contents of the tabbouleh package in a medium bowl and add boiling water as indicated on the package. Stir, then cover with plastic wrap and let sit at room temperature for 20 minutes.
2. Add the remaining ingredients and mix gently. Adjust the seasoning and serve.

Approximate Nutritional Information: Serving size: 1 cup terrific tabbouleh; Calories: 270 cals, 13%; Protein: 8 g, 17%; Total fat: 10 g, 15%; Saturated fat: 0.9 g, 5%; Cholesterol: 0 mg, 0%; Carbohydrates: 43 g, 14%; Fiber: 11 g, 43%; Sodium: 411 mg, 17%; Vitamin A: 1,292 IU, 26%; Vitamin C: 60 mg, 100%; Magnesium: 105 mg, 26%; Vitamin K: 14 mcg, 17%; Diabetic Exchange Values: 3 Starch, 2 Fat

Percentage of calories from fat: 30%

You Can Have Your Cheese and Eat It, Too

THIS DOES NOT mean indulging in a creamy slab of Brie or perfectly aged Stilton, but rather enjoying a reduced-fat piece of cheddar as a snack, a helping of low-fat feta in your salad, or some low-fat cottage cheese for breakfast. Basically, the rule of thumb is to choose a cheese that has a total fat of less than 5 grams per serving. Some examples of cheeses that fit into this category include:

Slices
- Kraft Fat Free Singles, 0 fat per slice
- Lactose Free Smart Beat Healthy Fat Free Non-Dairy Slices, 0 fat per slice
- Kraft 2% Milk Singles American Processed Cheese with Added Calcium, 3 grams total fat per slice
- Kraft Deli Deluxe 2% Milk Swiss Cheese, 4.5 grams total fat per slice
- Cabot All Natural 50% Light Cheddar Cheese Slices, 4.5 grams total fat per slice

String
- Frigo Cheese Heads 100% Natural String Cheese, 2.5 grams total fat per stick
- Kraft Poly-O Twist-Ums String Cheese (mozzarella and cheddar cheeses), 4 grams total fat per stick

Feta
- President Fat-Free Crumbled Feta, 0 total fat per ounce
- Miller's Feta Cheese, 4 grams total fat per ounce
- Athenos Reduced-Fat Crumbled Feta, 4.5 grams total fat per $1/4$ cup

Mozzarella
- Light low-moisture part-skim mozzarella cheese, 2.5 grams total fat per piece
- Sargento Reduced-Fat Mozzarella, 4.5 grams total fat per ounce

Other
- Cottage cheese, 1% fat, 1 gram total fat per $1/2$ cup
- Cabot Vermont Cheddar 75% Light, 2.5 grams total fat per ounce
- Friendship All Natural Farmer Cheese, 2.5 grams total fat per ounce
- Low-fat ricotta cheese, 3 grams total fat per $1/4$ cup
- Laughing Cow Original Creamy Swiss Cheese Flavor, 4 grams total fat per wedge
- Swiss Knight by Gerber Process Cheese Spread, 4 grams total fat per wedge
- Alouette Light Garlic and Herbs Spreadable Cheese, 4 grams total fat per 2 tablespoons
- Sargento Reduced-Fat Four Cheese Italian, 4.5 grams total fat per ounce

Greek Salad
with Whole Wheat Flat Bread

Heart-Health Benefits: Protein, vitamin C, B vitamins, folic acid, and fiber

Drizzling **the olive** oil over greens before adding the vinegar coats the leaves, which prevents the vinegar from wilting them too quickly. A squirt of lemon juice gives the salad a fresh citrus taste.

■ *Serves 2* ■

Salad

2 cups loosely packed sliced romaine lettuce

$1/3$ cup sliced cucumbers

1 small vine-ripened tomato, diced, or 12
   cherry tomatoes, halved

$1/4$ cup crumbled reduced-fat feta cheese

$1/4$ cup pitted black olives or green olives

A couple of slices of red onion (optional, see
   Cooking Tip below)

$1^1/2$ teaspoons olive oil

1 teaspoon red wine vinegar

1 teaspoon freshly squeezed lemon juice, or to
   taste

Dash of dried oregano, or to taste

Salt and freshly ground pepper, to taste

2 whole wheat flat breads or whole wheat pita
   pockets

1. Combine the salad ingredients in a bowl and toss gently.
2. Drizzle the olive oil over the salad and toss gently, then add the vinegar, lemon juice, and oregano and toss again. Adjust the seasoning and serve immediately with the flat bread.

▶ **Cooking Tip:** To temper the intense flavor of sliced or chopped raw onions, soak them in cold water for 10 minutes, then drain.

Approximate Nutritional Information: Serving size: one-half Greek salad and 1 whole wheat flat bread; Calories: 272 cals, 14%; Protein: 11 g, 22%; Total fat: 8.7 g, 14%; Saturated fat: 2.2 g, 11%; Cholesterol: 5 mg, 2%; Carbohydrates: 42 g, 14%; Fiber: 7 g, 29%; Sodium: 669 mg, 28%; Vitamin C: 24 mg, 39%; Thiamin: 0.3 mg, 19%; Folic acid: 112 mcg, 28%; Vitamin K: 67 mcg, 84%; Diabetic Exchange Values: 2 Starch, 3 Vegetable, 1 Fat

Percentage of calories from fat: 27%

Baby Spinach Salad with Asian Dressing

Heart-Health Benefits: Vitamins A and C, folic acid, and calcium; cholesterol free

This combination of baby spinach, Mandarin oranges, and toasted almonds, all bound together with an Asian dressing, is sure to become a salad staple in your home. Baby spinach wilts quickly, so add the dressing just a few minutes before serving.

■ *Serves 3* ■

Asian Dressing
1 teaspoon lite soy sauce
1 tablespoon seasoned rice vinegar
2 tablespoons canola oil
A few drops of toasted sesame oil
1 very small garlic clove, minced
Freshly ground pepper, to taste

Salad
One 6-ounce bag baby spinach (2 cups), washed and dried (see Timesaving Tip)
2 tablespoons sliced almonds, toasted (see Cooking Tip)
1/2 cup canned Mandarin oranges in juice (no added sugar), drained
A sprinkling of toasted sesame seeds (optional)

1. Combine the dressing ingredients in a small bowl and whisk to blend; set aside.
2. Combine the spinach, almonds, and Mandarin oranges in a salad bowl. Whisk the dressing to reblend it, add it to the salad, and toss gently. Sprinkle with the toasted sesame seeds, if using, and serve immediately.

▶ **Timesaving Tip:** Used packaged prewashed baby spinach leaves. Buy toasted almonds (they come in all different flavors; plain or wasabi works nicely in this salad), and toasted sesame seeds, often available in the Asian section of grocery store (spice racks).

▶ **Cooking Tip:** To toast almonds, place them in a small nonstick skillet over medium heat and stir or shake the pan until the almonds are golden brown. Or place the almonds on a baking sheet under the broiler for a minute or two. Watch them carefully, because they tend to burn quickly.

Approximate Nutritional Information: Serving size: one-third baby spinach salad (no dressing); Calories: 79 cals, 4%; Protein: 4 g, 7%; Total fat: 3 g, 5%; Saturated fat: 0.2 g, 1%; Cholesterol: 0 mg, 0%; Carbohydrates: 12 g, 4%; Fiber: 4 g, 15%; Sodium: 24 mg, 1%; Vitamin A: 10,253 IU, 205%; Vitamin C: 139 mg, 231%; Folic acid: 165 mcg, 41%; Calcium: 226 mg, 23%; Diabetic Exchange Values: 2 Vegetable, 1/2 Fat

Percentage of calories from fat: 31%

Approximate Nutritional Information: Serving size: one-third Asian dressing; Calories; 82 cals, 4%; Protein: 0 g, 0%; Total fat: 9 g, 14%; Saturated fat: 0.6 g, 3%; Cholesterol: 0 mg, 0%; Carbohydrates: 0 g, 0%; Fiber: 0 g, 0%; Sodium: 64 mg, 3%; Vitamin K: 11 mcg, 14%; Diabetic Exchange Values: 2 Fat

Percentage of calories from fat: 98%. **Note:** It is more important to focus on the total fat value of this dressing recipe, which is 9 grams, or 14% Daily Value, per serving, than on the percentage of calories from fat.

Romaine Lettuce with Chickpeas, Feta, and Lemon-Shallot Vinaigrette

Heart-Health Benefits: Vitamins A and C, folic acid, and fiber; cholesterol free

A **light, fresh green** salad that goes with everything. If you are not on a low-calorie diet, the avocado gives the salad a wonderful texture and flavor.

■ *Serves 3* ■

Lemon-Shallot Vinaigrette

1¹/₂ tablespoons freshly squeezed lemon juice, or to taste

1 teaspoon Dijon mustard

1 tablespoon minced shallot

1¹/₂ tablespoons olive oil

Salad

4 cups loosely packed sliced romaine lettuce

¹/₂ cup canned chickpeas, rinsed and drained

1 ripe avocado, peeled, pitted, quartered, and sliced crosswire (optional)

¹/₃ cup crumbled reduced-fat feta cheese

1 tablespoon chopped fresh dill

Salt and freshly ground pepper, to taste

1. Combine the vinaigrette ingredients in a small bowl and whisk to blend; set aside.
2. Combine the salad ingredients in a salad bowl. Whisk the vinaigrette to reblend it, add it to the salad, and toss gently. Adjust the seasoning and serve immediately.

Approximate Nutritional Information: Serving size: one-third romaine salad with chickpeas and feta cheese (no avocado and no dressing); Calories: 84 cals, 4%; Protein: 6 g, 12%; Total fat: 2.6 g, 4%; Saturated fat: 1.2 g, 6%; Cholesterol: 4.4 mg, 1%; Carbohydrates: 10 g, 4%; Fiber: 4 g, 15%; Sodium: 188 mg, 8%; Vitamin A: 4,490 IU, 90%; Vitamin C: 18 mg, 31%; Folic acid: 149 mcg, 37%; Vitamin K: 77 mcg, 97%; Diabetic Exchange Values: 2 Vegetables, ¹/₂ Fat

Percentage of calories from fat: 27%

Approximate Nutritional Information: Serving size: one-third romaine salad with chickpeas, avocado, and feta cheese (no dressing); Calories: 178 cals, 9%; Protein: 7 g, 14%; Total fat: 11.4 g, 18%; Saturated fat: 2.4 g, 12%; Cholesterol: 4.4 mg, 1%; Carbohydrates: 15 g, 5%; Fiber: 7 g, 30%; Sodium: 193 mg, 8%; Vitamin A: 4,573 IU, 91%; Vitamin C: 232 mg, 39%; Folic acid: 184 mcg, 46%; Vitamin K: 89 mcg, 112%; Diabetic Exchange Values: 3 Vegetable, 2 Fat

Percentage of calories from fat: 54%. **Note:** This high percentage of calories from fat comes from the healthy monounsaturated fat in the avocado.

Approximate Nutritional Information: Serving size: one-third lemon-shallot vinaigrette; Calories: 66 cals, 3%; Protein: 0.4 g, 1%; Total fat: 6.8 g, 10%; Saturated fat: 0.4 g, 2%; Cholesterol: 0 mg, 0%; Carbohydrates: 1.5 g, 1%; Fiber: 0 g, 0%; Sodium: 40 mg, 2%; Vitamin K: 78 mcg, 97%; Diabetic Exchange Values: 1 Fat

Percentage of calories from fat: 86%. **Note:** It is more important to focus on the total fat value of this dressing recipe, which is 7 grams, or 10% Daily Value, per serving, than on the percentage of calories from fat.

Eat Your Beans

▶ Add all kinds of beans to salads, or make a bean salad (see Super Easy Bean Salad, page 83).

▶ Make soups with a bean base (see Easy Black Bean Soup with Fresh Cilantro, page 59), or add beans to soups such as Classic Minestrone, page 70.

▶ Mix beans with grains such as rice or couscous (see Mediterranean-Style Couscous Salad, page 99).

▶ Add beans to vegetable dishes, including cooked greens (see Sautéed Kale with Black-Eyed Peas, page 123) and potatoes (see Baked Sweet Potatoes with Black Beans and Chili Dressing, page 128).

▶ Add beans or refried beans to burritos (see Lynn Rudolf's Southwestern-Style Breakfast Burrito, page 40), tacos, fajitas, or quesadillas.

▶ Add beans to chilis (see Bean, Mushroom, and Tofu Chili, page 148), ragouts, or stews.

▶ Make dips with beans (see Four Hummus Variations, page 90).

Attention Parents: Make beans part of your child's diet from a young age. Beans are fun to eat, and they lend themselves to counting games.

NON-DAIRY CHEESE ALTERNATIVES

NON-DAIRY CHEESES comprise the "fake cheese" category, and unless you are a vegan, you probably don't have much interest in them. But if you are curious about cholesterol-free and low-fat cheeses made from tofu or rice milk, look for the following brands in whole food and health food stores, and in some grocery stores: Soya Kaas Tofu Cheese (Mild Cheddar Style fat-free, Mozzarella Style, Jalapeno Mexi–Kaas Fat Free, or Monterey Jack Style), Vegan Singles, Soy Company Foods Low-Fat Veggy Singles (Rice Slice or Vegan Singles), and Soyco Foods Rice Shreds Cheddar Flavor (made with wholesome brown rice, not soy).

Four Hummus Variations

Once you've discovered how delicious and simple hummus is to prepare, you'll think twice about buying ready-made hummus again. Enjoy it with whole wheat flat bread, whole wheat pita bread, whole wheat crackers (see Wise Crackers, page 240), or cut-up raw vegetables. Use the procedure for Traditional Hummus (below) for the hummus variations that follow.

Traditional Hummus

Heart-Health Benefits: Protein, folic acid, and fiber; cholesterol free

---

■ *Each of the hummus recipes makes about 2 cups* ■

One 15-ounce can chickpeas, rinsed and drained

1 small garlic clove, minced

$^1/_2$ teaspoon ground cumin

2 to 3 tablespoons freshly squeezed lemon juice, to taste

1 tablespoon canola oil or olive oil

1 tablespoon tahini

About $^1/_4$ cup water (add more or less for the desired consistency)

Salt, to taste

Combine all of the ingredients in the bowl of a food processor or in a blender and process until smooth, stopping to scrape down the sides as needed. Adjust the seasoning and serve. Refrigerate any leftovers for up to 5 days.

▶ **Cooking Tip:** If serving this hummus as an appetizer for guests, garnish it with 2 tablespoons chopped fresh parsley, a dash of cayenne pepper, or toasted pine nuts.

Approximate Nutritional Information: Serving size: $^1/_2$ cup traditional hummus; Calories: 231 cals, 12%; Protein: 10 g, 20%; Total fat: 8.1 g, 13%; Saturated fat: 0.8 g, 4%; Cholesterol: 0 mg, 0%; Carbohydrates: 31 g, 10%; Fiber: 8 g, 34%; Sodium: 155 mg, 6%; Folic acid: 188 mcg, 47%; Vitamin K: 8 mcg, 11%; Diabetic Exchange Values: 2 Starch, 2 Fat

Percentage of calories from fat: 31%

Roasted Red Bell Pepper Hummus

Heart-Health Benefits: Protein, folic acid, and fiber; cholesterol free

One 15-ounce can chickpeas, rinsed and drained

$1/3$ cup jarred roasted red bell peppers

1 small garlic clove, minced

$1/2$ teaspoon ground cumin

1 tablespoon freshly squeezed lemon juice, or to taste

1 tablespoon canola oil

1 tablespoon tahini

About 3 tablespoons water (add more or less for the desired consistency)

Salt, to taste

Approximate Nutritional Information: Serving size: $1/2$ cup roasted red bell pepper hummus; Calories: 231 cals, 12%; Protein: 10 g, 20%; Total fat: 8.1 g, 13%; Saturated fat: 0.8 g, 4%; Cholesterol: 0 mg, 0%; Carbohydrates: 31 g, 10%; Fiber: 8 g, 34%; Sodium: 312 mg, 13%; Folic acid: 189 mcg, 47%; Vitamin K: 8 mcg, 11%; Diabetic Exchange Values: 2 Starch, 2 Fat

Percentage of calories from fat: 31%

Parsley and Scallion Hummus

Heart-Health Benefits: Protein, iron, vitamin C and K, folic acid, and fiber; cholesterol free

One 15-ounce can chickpeas, rinsed and drained

$3/4$ cup packed fresh parsley leaves

1 scallion, trimmed and sliced

1 small garlic clove, minced

$1/2$ teaspoon ground cumin

2 to 3 tablespoons freshly squeezed lemon juice, to taste

1 tablespoon canola oil or olive oil

1 tablespoon tahini

About $1/4$ cup water (add more or less for the desired consistency)

Salt, to taste

Approximate Nutritional Information: $1/2$ cup parsley and scallion hummus; Calories: 234 cals, 12%; Protein: 10 g, 21%; Total fat: 8.2 g, 13%; Saturated fat: 0.8 g, 4%; Cholesterol: 0 mg, 0%; Carbohydrates: 32 g, 11%; Fiber: 9 g, 35%; Sodium: 159 mg, 7%; Iron: 4 mg, 21%; Vitamin C: 16 mg, 27%; Folic acid: 201 mcg, 50%; Vitamin K: 134 mg, 168%; Diabetic Exchange Values: 2 Starch, 2 Fat

Percentage of calories from fat: 31%

Roasted Garlic Hummus

Heart-Health Benefits: Protein, folic acid, and fiber; cholesterol free

6 large garlic cloves, skins left on

One 15-ounce can chickpeas, rinsed and drained

$1/2$ teaspoon ground cumin

2 tablespoons freshly squeezed lemon juice, or to
    taste

1 tablespoon canola oil or olive oil

1 tablespoon tahini

About $1/4$ cup water (add more or less for the
    desired consistency)

Salt, to taste

To roast the garlic, preheat the oven to 425° F. Wrap the garlic in foil and bake for about 30 minutes, or until the inside of the garlic is soft and oozing.

Approximate Nutritional Information: Serving size: $1/2$ cup roasted garlic hummus; Calories: 235 cals, 12%; Protein: 10 g, 21%; Total fat: 8.1 g, 13%; Saturated fat: 0.8 g, 4%; Cholesterol: 0 mg, 0%; Carbohydrates: 32 g, 11%; Fiber: 8 g, 34%; Sodium: 155 mg, 6%; Folic acid: 188 mcg, 47%; Vitamin K: 8 mcg, 11%; Diabetic Exchange Values: 2 Starch, 2 Fat

Percentage of calories from fat: 30%

Go Nuts for Nuts

MANY STUDIES FROM around the world have shown that people who eat nuts regularly cut their risk of heart disease by as much as half compared to those who rarely or never eat nuts. In the last few years, several studies have found that 1 to 3 ounces a day of walnuts or almonds, in particular, can lower blood cholesterol levels, as well as levels of other substances in the blood (including apolipoprotein B) that have been linked to heart disease.

Why are nuts so good for your heart?

▶ They contain monounsaturated and polyunsaturated fats that can lower blood cholesterol and raise good (HDL) cholesterol, especially when substituted for foods high in saturated fats, such as meat or cheese.

▶ They are rich in folate and other B vitamins that may reduce the risk of heart disease by lowering blood levels of homocysteine (see Folic Acid for a Healthy Heart, page 121).

▶ They contain copper, potassium, and magnesium, which are all linked to heart health.

▶ They contain arginine, an amino acid that helps relax blood vessels and inhibits blood clotting.

▶ They are high in fiber, which has numerous heart and other benefits.

▶ They are rich in phytochemicals that may act as antioxidants and lower cholesterol.

▶ They are an excellent source of plant protein.

▶ They are cholesterol free.

Most nuts have between 160 and 190 calories and 13 to 18 grams of fat per 1-ounce serving. At least three-quarters of the calories come from fat, but that fat is from heart-healthy oils. Walnuts are richest in heart-healthy alpha-linolenic acid (an omega-3 fatty acid). Almonds are richest in calcium and vitamin E. Brazil nuts are the best dietary source of selenium. Macadamia nuts have the most calories and fat, chestnuts the least (just 70 calories and 1 gram of fat). Peanuts are legumes (like dried beans), not nuts, but they are similar nutritionally to nuts. They contain some resveratrol, a beneficial compound also found in red grapes; see Red Wine and Resveratrol, page 217.

Nuts are high in calories—a handful can pack as many calories as a piece of cake. Dry-roasted nuts are just as caloric as oil-roasted ones. The good news is that nuts tend to be satisfying and, according to some studies, help reduce hunger longer than many other foods. But be sure to eat nuts in place of other foods, not in addition to your regular diet.

For a list of mail-order companies that sell nuts and seeds, see Sources, page 268.[2]

Hearts of Palm, Tomato, and Asparagus Salad

Heart-Health Benefits: Vitamins A and C and iron; cholesterol free

---

A lovely salad, especially when asparagus and tomatoes are in season. To save time, use presliced hearts of palm.

■ *Serves 4* ■

Salad

1 pound asparagus, washed, tough stalks cut off, and cut into 1¹/₂-inch pieces

1 cup canned sliced hearts of palm

1 vine-ripened tomato, diced

Dressing

2 teaspoons red wine vinegar

1 teaspoon Dijon mustard

¹/₂ teaspoon minced garlic

1 tablespoon olive oil or canola oil

Salt and freshly ground pepper, to taste

1. Boil, steam, or microwave the asparagus until crisp-tender; the cooking time will depend on the cooking method, but the average time is about 5 minutes. If boiling the asparagus, drain, then run under cold water to stop the cooking, and drain again.
2. Arrange the asparagus, hearts of palm, and tomatoes on a platter, or in a serving bowl; set aside.
3. In a small bowl, mix the vinegar, mustard, and garlic. Add the olive oil and whisk until well blended. Drizzle the dressing evenly over the salad, season with salt and pepper, and serve immediately.

Approximate Nutritional Information: Serving size: one-quarter hearts of palm, tomato, and asparagus salad (no dressing); Calories: 38 cals, 2%; Protein: 4 g, 7%; Total fat: 0.4 g, 1%; Saturated fat: 0.1 g, 1%; Cholesterol: 0 mg, 0%; Carbohydrates: 7 g, 2%; Fiber: 4 g, 15%; Sodium: 159 mg, 7%; Vitamin A: 1,113 IU, 22%; Vitamin C: 13 mg, 22%; Iron: 4 mg, 20%; Vitamin K: 50 mcg, 62%; Diabetic Exchange Values: 2 Vegetable

Percentage of calories from fat: 8%

Approximate Nutritional Information: Serving size: one-quarter dressing; Calories: 32 cals, 2%; Protein: 0.2 g, 1%; Total fat: 3.4 g, 5%; Saturated fat: 0.2 g, 1%; Cholesterol: 0 mg, 0%; Carbohydrates: 0 g, 0%; Fiber: 0 g, 0%; Sodium: 175 mg, 7%; Vitamin K: 4 mcg, 5%; Diabetic Exchange Values: 1 Fat

Percentage of calories from fat: 92%. **Note:** It is more important to focus on the total fat value of this dressing recipe, which is 3 grams, or 5% Daily Value, per serving, than on the percentage of calories from fat.

Portion Sizes and Nutritional Information for Popular Unsalted Nuts

	CALORIES	PROTEIN	TOTAL FAT	SATURATED FAT	FIBER	CARBOHYDRATE
Almonds: 1 ounce, about 3 tablespoons	169	6 g	15 g	1 g	3 g	5 g

Excellent source of vitamin E, magnesium, and manganese
Good source of calcium, phosphorous, and copper

	CALORIES	PROTEIN	TOTAL FAT	SATURATED FAT	FIBER	CARBOHYDRATE
Cashews: 1 ounce, about 3 tablespoons	163	4 g	13 g	2.5 g	0.8 g	9 g

Excellent source of copper
Good source of phosphorous, magnesium, zinc, and manganese

	CALORIES	PROTEIN	TOTAL FAT	SATURATED FAT	FIBER	CARBOHYDRATE
English Walnuts: 1 ounce, about 1/4 cup	185	4 g	18 g	2 g	2 g	4 g

Excellent source of copper and manganese
Good source of phosphorous and magnesium

	CALORIES	PROTEIN	TOTAL FAT	SATURATED FAT	FIBER	CARBOHYDRATE
Peanuts: 1 ounce, about 3 tablespoons	166	7 g	14 g	2 g	2 g	6 g

Excellent source of manganese
Good source of vitamin E, niacin, folate, phosphorous, magnesium, and copper

	CALORIES	PROTEIN	TOTAL FAT	SATURATED FAT	FIBER	CARBOHYDRATE
Pistachios: 1 ounce, about 3 tablespoons	162	6 g	13 g	1.5 g	3 g	8 g

Good source of thiamin, vitamin B_6, phosphorous, manganese, and copper

Green Bean, Tomato, and Feta Salad

Heart-Health Benefits: Vitamins A and C

Because this salad makes a stunning presentation, you might want to wait until you get to the table before mixing it.

■ *Serves 5* ■

Salad

1 pound green beans, ends trimmed

1 cup halved cherry tomatoes

¹/₃ cup crumbled reduced-fat feta cheese

Dressing

2 teaspoons red wine vinegar

¹/₄ teaspoon minced garlic

1 teaspoon Dijon mustard

1 tablespoon olive oil

Salt and freshly ground pepper, to taste

3 tablespoons chopped fresh dill (optional)

1. Bring a large pot of water to a boil. Add the green beans and cook until crisp-tender, about 5 minutes. Drain, run under cold water to stop the cooking and drain again.
2. Place the green beans in a serving bowl or on a platter. Scatter the tomatoes on top of the beans and top with the feta cheese; set aside.
3. In a small bowl, mix the vinegar, garlic, and mustard. Add the olive oil and whisk until well blended. Drizzle the dressing over the beans, then mix gently. Adjust the seasoning, garnish with the dill, if using, and serve.

Approximate Nutritional Information: Serving size: one-fifth green bean, tomato, and feta salad (no dressing); Calories: 53 cals, 3%; Protein: 4 g, 7%; Total fat: 1.3 g, 2%; Saturated fat: 0.7 g, 4%; Cholesterol: 2.6 mg, 1%; Carbohydrates: 9 g, 3%; Fiber: 4 g, 14%; Sodium: 118 mg, 5%; Vitamin A: 985 IU, 20%; Vitamin C: 23 mg, 38%; Vitamin K: 16 mcg, 19%; Diabetic Exchange Values: 2 Vegetable

Percentage of calories from fat: 19%

Approximate Nutritional Information: Serving size: one-fifth dressing; Calories: 25 cals, 1%; Protein: 0 g, 0%; Total fat: 2.7 g, 4%; Saturated fat: 0.1 g, 1%; Cholesterol: 0 mg, 0%; Carbohydrates: 0 g, 0%; Fiber: 0 g, 0%; Sodium: 140 mg, 6%; Vitamin K: 3 mcg, 4%; Diabetic Exchange Values: ¹/₂ Fat

Percentage of calories from fat: 92%. **Note:** It is more important to focus on the total fat value of this dressing recipe, which is 3 grams, or 4% Daily Value, per serving, than on the percentage of calories from fat.

Healthy Seeds

SEEDS ARE RICH in vitamins, minerals, and fiber. Ounce for ounce they are high in calories and (healthy) monounsaturated and polyunsaturated fats, and they have zero cholesterol. Seeds also contain phytochemicals, some of which may have cardio-protective or anticancer effects.

So, the message is, eat seeds! Grab a handful for a snack, put them in salads (fruit and vegetable) and soups, add them to baked goods (especially muffins and breads), sprinkle them on cereal (hot or cold), or add them to grains, stir-fries, or pasta dishes.

Seed Facts

Flaxseeds: 59 calories and 4 grams of fat per tablespoon (about $1/2$ ounce). Excellent source of heart-healthy alpha-linolenic acid and omega-3 fatty acid. Whole seeds pass through the body undigested; buy them milled or grind them at home.

Sesame Seeds: 55 calories and 5 grams of fat per tablespoon (about $1/3$ ounce). Supply some vitamin E, iron, and zinc.

Poppy Seeds: 47 calories and 4 grams of fat per tablespoon (about $1/3$ ounce). Good source of calcium (127 milligrams per tablespoon) and iron.

Pumpkin Seeds: 148 calories and 12 grams of fat per ounce (about 3 tablespoons). Good source of vitamin E, iron, magnesium, potassium, zinc, selenium, and fiber.

Sunflower Seeds: 165 calories and 14 grams of fat per ounce (about $1/4$ cup). One ounce has 14 milligrams of vitamin E (93% of RDA), lots of thiamin, magnesium, iron, zinc, and folic acid, plus 3 grams of fiber.[3]

Sesame-Ginger Noodle Salad

Heart-Health Benefits: Protein, vitamins A and C, folic acid, and magnesium; cholesterol free

*A*side dish the whole family will enjoy. If serving this salad to kids, you might replace the red bell peppers and the spinach with their favorite vegetables (such as shredded carrots from a salad bar or quick-cooked broccoli florets). If the whole wheat noodles drink up too much of the dressing, add a little sesame oil or canola oil to moisten them.

■ *Serves 4* ■

8 ounces whole wheat thin linguine or thin spaghetti

1½ tablespoons toasted sesame oil

2 tablespoons lite soy sauce, or to taste

1 tablespoon seasoned rice vinegar, or to taste

½ cup thinly sliced red bell pepper

1½ cups packed baby spinach leaves or 1 bunch watercress, trimmed (use top leafy part only), washed, and dried

½ teaspoon minced garlic

1 teaspoon minced fresh ginger (optional)

Dash of toasted sesame seeds (optional)

1. Cook the pasta according to the package directions. Drain and rinse quickly under cold water. Drain again, then place in a large bowl.
2. Add the sesame oil, soy sauce, and rice vinegar to the pasta and toss to coat. Add the remaining ingredients and toss gently until well combined. Adjust the seasoning and serve.

Approximate Nutritional Information: Serving size: one-quarter sesame ginger noodle salad; Calories: 271 cals, 14%; Protein: 11 g, 21%; Total fat: 6.1 g, 9%; Saturated fat: 0.8 g, 4%; Cholesterol: 0 mg, 0%; Carbohydrates: 48 g, 16%; Fiber: 2 g, 8%; Sodium: 294 mg, 12%; Vitamin A: 6,152 IU, 123%; Vitamin C: 109 mg, 181%; Folic acid: 125 mg, 31%; Magnesium: 90 mg, 23%; Vitamin K: 2 mcg, 2%; Diabetic Exchange Values: 3 Starch, 1 Fat

Percentage of calories from fat: 19%

NUT BUTTERS

NUT BUTTERS HAVE the same nutritional advantages, with the exception of less fiber, as nuts do. When choosing a nut butter, look for one that does not contain partially hydrogenated oil. That will eliminate most of the big-name brands, although Smuckers, for example, has an all-natural peanut butter that is excellent. But don't stop with peanut butter. There is a whole word of nut butters worth trying—cashew, almond, hazelnut, and soy nut butters, among others.

Mediterranean-Style Couscous Salad

Heart-Health Benefits: Fiber; cholesterol free

This salad is always a winner. For a really fun and different salad, use Middle Eastern couscous (also called Israeli couscous), which comes in the shape of tiny pearls.

■ *Serves 5* ■

Dressing

- 1 tablespoon red wine vinegar
- 1 small garlic clove, minced
- 1 teaspoon Dijon mustard
- 2 tablespoons olive oil or canola oil

Couscous Salad

- 3 cups cooked whole wheat couscous (about ³⁄₄ cup uncooked couscous)
- 2 vine-ripened tomatoes, cut into wedges, or 15 cherry tomatoes, halved
- ²⁄₃ cup (one 7³⁄₄-ounce can) chickpeas, rinsed and drained
- ¹⁄₃ cup canned or jarred artichoke hearts (in brine), quartered
- ¹⁄₂ cup pitted black olives or green olives
- ¹⁄₄ cup pine nuts, toasted, or pistachio nuts
- ¹⁄₄ cup chopped fresh parsley
- ¹⁄₄ cup thinly sliced scallions
- Squeeze of fresh lemon juice, or to taste
- Salt and freshly ground pepper, to taste

1. In a small bowl, mix the red wine vinegar, garlic, and mustard until well blended. Add the olive oil and whisk until well blended; set aside.
2. Cook the couscous according to the package directions. Transfer the couscous to a large bowl and allow to cool, then fluff with a fork to separate the grains.
3. Add the remaining ingredients to the couscous, then add the dressing and mix gently until well combined. Adjust the seasoning and serve.

Approximate Nutritional Information: Serving size: 1 cup Mediterranean-style couscous salad (no dressing): Calories: 143 cals, 7%; Protein: 5 g, 11%; Total fat: 5.5 g, 9%; Saturated fat: 0.4 g, 2%; Cholesterol: 0 mg, 0%; Carbohydrates: 21 g, 7%; Fiber: 5 g, 19%; Sodium: 175 mg, 7%; Vitamin K: 51 mcg, 63%; Diabetic Exchange Values: 1 Starch, 1 Vegetable, 1 Fat

Percentage of calories from fat: 33%

Approximate Nutritional Information: Serving size: one-fifth dressing; Calories: 42 cals, 2%; Protein: 0 g, 0%; Total fat: 4.5 g, 7%; Saturated fat: 0.3 g, 2%; Cholesterol: 0 mg, 0%; Carbohydrates: 0 g, 0%; Fiber: 0 g, 0%; Sodium: 20 mg, 1%; Vitamin K: 6 mcg, 7%; Diabetic Exchange Values: 1 Fat

Percentage of calories from fat: 95%. **Note:** It is more important to focus on the total fat value of this dressing recipe, which is 5 grams, or 7% Daily Value, per serving, than on the percentage of calories from fat.

Buying, Storing, and Using
Nuts and Seeds

THE HIGH FAT content of nuts and seeds makes them prone to rancidity, and therefore they require careful storage. Buy nuts and seeds from a source that you know has a good turnover. Choose nuts and seeds in airtight packaging, as opposed to those in open bins. When buying nuts and seeds in their shells, look for uniformly colored shells without cracks or holes. Nuts should feel heavy in their shells, not light—which may indicate a shriveled nut inside.

Store shelled nuts and seeds in airtight containers away from light. Pine nuts and other nuts with a high oil content are best kept refrigerated or frozen. Because chestnuts have a high water content they should be refrigerated or they may spoil. All shelled nuts and seeds can be frozen for up to one year. Always taste nuts that have been frozen before using them. If they are bitter or sour, or if they have lost their crunch, discard them.

Nuts and seeds can be eaten on their own, or added to baked goods (from breads and muffins to crisps and cobblers); breakfast cereals (hot and cold); trail mixes; grains (all types, from rice to kasha); stir-fries; vegetables; salads; pilafs and other rice dishes; soups; pasta dishes; stuffings; fish, chicken, and/or meat dishes; fruit salads; yogurt; cottage cheese; ice cream or frozen yogurt—basically everything!

ROASTING NUTS AND SEEDS

ROASTING NUTS AND seeds may seem like extra work, but the taste benefits are well worth the trouble, especially with pecans, walnuts, and pine nuts. To roast nuts or seeds, place them in a dry nonstick skillet over medium heat and cook until fragrant and light golden, stirring or shaking the pan frequently. Or, preheat the oven to 300 degrees F, place the nuts or seeds on a baking sheet, and bake for 10 to 15 minutes, turning once, until fragrant and light golden. Nuts tend to burn quickly, so watch them carefully.

Baby Greens with Shrimp and Curry Vinaigrette

Heart-Health Benefits: Protein, vitamins A and C, and fiber

$\mathcal{A}$ **delicious lunch or** light dinner. The shrimp can be replaced with sautéed or grilled scallops, chicken, or extra-firm tofu. The avocado gives this salad a wonderful texture and flavor and adds healthy monounsaturated fats.

■ *Serves 3* ■

Curry Vinaigrette

- 1 teaspoon Dijon mustard
- 1¹/₂ teaspoons freshly squeezed lemon juice, or to taste
- 1¹/₂ teaspoons seasoned rice vinegar
- 1 teaspoon curry powder, or to taste
- 1¹/₂ tablespoons canola oil

Salad

- 4 cups loosely packed mixed baby greens
- About 6 ounces cooked peeled shrimp
- 1 ripe avocado, peeled, pitted, quartered, and sliced crosswise (optional)
- ¹/₂ cup halved cherry tomatoes
- 1 tablespoon chopped fresh cilantro
- 1 tablespoon finely sliced scallion greens or fresh chives

1. Combine the vinaigrette ingredients in a small bowl and whisk to blend; set aside.
2. Arrange a bed of mixed baby greens on each of three plates. Top with the shrimp, avocado slices, if using, tomatoes, cilantro, and scallions. Whisk the dressing to reblend it, then drizzle it over the salads and serve.

Approximate Nutritional Information: Serving size: one-third baby greens with shrimp (no avocado and no vinaigrette); Calories: 73 cals, 4%; Protein: 13 g, 26%; Total fat: 0.8 g, 1%; Saturated fat: 0.2 g, 1%; Cholesterol: 110 mg, 37%; Carbohydrates: 3 g, 1%; Fiber: 1 g, 5%; Sodium: 140 mg, 6%; Vitamin A: 1,108 IU, 22%; Vitamin C: 12 mg, 21%; Vitamin K: 63 mcg, 79%; Diabetic Exchange Values: 2 Very Lean Meat

Percentage of calories from fat: 11%

Approximate Nutritional Information: Serving size: one-third baby greens with shrimp and avocado (no vinaigrette); Calories: 168 cals, 8%; Protein: 14 g, 28%; Total fat: 9.5 g, 15%; Saturated fat: 1.4 g, 7%; Cholesterol: 110 mg, 37%; Carbohydrates: 8 g, 3%; Fiber: 5 g, 21%; Sodium: 145 mg, 6%; Vitamin A: 1,191 IU, 24%; Vitamin C: 17 mg, 29%; Folic acid: 96 mcg, 24%; Vitamin K: 75 mcg, 94%; Diabetic Exchange Values: 2 Very-Lean Meat, 1 Vegetable, 2 Fat

Percentage of calories from fat: 49%. **Note:** This high percentage of calories from fat comes from the healthy monounsaturated fat in the avocado.

Approximate Nutritional Information: Serving size: one-third curry vinaigrette: Calories: 65 cals, 3%; Protein: 0.4 g, 1%; Total fat: 6.8 g, 11%; Saturated fat: 0.4 g, 2%; Cholesterol: 0 mg, 0%; Carbohydrates: 0 g, 0%; Fiber: 0 g, 0%; Sodium: 40 mg, 2%; Vitamin K: 9 mcg, 11%; Diabetic Exchange Values: 1 Fat

Percentage of calories from fat: 92%. **Note:** It is more important to focus on the total fat value of this dressing recipe, which is 7 grams, or 11% Daily Value, per serving, than on the percentage of calories from fat.

Red Potatoes
with Feta Cheese and Olives

Heart-Health Benefit: Vitamin C

The olives and feta cheese add a wonderful Mediterranean touch. Leave the skin on the potatoes for added fiber.

■ *Serves 6* ■

1¼ pounds baby red potatoes, scrubbed

¼ cup crumbled reduced-fat feta cheese

¼ cup coarsely chopped pitted green olives or
    black olives

½ teaspoon minced garlic

⅓ cup thinly sliced scallions

2 tablespoons chopped fresh dill

2 to 3 tablespoons olive oil or canola oil

2 tablespoons red wine vinegar, or to taste

Salt and freshly ground pepper, to taste

1. Place the potatoes in a pot of water and bring to a boil. Cook 10 to 12 minutes, or just until tender; do not overcook. Check the potatoes periodically by piercing them with the tip of a knife. Drain the potatoes and allow them to cool. Slice them in half, or into quarters if they are large.
2. Combine the potatoes, feta cheese, olives, garlic, scallions, and dill in a large bowl. Drizzle the olive oil on top and toss, then sprinkle with the red wine vinegar and toss again. Adjust the seasoning and serve immediately.

Approximate Nutritional Information: Serving size: one-sixth red potatoes with feta cheese and olives; Calories: 158 cals, 8%; Protein: 4 g, 7%; Total fat: 6.1 g, 9%; Saturated fat: 0.8 g, 4%; Cholesterol: 1.6 mg, 1%; Carbohydrates: 24 g, 8%; Fiber: 2 g, 9%; Sodium: 235 mg, 10%; Vitamin C: 15 mg, 24%; Vitamin K: 6 mcg, 8%; Diabetic Exchange Values: 1 Starch, 1 Vegetable, 1 Fat

Percentage of calories from fat: 34%

High-Fiber Foods

FOOD	SERVING SIZE	FIBER (G)
General Mills Fiber One Cereal	½ cup	14
Kellogg's All Bran Cereal	½ cup	10
Raspberries	1 cup	8
Cooked lentils	½ cup	8
Cooked black beans	½ cup	7
Thomas' Whole Wheat Bagels	1 bagel	7
Cooked chickpeas	½ cup	5
Potato with skin	1 medium	5
Canned kidney beans	½ cup	5
Cooked green peas	⅓ cup	4
Quick-cooking oatmeal	1 cup	4
Blueberries	1 cup	4
Apple with skin	1 medium	4
Whole wheat bread	2 slices	3
Strawberries	1 cup	3
Orange	1 medium	3
Wheat germ	¼ cup	3
Dried dates	5	3
Almonds	3 tablespoons	3
Broccoli	½ cup	2
Whole wheat crackers	5	2
Brussels sprouts	½ cup	2

For comparison, the Recommended Daily Allowance for fiber is 25 grams.

Roasted Beet Salad
with Balsamic-Shallot Vinaigrette

Heart-Health Benefits: Vitamins A and K and folic acid

---

*R*oasted beets liven up any salad. Try to choose small beets, which will cook faster than larger ones. If you're in a hurry, use jarred or canned beets. Also, feel free to add your favorite greens—endive, watercress, or frisée—in place of the baby greens.

■ *Serves 4* ■

4 small beets (about ³/₄ pound), leaves and roots trimmed, scrubbed

Balsamic-Shallot Vinaigrette

2 teaspoons balsamic vinegar

¹/₂ teaspoon Dijon mustard

2 teaspoons minced shallot

1¹/₂ tablespoons olive oil or canola oil

4 cups baby greens, washed and dried

¹/₃ cup crumbled reduced-fat feta cheese

1 tablespoon coarsely chopped walnuts

Salt and freshly ground pepper, to taste

1. Preheat the oven to 425 degrees F.
2. Wrap each beet in foil. Bake for 45 minutes to 1 hour, or until tender. Check for tenderness by inserting the tip of the knife (through the foil) into the middle of a beet. Remove the foil and let cool slightly.
3. When the beats are cool enough to handle, remove the skin. Slice the beets into matchsticks and place them in a bowl (be careful not to stain your clothing with the beet juice).
4. Mix the balsamic vinegar, mustard, and shallot in a small bowl, then whisk in the olive oil; set aside.
5. Arrange the baby greens in a serving bowl or on a platter. Place the beets on top. Drizzle the dressing evenly over the salad, then garnish with the feta cheese and walnuts. Adjust the seasoning and serve immediately.

Approximate Nutritional Information: Serving size: one-quarter roasted beet salad (no dressing); Calories: 77 cals, 4%; Protein: 5 g, 9%; Total fat: 2.8 g, 4%; Saturated fat: 0.9g, 5%; Cholesterol: 3.3 mg, 1%; Carbohydrates: 10 g, 3%; Fiber: 3 g, 10%; Sodium: 385 mg, 16%; Vitamin A: 8,360 IU, 167%; Folic acid: 108 mcg, 27%; Vitamin K: 536 mg, 670%; Diabetic Exchange Values: 2 Vegetable, ¹/₂ Fat

Percentage of calories from fat: 30%

Approximate Nutritional Information: Serving size: one-quarter balsamic-shallot vinaigrette; Calories: 49 cals, 2%; Protein: 0 g, 0%; Total fat: 5.1 g, 8%; Saturated fat: 0.3g, 2%; Cholesterol: 0 mg, 0%; Carbohydrates: 0 g, 0%; Fiber: 0 g, 0%; Sodium: 15 mg, 1%; Vitamin K: 6 mcg, 8%; Diabetic Exchange Values: 1 Fat

Percentage of calories from fat: 93%. **Note:** It is more important to focus on the total fat value of this dressing recipe, which is 5 grams, or 8% Daily Value, per serving, than on the percentage of calories from fat.

Black and White
Gazpacho Salad

Heart-Health Benefits: Vitamins A and C, thiamin, folic acid, and fiber; cholesterol free

Black beans and barley are the black and white in this salad. For a zing, add red pepper flakes or finely chopped jalapeño pepper. Ideally, cut all of the vegetables into small dice of equal size.

■ *Serves 4* ■

¹/₂ cup uncooked whole barley (not quick-cooking barley) or about 2 cups cooked barley

1 cup canned black beans, rinsed and drained

¹/₂ cup finely diced cucumber (peeled or unpeeled)

³/₄ cup finely diced tomatoes

¹/₂ cup finely diced celery

¹/₄ cup finely diced red bell pepper or green banana pepper

¹/₄ cup chopped fresh cilantro

¹/₄ cup thinly sliced scallions

¹/₂ teaspoon minced garlic

2 tablespoons freshly squeezed lime juice, or to taste

1 tablespoon olive oil

¹/₄ cup low-sodium tomato juice

Salt and freshly ground pepper, to taste

1. To cook the barley, bring 4 cups water to a boil in a medium saucepan. Add the barley, reduce the heat, and simmer for 45 minutes, or until the barley is tender. Drain and briefly rinse the barley under cold running water; drain again.
2. Combine the barley and all of the remaining ingredients in a serving bowl and mix gently. Adjust the seasoning and serve. Refrigerate leftovers.

Approximate Nutritional Information: Serving size: one-quarter black and white gazpacho salad; Calories: 186 cals, 9%; Protein: 8 g, 15%; Total fat: 4.3 g, 7%; Saturated fat: 0.6 g, 3%; Cholesterol: 0 mg, 0%; Carbohydrates: 31 g, 10%; Fiber: 9 g, 35%; Sodium: 348 mg, 15%; Vitamin A: 1,013 IU, 20%; Vitamin C: 31 mg, 52%; Thiamin: .3 mg, 20%; Folic acid: 90 mcg, 22%; Vitamin K: 11 mcg, 14%; Diabetic Exchange Values: 2 Starch, 1 Fat

Percentage of calories from fat: 20%

A Guide to Cooking Healthy Grains

Barley (hulled, or pearled)

Uses: Soups, casseroles, side dishes, salads, hot cereal, stuffings (see Black and White Gazpacho Salad, page 105)

Basic Cooking Instructions: *Ratio: 3 cups water to $1/2$ cup barley.* Add directly to soups. To use cooked barley in salads or side dishes, bring 3 cups water to a boil, add $1/2$ cup barley, and simmer, uncovered, for 45 minutes, or until the grains are soft. Drain, rinse under cold running water, and drain again. (Note: A $1/2$ cup of raw barley makes about 2 cups cooked barley.)

Tips: Quick-cooking barley, such as Quaker Oats Mother's Quick Cooking Barley, cooks in about 10 minutes. Barley flakes, which resemble rolled oats, can be made into hot cereal. Barley grits, a fine grind of the grain, are used for hot cereal.

Brown Rice

Uses: Side dishes, salads, soups, risottos, pilafs, stuffings (see Brown Rice with Tofu and Shiitake Mushroom Pilaf, page 130)

Basic Cooking Instructions: *Ratio: 2 cups water to 1 cup rice.* Stove-top cooking method: Bring the water to a boil in a large saucepan. Add the rice and return to a boil, then reduce the heat to a simmer, cover, and cook for 45 minutes, or until the grains are tender and the water has evaporated. (Note: The grains will not be as soft as white rice, but they should not be too hard.) Oven method: Preheat the oven to 400 degrees F. Bring the water to a boil. Place the rice in an 8-inch baking dish, add the water, and cover with foil. Bake for 45 minutes, or until the grains are tender.

Tips: Brown rice comes in short, medium, or long grains; brown basmati rice is also available. The outer hull, or bran, is left on the rice grain, which means brown rice has twice as much fiber as white rice, as well as vitamin E. Lundberg Family Farms produces fabulous brown rice in an assortment of varieties and mixtures.

Buckwheat Groats (also known as kasha)

Uses: Side dishes, breakfast cereal, pilafs, stuffings

Basic Cooking Instructions: *Ratio: 2 cups water to 1 cup kasha.* Bring the water to a boil; set aside. In a medium nonstick saucepan, heat 2 teaspoons canola oil over medium-high heat. Add the kasha and stir until the grains are slightly toasted and aromatic, about 3 minutes. Add the hot water, stir, and return to a boil. Reduce the heat to a simmer, cover, and cook for 10 to 12 minutes (cooking time depends on the grind; see below), or until the grains are tender and the water is absorbed.

Tips: Whole or coarse buckwheat groats retain their shape best when cooked. The fine or medium grains have a shorter cooking time and tend to get a bit mushy.

Bulgur (also known as tabbouleh, or tabouli)

Uses: Salads, pita pockets sandwiches with hummus, stuffings (see Terrific Tabbouleh, page 84)

Basic Cooking Instructions: *Ratio: 1 1/2 cups water to 1 cup bulgur* (The amount of water absorbed will depend on the size of the grain; drain off any water that is not absorbed after 25 minutes of soaking.) Bulgur grains are softened, not cooked. Bring the water to a boil. Place the grains in a heatproof bowl, add the boiling water, stir, and cover with plastic wrap. Let sit at room temperature for 20 to 25 minutes, or until the grains are soft; drain if necessary.

Tips: Boxed tabbouleh mixes that contain spice packets are quick and easy to prepare. Near East Taboule Mix Wheat Salad seems to have the perfect balance of spice to grain. To make your own tabbouleh salad, soften the grains (as above), then add freshly squeezed lemon juice, olive oil, garlic, chopped fresh parsley and mint, finely sliced scallions, diced tomatoes, and salt and pepper, all to taste. Feel free to experiment by adding other grains (brown rice or wheat berries), shredded or chopped vegetables (carrots, cucumbers, bell peppers, or olives), crumbled cheese (fat-free feta), nuts (toasted pine nuts or pistachios), or fresh herbs (basil or cilantro). (See Terrific Tabbouleh, page 84.)

Quinoa (pronounced "KEEN-wah")

Uses: Salads, side dishes, stuffings (see Quinoa with Chicken and Hoisin Dressing, page 108.)

Basic Cooking Instructions: *Ratio: 2 cups water to 1 cup quinoa.* Rinse the quinoa in a fine-mesh strainer under cold running water for about 1 minute, then drain. Combine the quinoa with the water in a saucepan and bring to a boil. Reduce the heat and simmer, covered, for 15 to 20 minutes, or until the grains look translucent and the spiral-like germ has separated. Remove from the heat and let stand for 5 minutes, then fluff with a fork.

Tips: It is advisable to purchase boxed quinoa (such as Ancient Harvest) rather than buying it in bulk from bins. Boxed grains tend to be larger, cleaner, sweeter, and fluffier when cooked. It is essential to rinse quinoa before cooking it to remove the bitter natural outer coating on each grain. Although most of this coating is removed before sale, there may be a small residue left. This grain is a complete protein, comparable to the protein found in meat and eggs.

Whole Wheat Couscous

Uses: Salads, side dishes, stuffings (See Mediterranean-Style Couscous Salad, page 99.)

Basic Cooking Instructions: *Ratio: 1 1/2 cups water to 1 cup couscous.* Bring the water to a boil in a saucepan. Add the couscous, stir, and return to a boil. Cover, remove from the heat, and let sit, covered, for 7 minutes. Fluff with a fork.

Tips: Whole wheat couscous contains more fiber and iron than regular couscous. Israeli, Mediterranean, or Middle Eastern couscous (all the same thing) is perfectly round grains of toasted pasta that have no fiber or iron, but they make a fun salad (kids might like these tiny balls as a salad).

Quinoa with Chicken and Hoisin Dressing

Heart-Health Benefits: Protein, iron, vitamins A and C, B vitamins, folic acid, magnesium, and fiber

Quinoa is an easy-to-cook, high-protein grain with an earthy taste and a pop-in-your-mouth texture. Use it as you would couscous. Purchase boxed quinoa (such as Ancient Harvest Quinoa), which tends to have larger, cleaner, sweeter, and fluffier grains than quinoa from an open bin. You can substitute tofu for the chicken here, and you can vary the vegetables to suit your taste (use about 3 cups total of vegetables).

■ *Serves 4* ■

Salad

½ cup uncooked quinoa, thoroughly rinsed (see Cooking Tip on page 109)

8 ounces chicken tenders or boneless, skinless chicken breasts

1 cup frozen edamame (shelled soy beans), cooked according to package directions

4 ounces (about 1 heaping cup) snow peas, cooked in boiling water until crisp-tender

⅔ cup thinly sliced red bell peppers

¼ cup thinly sliced scallions

Hoisin Dressing

1 tablespoon hoisin sauce

1 tablespoon peanut sauce

1 tablespoon seasoned rice vinegar

1 tablespoon water

Dash of toasted sesame oil

Dash of lite soy sauce

Dash of hot chili oil or hot pepper flakes (optional)

1. Prepare the quinoa according to the package directions. (Or, if you do not have a package with directions, rinse the quinoa in a fine-mesh strainer under cold running water for 1 minute. In a medium saucepan, bring 1 cup water to a boil. Add the quinoa and return to a boil, then reduce the heat and simmer, covered, for 15 to 20 minutes, or until the water is absorbed, the grains look translucent, and the spiral-like germ has separated.) Remove from the heat and let stand for 5 minutes. Fluff with a fork, then transfer to a large bowl; set aside.

2. While the quinoa is cooking, prepare the chicken. Bring a medium saucepan of water to a boil. Add the chicken, reduce the heat to a simmer, and cook for 7 minutes, or until the chicken is thoroughly cooked. (Note: Chicken breasts will take longer to cook than the chicken tenders.) Drain and cool, then slice the chicken into ½-inch pieces.

3. Add the chicken and the remaining salad ingredients to the quinoa. Mix gently until well incorporated; set aside.

4. Combine the hoisin dressing ingredients in a small bowl and mix. Add the dressing to the salad, mix gently, and adjust the seasoning. Serve at room temperature or chilled.

▶ **Cooking Tip:** It is essential to rinse quinoa before cooking it to remove the bitter natural outer coating on each grain. Although this coating is removed during processing, there may be a small residue left. Rinse the quinoa in a fine-mesh strainer under running water for about 1 minute. Or place it in the saucepan you plan to cook it in, add water to cover, and swish the grains with your hands for about 1 minute; drain.

Approximate Nutritional Information: Serving size: one-quarter quinoa with chicken and hoisin dressing; Calories: 305 cals, 15%; Protein: 30 g, 60%; Total fat: 8.6 g, 13%; Saturated fat: 1.4 g, 7%; Cholesterol: 48 mg, 16%; Carbohydrates: 28 g, 9%; Fiber: 5 g, 21%; Sodium: 206 mg, 9%; Iron: 5 mg, 30%; Vitamin A: 1,003 IU, 20%; Vitamin C: 76 mg, 126%; Niacin: 10 mg, 49%; B_6: 0.53 mg, 27%; Folic acid: 134 mcg, 33%; Magnesium: 112 mg, 28%; Vitamin K: 6 mcg, 8%; Diabetic Exchange Values: 1 Starch, 3 Vegetable, 3 Very Lean Meat, 1 Fat

Percentage of calories from fat: 25%

Tips for Preparing Grains

▶ Substitute fat-free low-sodium stock for water in savory recipes.

▶ Use olive oil, canola oil, or heart-healthy margarine in place of butter to moisten grains during or after cooking.

▶ Make long-cooking grains (such as whole pearl barley or wheat berries) in advance and freeze them.

▶ Mix grains to create different textures and flavors in side dishes and stuffings.

▶ Use cooked grains to stuff vegetables (peppers or tomatoes) and poultry (chicken or turkey).

▶ Liven up grains with raw or cooked vegetables, nuts, dried fruit, spices, and herbs.

▶ Sweeten grains for breakfast with brown sugar, maple syrup, honey, molasses, fruit compote, dried fruits, or jam.

▶ Add grains such as wheat germ and whole oats to batters for muffins or breads.

FOUR

VEGETABLE AND SOY DISHES

HEART-HEALTH TIPS AT A GLANCE

Vegetable Dishes

▶ Eat five servings of vegetables and fruits per day. This is not as hard as you think if you consider the following ready-to-eat or drink sources: fresh or frozen fruits and vegetables; dried fruits such as apricots and prunes; low-sodium tomato juice and other vegetable juices; fruit juice (preferably with pulp); salads and vegetables from a salad bar; canned fruit cups in light syrup; Mandarin oranges in natural or light syrup; unsweetened apple-sauce or other unsweetened fruit purees; canned pineapple and peaches; canned or jarred beets; baby carrots; grape tomatoes; prewashed bagged spinach leaves and other lettuce greens; and vegetable soups.

▶ Remember that the healthiest fruits and vegetables are also the most colorful (see The Top 15 High-Antioxidant Fruits and Vegetables, page 113). Leave skins and peels on whenever possible for added fiber and antioxidants.

▶ Use heart-healthy oils in place of saturated fats, such as butter or cream. Ideally, include in your diet oils that contain omega-3 fatty acids, such as soybean oil, walnut oil, and pumpkin seed oil. Other popular heart-healthy oils are olive oil, canola oil, and safflower oil (see Understanding Heart-Healthy Oils, page 116, and Storing and Cooking Heart-Healthy Oils, page 118).

▶ Get folic acid (also called folate) into your diet to lower your homocysteine level in the blood (homocysteine is a byproduct formed from protein metabolism). See Folic Acid for a Healthy Heart, and Good Sources of Folic Acid, page 121.

▶ Increase your consumption of fiber. There are basically two types of fiber, soluble and insoluble, and both are good for you, for different reasons. Soluble fiber, in the form of whole grains, barley, oat bran, psyllium seed husks, ground flaxseeds, and whole oats, has been found to be effective in lowering LDL (bad) cholesterol levels. Insoluble fiber, from fruits and vegetables, contains vitamins and minerals, and fiber, which help to maintain a healthy body and digestive tract (see Soluble Fiber Reduces LDL Cholesterol, page 141, and Adding Ground Flaxseed to Your Diet, page 127).

Soy Dishes

▶ For many people around the globe, especially in Asia, soy is a dietary staple. It is a cholesterol-free, low-fat, nutrient-dense source of protein. As a matter of fact, the U.S. Food and Drug Administration has claimed that soy products may decrease your levels of both overall cholesterol and LDL (bad) cholesterol, as well as triglycerides (see Soy Power, page 129).

▶ Don't be scared to buy, cook, and eat soy products. Soy is not just part of a health-food craze embraced by "crunchy" people—it's been around for centuries and it has been proven to be good for your health (see Uses for Tofu, page 136, and Welcome to the World of Soy, page 131).

▶ Soy products, such as soy milk, yogurt, sour cream, silken tofu, and cream cheese, can be substituted for traditional dairy products, eaten on their own or used in recipes. There are many different brands of soy products on the market, so shop around until you find your favorites.

▶ Low-fat or fat-free dairy products (not full fat) are good for you, especially if you are trying to lose weight. Studies show that consuming high-calcium dairy foods plays a key role in a healthy metabolism and decreases the likelihood of gaining weight (see High Calcium Intake from Dairy Sources Boosts Weight Loss, page 143).

▶ Calcium is an essential tool in the fight against osteoporosis, for both men and women (see Preventing Osteoporosis, page 146). It is also vital for healthy growing bones in children.

The Top 15
High-Antioxidant Fruits and Vegetables

SOME OF THE healthiest fruits and vegetables are also the most colorful. As a rule, the amount of color corresponds to the amount of antioxidants, which help prevent heart disease and cancer. Keep those colorful skins on whenever possible. The skins of fruits and vegetables are a good source of fiber and antioxidants.

Beets
Blackberries
Blueberries
Broccoli
Brussels sprouts
Cherries
Kale
Kiwifruit
Oranges
Pink grapefruit (but see The Dangers of Grapefruit, page 30)
Plums
Red grapes
Red peppers
Spinach
Strawberries

Simply Perfect Zucchini

Heart-Health Benefits: Vitamin C; cholesterol free

Boiling or steaming zucchini and yellow summer squash before sautéing it brings out its subtle flavor and buttery consistency. You can add any additional flavoring to the cooked zucchini you like, such as chopped fresh herbs, minced garlic, or soy sauce. For a festive presentation, combine the yellow and green squash with a handful of chopped red peppers.

■ *Serves 4* ■

1 pound small zucchini, washed, halved and cut into ³/₄-inch slices

1 tablespoon olive oil or canola oil

Salt and freshly ground pepper, to taste

1. Place about 2 inches of water in a large nonstick skillet and bring to a boil. Add the zucchini and cook for 1 minute; do not overcook. Drain; leave the zucchini in the strainer. (Do not rinse the skillet.)
2. Place the skillet over medium-high heat. As soon as it is dry, add the olive oil and heat until hot. Add the drained zucchini and sauté for 2 minutes, stirring occasionally. Adjust the seasoning, transfer the zucchini to a serving dish, and serve immediately.

Approximate Nutritional Information: Serving size: one-quarter simply perfect zucchini; Calories: 48 cals, 2%; Protein: 1 g, 3%; Total fat: 3.5 g, 6%; Saturated fat: 0.4 g, 2%; Cholesterol: 0 mg, 0%; Carbohydrates: 4 g, 7%; Fiber: 1 g, 5%; Sodium: 157 mg, 7%; Vitamin C: 19 mg, 32%; Vitamin K: 7 mcg, 9%; Diabetic Exchange Values: 1 Vegetable, ¹/₂ Fat

Percentage of calories from fat: 61%. **Note:** It is more important to focus on the total fat value of this low-calorie recipe, which is 4 grams, or 6% Daily Value, per serving, than on the percentage of calories from fat.

Cauliflower with Lemon, Parsley, and Garlic

Heart-Health Benefits: Vitamin C, folic acid, and fiber; cholesterol free

---

The **combination of** olive oil, lemon juice, parsley, and garlic works on just about any steamed or boiled vegetable.

■ *Serves 4* ■

6 cups cauliflower florets (about 1 pound florets)

2 tablespoons olive oil or canola oil

1¹/₂ tablespoons freshly squeezed lemon juice, or to taste

Pinch of minced garlic (optional)

2 tablespoons chopped fresh parsley

Salt and freshly ground pepper, to taste

1. Bring a large saucepan of water to a boil. Add the cauliflower florets, return to a boil, and cook for about 2 minutes, or until the florets are crisp-tender. Drain well, then place in a serving bowl.
2. Drizzle the olive oil over the cauliflower. Add the lemon juice, garlic, if using, and parsley, and mix gently. Adjust the seasoning and serve.

Approximate Nutritional Information: Serving size: one-quarter cauliflower with lemon, parsley, and garlic; Calories: 105 cals, 5%; Protein: 3 g, 7%; Total fat: 7.5 g, 12%; Saturated fat: 1.0 g, 5%; Cholesterol: 0 mg, 0%; Carbohydrates: 8 g, 3%; Fiber: 5 g, 20%; Sodium: 174 mg, 7%; Vitamin C: 86 mg, 143%; Folic acid: 84 mcg, 21%; Vitamin K: 45 mcg, 56%; Diabetic Exchange Values: 2 Vegetable, 1 Fat

Percentage of calories from fat: 59%. **Note:** It is more important to focus on the total fat value of this low-calorie recipe, which is 8 grams, or 12% Daily Value per serving, than on the percentage of calories from fat.

Understanding Heart-Healthy Oils

SCIENTIFIC EVIDENCE SHOWS that replacing saturated fats with heart-healthy unsaturated fats will lower both total cholesterol and LDL (bad) cholesterol while maintaining HDL (good) cholesterol, or even boosting it slightly. So, what are saturated fats and unsaturated fats, and where are they found?

Saturated fatty acids, which carry the maximum number of hydrogen atoms, are solid at room temperature. They come mainly from animal sources and include foods such as butter, cheese, whole milk, cream, lard, and meats. These animal fats are also high in cholesterol. Three vegetable oils—coconut, palm, and palm kernel—are highly saturated, but these tropical oils do not act exactly like other saturated fats in the body. They are cholesterol free, and they may not be as unhealthy as once thought.

Trans fatty acids, such as partially hydrogenated oil and hydrogenated oil, are particularly harmful man-altered fats that are produced by passing hydrogen bubbles through heated oil. Trans fats are found in hard margarines, vegetable shortening, and many other processed products, from breakfast cereals and cookies to frozen foods and hot cocoa mix. (For more information, see What Is Partially Hydrogenated Oil and Why Is It Bad for You?, page 61). Conjugated linoleic acid (CLA) is a naturally occurring trans fatty acid found in food products derived from ruminants, such beef from cows (see Conjugated Linoleic Acid: A Natural Trans Fatty Acid, page 63.)

Unsaturated fatty acids, primarily from plants and fish, remain liquid at room temperature. Some of the hydrogen atoms in each molecule in these fatty acids have been replaced by double bonds. Monounsaturated fatty acids are missing one pair of hydrogen atoms. Olive, canola, peanut, and sesame oils contain mostly monounsaturated fatty acids. Polyunsaturated fatty acids are missing two or more pairs of hydrogen atoms. Safflower, flaxseed, walnut, grape seed, corn, and soybean oils are primarily polyunsaturated.

All vegetable oils are combinations of saturated, monounsaturated, and polyunsaturated fatty acids. They are categorized according to the predominant type of fatty acid they contain. Canola oil, for instance, is called monounsaturated because it contains 8 grams of monounsaturated fat, 4 grams of polyunsaturated fat, and 0.9 gram of saturated fat. Corn oil is classified as polyunsaturated because it contains 8 grams of polyunsaturated fat, 3 grams of monounsaturated fat, and 1.7 grams of saturated fat.

It does not really matter which of these monounsaturated or polyunsaturated oils you choose. The most important thing is that heart-healthy oils replace saturated fats in your diet and ideally that they include some vegetable oils with omega-3 fatty acid.

Monounsaturated oils	Polyunsaturated oils	Vegetable oils with omega-3 fatty acids
Almond	Corn	Canola
Avocado	Flaxseed	Pumpkin seed
Canola	Grape seed	Soybean
Olive	Pumpkin seed	Walnut
Peanut	Safflower	
Sesame	Soybean	
	Sunflower	
	Walnut	

Roasted Asparagus with Lime Zest

Heart-Health Benefits: Vitamin A and folic acid; cholesterol free

Asparagus is one of those vegetables that can be cooked a million different ways with consistently excellent results. When roasting, be sure to coat the asparagus spears in oil, otherwise, they tend to get a bit dry. Add your favorite chopped fresh herbs for a special touch.

■ *Serves 3* ■

1 pound asparagus: cut off tough part of stalks and wash remaining spears

Canola oil cooking spray or 1 tablespoon canola oil

Salt and freshly ground pepper, to taste

1/2 teaspoon grated lime zest or lemon zest (avoid the bitter white pith)

1. Preheat the oven to 400 degrees F. Line a baking sheet with foil.
2. Place the asparagus spears on the baking sheet and spray with the cooking spray or drizzle the canola oil over them. Toss the spears with your hands until they are completely coated in the oil and the foil is greased. Line up the spears in a single row and season with salt and pepper. Roast for about 5 minutes, or just until crisp-tender. (Note: The cooking time will depend on the thickness of the asparagus spears.)
3. Transfer the asparagus to a serving platter, adjust the seasoning, and sprinkle with the lime zest. Serve immediately.

Approximate Nutritional Information: Serving size: one-third roasted asparagus with lime zest; Calories: 51 cals, 3%; Protein: 3 g, 7%; Total fat: 2.4g, 4%; Saturated fat: 0.2 g, 1%; Cholesterol: 0 mg, 0%; Carbohydrates: 6 g, 2%; Fiber: 3 g, 13%; Sodium: 197 mg, 8%; Vitamin A: 1,144 mg, 23%; Folic acid: 79 mcg, 20%; Vitamin K: 66 mcg, 82%; Diabetic Exchange Values: 1 Vegetable, 1/2 Fat

Percentage of calories from fat: 37%. **Note:** It is more important to focus on the total fat value of this low-calorie recipe which is 2 grams, or 4% Daily Value, per serving than on the percentage of calories from fat.

Storing and Cooking
Heart-Healthy Oils

Storing

Polyunsaturated oils, including those high in heart-healthy omega-3 fatty acids, such as flaxseed, pumpkin seed, soybean, and walnut oil, are very susceptible to damage from heat, light, and oxygen. When overexposed to these elements, the fatty acids in the oil become oxidized or rancid, which can be detected by a slightly bitter or chalky taste and smell. Rancidity not only alters the taste and flavor of the oils, but it also diminishes their nutritional values.

Oils rich in polyunsaturated fatty acids; some of the less refined monosaturated oils, such as almond and avocado oil, should be stored in tightly closed dark glass containers in the refrigerator. These oils are ideal for salad dressings (see Omega-3 Power Dressing, page 74), and they can be drizzled over cooked fish, meat, and poultry; soups; cooked vegetables; or composed salads for added flavor. If they are heated, they should only be warmed over a low flame.

Cooking

The best heart-healthy oils for cooking are those that have a smoking point of between 320 and 500 degrees F (a normal cooking temperature is between 350 and 375 degrees F). Refined oils that fit into this category include canola, safflower, peanut, and corn oil. Olive oil should only be used with medium heat—for example, when sautéing fish or shellfish. Deep-frying should be avoided, and a minimal amount of oil or canola oil cooking spray and a nonstick pan should be used for sautéing and other cooking.

Green Beans with Red Bell Peppers, Pine Nuts, and Fresh Basil

---

Heart-Health Benefits: Vitamins A and C; cholesterol free

S tunning, crowd-pleasing, easy, and delicious—what more could you ask for?

■ *Serves 5* ■

1 pound fresh green beans, ends trimmed, or frozen haricots verts

2 tablespoons olive oil or canola oil

1 cup thinly sliced red bell peppers

2 tablespoons pine nuts, toasted

2 tablespoons finely sliced fresh basil leaves

Salt and freshly ground pepper, to taste

1. Bring a large saucepan of water to a boil. Add the green beans, return to a boil, and cook for about 2 minutes, or until crisp-tender (the beans will be sautéed later, so do not overcook them). Drain well and set aside.
2. Heat the olive oil in a large skillet over medium-high heat. Add the red bell peppers and sauté for 2 minutes. Add the green beans and sauté for 2 minutes more. Transfer to a serving dish.
3. Add the pine nuts and basil and gently mix. Adjust the seasoning and serve immediately, or cool and serve at room temperature.

Approximate Nutritional Information: Serving size: one-fifth green beans with red bell peppers, pine nuts, and fresh basil; Calories; 83 cals, 4%; Protein: 2 g, 5%; Total fat: 5.2 g, 8%; Saturated fat: 0.4 g, 2%; Cholesterol: 0 mg, 0%; Carbohydrates: 9 g, 3%; Fiber: 4 g, 15%; Sodium: 122 mg, 5%; Vitamin A: 1,560 IU, 31%; Vitamin C: 71 mg, 119%; Vitamin K: 20 mcg, 25%; Diabetic Exchange Values: 1 Vegetable, 1 Fat

Percentage of calories from fat: 52%. **Note:** It is more important to focus on the total fat value of this low-calorie recipe, which is 5 grams, or 8% Daily Value, per serving, than on the percentage of calories from fat.

Asian-Style Broccoli

Heart-Health Benefits: Vitamins A and C; cholesterol free

This is a great way to serve broccoli. Try to keep the florets about the same size so they cook evenly. If you are serving this dish to kids, you may want to leave out the red pepper flakes. If you are not on a low-calorie diet, the cashew nuts are a delicious addition.

■ *Serves 5* ■

2 tablespoons lite soy sauce

1 tablespoon reduced-fat smooth peanut butter

1 tablespoon hoisin sauce

Pinch of red pepper flakes (optional)

1 tablespoon canola oil

6 cups broccoli florets (about 1 pound florets)

1 garlic clove, minced

2 tablespoons chopped cashew nuts (optional)

1. In a small bowl, combine the soy sauce, peanut butter, hoisin sauce, and pepper flakes, if using, and mix until smooth. Set aside.
2. Heat the canola oil in a large skillet over medium-high heat. Add the broccoli florets and sauté for 2 minutes. Add the garlic and sauté for 30 seconds, then add 3 tablespoons water and cook, stirring, for 2 minutes. (Note: The florets should still be slightly crisp; do not overcook.) Add the reserved soy sauce mixture and cook for 1 minute more. Adjust the seasoning.
3. Transfer the broccoli and sauce to a serving dish, garnish with the cashew nuts, if using, and serve.

▶ **Substitutions:** Use frozen broccoli florets and cook in the canola oil just until defrosted. Proceed as directed.

Approximate Nutritional Information: Serving size: one-fifth Asian-style broccoli (no cashew nuts); Calories: 58 cals, 3%; Protein: 3 g, 7%; Total fat: 2.3 g, 4%; Saturated fat: 0.2 g, 1%; Cholesterol: 0 mg, 0%; Carbohydrates: 7 g, 2%; Fiber: 0.2 g, 1%; Sodium: 317 mg, 13%; Vitamin A: 2,579 IU, 52%; Vitamin C: 80 mg, 133%; Vitamin K: 176 mcg, 220%; Diabetic Exchange Values: 1 Vegetable, 1 Fat

Percentage of calories from fat: 33%

FOLIC ACID FOR A HEALTHY HEART

FOLIC ACID PLAYS a vital role in maintaining a healthy heart (it is also important in preventing neural tube birth defects in pregnancy). Folic acid and other B vitamins help lower homocysteine levels in the blood. Homocysteine is a by-product formed in protein metabolism. Certain vitamins help break down homocysteine, so increased homocysteine levels may indicate a deficiency of folic acid, vitamin B_6, and/or vitamin B_{12}. A normal homocysteine level is less than 12 µmol/L; a level greater than 12 is considered high.

The American Heart Association (AHA) has not yet called hyperhomocysteinemia, or a condition of high homocysteine levels in the blood, a major risk factor for cardiovascular disease, and the AHA does not recommend widespread use of folic acid and B-vitamin supplements to reduce the risk of heart disease and stroke. Instead, it advises a healthy, balanced diet that includes at least five servings of fruits and vegetables a day. For folic acid, the recommended daily value is 400 micrograms (mcg). Fortified breakfast cereals and breads, lentils, romaine lettuce, chickpeas, legumes, asparagus, citrus fruits, and green vegetables are all good sources of folic acid (see Good Sources of Folic Acid, below). Since January 1998, flour has been fortified with folic acid to add an estimated 100 micrograms (mcg) per day to the average diet.[1]

Apart from a diet deficient in folic acid, other factors that may increase homocysteine levels include smoking, excessive alcohol intake, and high coffee consumption, all of which break down vitamins and reduce their absorption. Lack of physical exercise, obesity, and stress are all associated with higher levels of homocysteine in the blood as well.[2]

Good Sources of Folic Acid

FOOD	SERVING SIZE	FOLIC ACID (MCG)
All Bran Cereal	½ cup	400
Cooked lentils	½ cup	179
Romaine lettuce (sliced)	2 cups	152
Chickpeas	½ cup	141
Asparagus	½ cup	131
Cooked spinach	½ cup	131
Cooked black beans	½ cup	128
Brewer's yeast	1 teaspoon	104
Sunflower seeds	¼ cup	76
Orange juice	1 cup	74
Canned kidney beans	½ cup	64
Avocado	½ medium	56
Wheat germ	2 tablespoons	51
Tomato juice	1 cup	49
Calcium-fortified white bread	2 slices	48
Brussels sprouts	½ cup	47
Roasted peanuts	¼ cup	45
Orange	1 medium	39
Cooked broccoli	½ cup	39

Brussels Sprouts with Walnuts and Walnut Oil

Heart-Health Benefits: Vitamin C; cholesterol free

This dish might make a sprouts convert out of you yet! Cut the sprouts in halves or quarters so they can absorb the heart-healthy walnut oil. Use fresh sprouts if at all possible—they have a crisper texture and better flavor than the frozen.

■ *Serves 6* ■

¹/₄ cup chopped walnuts

4 cups Brussels sprouts (about 1 pound), washed, bottoms trimmed, loose or damaged outer leaves removed, and cut in half, or into quarters if large (see Cooking Tip below for frozen Brussels sprouts)

2 tablespoons walnut oil

Salt and freshly ground pepper, to taste

1. To toast the walnuts, place them in a small nonstick skillet over medium-high heat. Toast for about 5 minutes, periodically shaking the skillet, until they are brown in spots. Watch carefully to avoid burning. Set aside.
2. Bring a large saucepan of water to a boil. Add the sprouts and cook for 5 minutes, or until crisp-tender; do not overcook. Drain the sprouts and place them in a serving dish.
3. Drizzle the walnut oil over the sprouts, add the toasted walnuts, season with salt and pepper, and stir gently. Serve immediately, or cool and serve at room temperature.

▶ **Cooking Tip:** Cook frozen Brussels sprouts according to the package directions. When the sprouts are cool enough to handle, cut them into halves or quarters, and proceed with the recipe.

Approximate Nutritional Information: Serving size: one-sixth Brussels sprouts with walnuts and walnut oil; Calories: 98 cals, 5%; Protein: 3 g, 5%; Total fat: 7.9 g, 12%; Saturated fat: 0.7 g, 4%; Cholesterol: 0 mg, 0%; Carbohydrates: 6 g, 2%; Fiber: 3 g, 10%; Sodium: 112 mg, 5%; Vitamin C: 50 mg, 83%; Vitamin K: 105 mcg, 131%; Diabetic Exchange Values: 1 Vegetable, 1¹/₂ Fats

Percentage of calories from fat: 67%. **Note:** It is more important to focus on the total fat value of this low-calorie recipe, which is 8 grams, or 12% Daily Value, per serving, than on the percentage of calories from fat.

Sautéed Kale with Black-Eyed Peas

Heart-Health Benefits: Vitamins A and C; cholesterol free

f you are a kale fan, you'll love this dish. If you've never tried kale, this is a good introduction.

■ *Serves 4* ■

1 tablespoon canola oil

1 small onion, finely diced

1 garlic clove, minced

³/₄ pound kale, washed, stems trimmed, leaves sliced into 1-inch strips (if the leaves are large, cut them lengthwise in half before slicing them)

¹/₄ cup water

1 cup canned black-eyed peas, rinsed and drained

1 tablespoon red wine vinegar or balsamic vinegar, or to taste

Salt and freshly ground pepper, to taste

1. In a large nonstick skillet, heat the canola oil over medium-high heat. Add the onion and garlic and sauté for 1 minute. Reduce the heat to medium, add the kale and water, and cook, stirring occasionally, until the kale is wilted, about 10 minutes; add more water if it evaporates too quickly. (Note: You may need to add the kale in batches—as one batch wilts, add the next.)
2. Add the black-eyed peas and vinegar and cook for 2 minutes, or until heated through. Adjust the seasoning and serve immediately, or cool and serve at room temperature.

Approximate Nutritional Information: Serving size: one-quarter sautéed kale with black-eyed peas; Calories: 103 cals, 5%; Protein: 3 g, 6%; Total fat: 3.9 g, 6%; Saturated fat: 0.3 g, 2%; Cholesterol: 0 mg, 0%; Carbohydrates: 15 g, 5%; Fiber: 4 g, 16%; Sodium: 167 mg, 7%; Vitamin A: 11,911 IU, 238%; Vitamin C: 37 mg, 62%; Vitamin K: 710 mcg, 888%; Diabetic Exchange Values: 1 Starch, 1 Fat

Percentage of calories from fat: 32%

Tips for Coping with Gas

IF EATING HEART-HEALTHY doses of fiber, dairy products, beans, or legumes leave you with gas, here are some tips for relief and prevention.

- ▶ Try to identify the culprits. Some common ones include fiber, beans, dairy products, dried fruit, and raw vegetables such as cucumbers, peppers, cabbage, onions, and cauliflower.
- ▶ Take Beano or a similar product to help with gas from beans.
- ▶ Take Lactaid Original Ultra, or Fast Act to help with gas from lactose intolerance. Or buy lactose-free milk or soy milk (see Tips for Dealing with Lactose Intolerance, page 145).
- ▶ Eat cooked vegetables, not raw ones.
- ▶ Eat fresh fruit instead of dried.
- ▶ Take a walk after meals.
- ▶ Eat smaller, more frequent meals.
- ▶ Eat slowly, and chew foods well.
- ▶ Don't eat and drink at the same time.

Bok Choy with Soy Sauce and Garlic

Heart-Health Benefits: Vitamins A, C, and K; cholesterol free

*U*se tender baby bok choy if you can find it. Feel free to drizzle a little more sesame oil over the finished dish for a stronger sesame flavor.

■ *Serves 4* ■

1 tablespoon canola oil

1 teaspoon toasted sesame oil

1 small onion, finely sliced

1 large garlic clove, minced

1 pound bok choy, washed, stems trimmed, and
 sliced into ¹/₂-inch-wide slices (slice both
 leaves and stalks)

1 tablespoon lite soy sauce

1 teaspoon seasoned rice vinegar

Toasted sesame seeds, for garnish (optional)

1. In a large nonstick skillet, heat the canola oil and sesame oil over medium-high heat. Add the onion and sauté for 1 minute. Add the garlic and bok choy and sauté, stirring occasionally, for 3 minutes, or until the bok choy stalks are crisp-tender; do not overcook. Add the soy sauce and rice vinegar, stir, and cook for 30 seconds longer.
2. Transfer the bok choy to a serving dish, adjust the seasoning, and garnish with sesame seeds, if using. Serve immediately, or cool and serve at room temperature.

Approximate Nutritional Information: Serving size: one-quarter bok choy with soy sauce and garlic; Calories: 40 cals, 2%; Protein: 2 g, 4%; Total fat: 1.9 g, 3%; Saturated fat: 0.1 g, 1%; Cholesterol: 0 mg, 0%; Carbohydrates: 5 g, 2%; Fiber: 1 g, 5%; Sodium: 220 mg, 9%; Vitamin A: 4,434 IU, 89%; Vitamin C: 46 mg, 77%; Vitamin K: 37 mcg, 46%; Diabetic Exchange Values: 1 Vegetable, ¹/₂ Fat

Percentage of calories from fat: 39%. **Note:** It is more important to focus on the total fat value of this low-calorie recipe, which is 1.9 grams, or 3% Daily Value per serving, than on the percentage of calories from fat.

Roasted Marinated Vegetables with Fresh Herbs

Heart-Health Benefits: Vitamins A and C and B vitamins; cholesterol free

---

These vegetables are a perfect match for pasta, brown rice, whole wheat couscous, quinoa, or any other whole grain. Add a bit of tomato sauce, and use them as a fabulous filling for lasagna. If you want to grill the vegetables instead of roasting them, cut them into large enough pieces so they don't fall through the grill, or use a metal grill basket; after grilling, cut the vegetables into bite-size pieces. Feel free to use your favorite vegetables instead of the ones called for.

■ *Serves 4 (makes about 4 cups)* ■

1 medium (about 8 ounces) purple eggplant, washed and cut into $^1/_2$-inch cubes (see Cooking Tip on page 127 for removing the bitterness from eggplant)

1 medium red bell pepper, washed, cored, seeded, and chopped

1 medium zucchini, washed, halved lengthwise, and cut into thick slices

1 medium yellow squash, washed, halved lengthwise, and cut into thick slices

8 ounces large button mushrooms or other large mushrooms such as shiitake or portobello, stems trimmed (discard if using shiitake), washed, and cut into large pieces

2 large garlic cloves, minced

Marinade

1 teaspoon dried oregano

1 teaspoon dried basil or Italian seasoning

$^1/_2$ teaspoon salt

3 tablespoons olive oil or canola oil

1 tablespoon balsamic vinegar

1 teaspoon sugar

Canola oil cooking spray or canola oil

2 tablespoons finely sliced fresh basil leaves

2 tablespoons chopped fresh parsley

Salt and freshly ground pepper, to taste

1. If desired, prepare the diced eggplant according to the Cooking Tip.
2. Place all of the vegetables and the garlic in a very large bowl. Add the marinade ingredients and toss gently until all of the vegetables are well coated. Allow the vegetables to marinate at room temperature for 20 to 40 minutes.
3. Preheat the oven to 450 degrees F. Line a large roasting pan or baking sheet with sides with foil and spray with cooking spray or lightly grease with canola oil.
4. Spread the marinated vegetables in the roasting pan or on the baking sheet and roast them for 20 minutes, or until crisp-tender.
5. Place the vegetables in a serving bowl, add the fresh basil and parsley, and mix

gently. Adjust the seasoning and serve immediately, or cool and serve at room temperature.

▶ **Cooking Tip:** Removing the moisture and bitterness from the eggplant with salt is an optional step that requires 20 minutes. Place the diced eggplant in a colander on a large plate with a rim, sprinkle it with 2 teaspoons salt, and toss gently. Allow to stand for 20 minutes. Rinse the eggplant quickly under cold water, then spread it out on a double thickness of paper towels and blot dry.

Approximate Nutritional Information: Serving size: one-quarter roasted marinated vegetables with fresh herbs (no marinade); Calories: 50 cals, 3%; Protein: 4 g, 8%; Total fat: 0.5 g, 1%; Saturated fat: 0.1 g, 1%; Cholesterol: 0 mg, 0%; Carbohydrates: 10g, 3%; Fiber: 4 g, 17%; Sodium: 14 mg, 1%; Vitamin A: 1,511 IU, 30%; Vitamin C: 90 mg, 151%; Riboflavin: 0.4 mg, 24%; Vitamin B_6: 0.4 mg, 20%; Vitamin K: 39 mcg, 48%; Diabetic Exchange Values: 2 Vegetable

Percentage of calories from fat: 9%

Approximate Nutritional Information: Serving size: one-quarter marinade; Calories: 100 cals, 5%; Protein: 0 g, 0%; Total fat: 10.2 g, 16%; Saturated fat: 0.7 g, 4%; Cholesterol: 0 mg, 0%; Carbohydrates: 2 g, 1%; Fiber: 0.3 g, 1%; Sodium: 291 mg, 12%; Vitamin K: 12 mcg, 16%; Diabetic Exchange Values: 2 Fat

Percentage of calories from fat: 90%. **Note:** It is not important to focus on the fat or calories in this marinade, as almost all of it will be discarded.

ADDING GROUND FLAXSEED TO YOUR DIET

Ground flaxseed—not whole—is a good source of heart-healthy omega-3 fatty acids, especially for those people who don't eat much fish. Ground flaxseed is preferable to flaxseed oil because in addition to omega-3 fatty acids, the seeds contain fiber, protein, vitamins, and minerals. While there is no official Recommended Dietary Allowance (RDA) or Recommended Daily Intake (RDI) for omega-3, 2 tablespoons of ground flaxseed per day, which provides about 3.5 grams of omega-3 fatty acids, is generally considered a good amount.

Ground flaxseed is available in whole foods and health food stores. It can be added to cold and hot cereals, oatmeal, batters, yogurts, salads, and just about anything else. For more information on the cardiac benefits of omega-3 fatty acids, see What Are Omega-3 Fatty Acids and Why Are They Good for You?, page 150; How Much Omega-3 Should You Consume?, page 155; Omega-3 Supplement Warning, page 157; and Omega-3 Sources, page 158.

Baked Sweet Potatoes with Black Beans and Chili Dressing

Heart-Health Benefits: Vitamins A and C, and fiber; cholesterol free

A **colorful dish packed** with vitamins. If you are serving this bright and flavorful side dish to kids, you may want to go easy on the chili powder.

■ *Serves 6* ■

1 pound (about 2 large) sweet potatoes, scrubbed

Chili Dressing

1 teaspoon chili powder, or to taste

1/2 teaspoon paprika

1/2 teaspoon ground cumin

2 tablespoons freshly squeezed lemon or lime juice, or to taste

3 tablespoons canola oil

1 cup canned black beans, rinsed and drained

3 tablespoons chopped fresh cilantro

3 tablespoons thinly sliced scallion greens

Salt, to taste

1. Preheat the oven to 425 degrees F. Line a baking sheet with foil.
2. Place the sweet potatoes on the foil-lined baking sheet and bake for about 1 hour, or until they are soft everywhere; check a few areas of each potato for doneness.
3. While the potatoes are cooking, make the dressing: Combine all of the ingredients in a small bowl and whisk. Set aside.
4. Remove the potatoes from the oven and allow them to cool briefly. As they cool, their skins will separate from their flesh, making them very easy to peel. (Note: If the skin does not separate easily from the flesh, the potato might not be fully cooked. Microwave any hard potato.)
5. Peel the potatoes, then cut them into 1/2-inch cubes. Place them in a serving bowl. Add the black beans, cilantro, scallions, and dressing, and mix gently. Adjust the seasoning and serve immediately or at room temperature.

Approximate Nutritional Information: Serving size: one-sixth baked sweet potatoes with black beans (no dressing); Calories: 96 cals, 5%; Protein: 4 g, 8%; Total fat: 0 g, 0%; Saturated fat: 0 g, 0%; Cholesterol: 0 mg, 0%; Carbohydrates: 20 g, 7%; Fiber: 5 g, 19%; Sodium: 205 mg, 9%; Vitamin A: 11,121 IU, 222%; Vitamin C: 18 mg, 30%; Vitamin K: 2 mcg, 3%; Diabetic Exchange Values: 1 Starch

Percentage of calories from fat: 2%

Approximate Nutritional Information: Serving size: one-sixth chili dressing; Calories: 64 cals, 3%; Protein: 0 g, 0%; Total fat: 6.9 g, 11%; Saturated fat: 0.4 g, 2%; Cholesterol: 0 mg, 0%; Carbohydrates: 0 g, 0%; Fiber: 0.3 g, 1%; Sodium: 0 mg, 0%; Vitamin K: 9 mcg, 11%; Diabetic Exchange Values: 1 1/2 Fat

Percentage of calories from fat: 94%. **Note:** It is more important to focus on the total fat value of this dressing recipe which is 7 grams or, 11% Daily Value, per serving, than on the percentage of calories from fat.

Soy Power

THREE GOOD REASONS to eat products high in soy protein:

- ▶ Soy is cholesterol free and low in fat.
- ▶ Soy helps decrease your levels of overall cholesterol, LDL cholesterol, and triglycerides.[3]
- ▶ Soy's high calcium content (especially in calcium-enriched soy products) may be beneficial in preventing osteoporosis.

In 1999, the Food and Drug Administration approved the heart-health claim that diets low in saturated fat and cholesterol that include 25 grams of soy protein a day may reduce the risk of heart disease. To qualify, foods must contain the following values per serving:

- ▶ 6.25 grams of soy protein
- ▶ Less than 3 grams of fat
- ▶ Less than 1 gram of saturated fat
- ▶ Less than 20 milligrams of cholesterol
- ▶ Sodium value of less than 480 milligrams for foods eaten on their own, less than 720 milligrams if served as a main dish, or less than 960 milligrams if an entire meal

Many researchers believe that the high intake of soy in Asian cultures helps explain the lower incidence of heart disease. But soy consumption is on the rise in the United States, and not only because of its latest heart-health claim. According to the Soy Foods Association of North America, the double-digit growth in Asian populations in the U.S. has fueled demand for traditional soy foods, and young people are choosing more plant-based foods. Americans have a long way to go before our consumption reaches Asian levels, but we've taken the first step of trying soy products, and supermarkets now stock them next to traditional foods instead of hiding them in the health food section. Soy-based burgers and sausages are found in the freezer case next to other meats, and soy milk is refrigerated next to cow's milk.[4]

PROTEIN VALUES FOR SOY FOODS[5]

$^1/_2$ cup tempeh = 19.5 grams

$^1/_4$ cup roasted soy nuts = 19 grams

$^1/_2$ cup fresh green soybeans (edamame) = 17 grams

1 soy protein bar = 14 grams

4 ounces firm tofu = 13 grams

1 soy burger = 10 to 12 grams

One 8-ounce glass plain soy milk = 10 grams

2 tablespoons soy nut butter = 7 grams

1 soy sausage link = 6 grams

8 ounces soy yogurt = 5 grams

Brown Rice with Tofu and Shiitake Mushrooms

Heart-Health Benefits: Protein, calcium, B vitamins, and magnesium; cholesterol free

The best brand of brown rice is Lundberg, which comes in a variety of blends. Accompanied by a fresh green salad or green vegetable, this pilaf makes a tasty light meal.

■ *Serves 4 as a main course* ■

2 cups fat-free low-sodium stock or water

1/2 teaspoon salt

2 tablespoons canola oil

2 tablespoons minced shallots

1 garlic clove, minced

4 ounces shiitake mushrooms, stems discarded, washed, and thinly sliced

15 ounces extra-firm tofu, drained and cut into 1/2-inch cubes

1 cup brown rice

2 teaspoons dried tarragon

1. Preheat the oven to 400 degree F. Have ready a 9-inch oval or square baking dish.
2. Bring the stock just to a boil. Remove from the heat, add the salt, and stir. Set aside.
3. In a medium nonstick skillet, heat the canola oil over medium-high heat. Add the shallots, garlic, and mushrooms and sauté, stirring occasionally, for 3 minutes. Add the tofu and sauté for 1 minute, then stir in the rice and tarragon and remove from the heat.
4. Transfer the mushroom-rice mixture to the baking dish, add the reserved stock, and stir. Cover with foil and bake for about 1 hour, or until the rice is soft. (Note: Different types of brown rice require different cooking times, so check the rice after 45 minutes.) Adjust the seasoning and serve immediately.

Approximate Nutritional Information: Serving size: one-quarter brown rice with tofu and shiitake mushrooms; Calories: 343 cals, 17%; Protein: 14 g, 29%; Total fat: 12.9 g, 20%; Saturated fat: 1.4 g, 7%; Cholesterol: 0 mg, 0%; Carbohydrates: 45 g, 15%; Fiber: 3 g, 11%; Sodium: 581 mg, 24%; Calcium: 200 mg, 20%; Thiamin: 0.3 mg, 20%; Vitamin B_6: 0.4 mg, 19%; Magnesium: 121 mg, 30%; Vitamin K: 11 mcg, 14%; Diabetic Exchange Values: 2 Starch, 2 Vegetable, 1 Medium-Fat Meat, 2 Fat

Percentage of calories from fat: 33%

Welcome to the World of Soy

Tofu: Tofu, or soybean curd, is a high-protein, low-fat staple of many Asian diets. The process of making tofu is similar to making cheese. Soybeans are first partially cooked, then pureed. Soy milk is extracted from the puree, poured into shaping containers, and solidified with one of two natural coagulants—nigari or calcium sulphate. The texture of tofu varies from silky (almost liquid) to extra firm. Tofu is sold in regular or plain, lite, seasoned, marinated, and baked varieties. If you buy tofu from a tub, make sure that the water is clear and odorless and that the store has a high turnover.

Tofu can be used in endless ways depending on its consistency and flavor. It is an excellent substitute for meat in dishes such as hamburgers, lasagna, meatballs, stir-fries, casseroles, and taco filling. For more suggestions, see Uses for Tofu, page 136.

Tempeh: Tempeh is a firm, nubbly, soy-based brick that is high in protein and fiber, low in fat, and a good source of calcium, iron, phosphorous, vitamin A, and B vitamins. To make tempeh, cooked and hulled soybeans (or a combination of soybeans and a grain such as brown rice, barley, wheat, or quinoa) are spread out on trays and inoculated with a beneficial mold culture called *Rhisopus oligosporous*. This mold causes a fermentation process to occur, during which the soybeans are bound together into firm cakes. Tempeh can be sautéed and used in salads, soups, or stews or in vegetable side dishes. It can be seasoned, panfried, and added to sandwiches in place of deli meats; breaded and panfried as cutlets and served with a sauce; or crumbled, cooked, and used in fillings and other dishes in place of ground beef.

Soy milk: Soy milk is extracted from soybeans that have been soaked and pureed. The flavor varies from brand to brand, but in general it is nutty and slightly sweet. Compared to cow's milk, soy milk has about the same amount of protein, half the calories and fat, and one-fifth the calcium, and it is lactose free. Soy milk is often enriched with calcium or protein and with vitamins, including A, D, and B_{12}. Beverages made from a soy milk base include smoothies and shakes; latte, mocha, and chai; and energy drinks. Flavored soy milk comes in vanilla, carob, strawberry, and chocolate varieties, which may be sweetened or unsweetened; fat-free, low fat, or 1% fat; and organic or nonorganic. Soy milk can be consumed straight or used as a substitute for dairy milk in cooking and baking.

Soy cheese, cream cheese, sour cream, yogurt, and coffee creamer—all of these products are excellent low-fat, cholesterol-free, lactose-free alternatives to dairy products.

Soy nuts: Soy nuts are whole soybeans that have been partially cooked, split, and dry-roasted. They come in all sorts of flavors, including barbecue, wasabi, and Cajun. They can be eaten as a high-protein snack or tossed in salads and soups.

Soy nut butter: Soy nut butter is made from ground soy nuts. It comes in a variety of textures, from pasty to creamy, and degrees of sweetness, depending on the brand.

Miso: Miso is a salty fermented soybean (sometimes a grain is added) paste with the texture of natural peanut butter. Natural-aged miso may be fermented for only a couple of weeks or as long as three years, depending on the type. The ingredient list on packages of naturally aged miso should include only soybeans (plus the grain if a grain is used), salt, water, and *Aspergillis orzyae* (a friendly mold). The three most commonly available types of miso are: soybean miso (also called hatcho miso, it has a dark brown color and a strong flavor); soybean and rice miso (the most popular miso, this may be white, red, or brown and has a sweet, mild flavor); and soybean and barley miso (also called mugi miso, it is yellow or brown, with a nubbly texture and balanced earthy flavor).

In most grocery stores, miso can be found near the tofu in resealable plastic tubs. It is best known as a base for simple, broth-type soups, but it can also be used in sauces, marinades, dips, and dressings. Miso serves as a salt or soy sauce substitute, so a little goes a long way. The fermentation process makes miso easily digestible, and the lactic-acid bacteria and enzymes it contains aid in general digestion (much as the cultures in yogurt do). When cooking with miso, do not boil it, as that destroys the beneficial enzymes.

Health note for people on salt-restricted diets: One tablespoon of hatcho or soybean miso contains 750 milligrams of sodium; for comparison, 1 tablespoon of table salt contains more than 7,000 milligrams of sodium.

Fresh green soybeans (edamame): Bright green fresh soybeans are usually sold shelled or unshelled and frozen, but they can also be found cooked in their fuzzy green pods, usually in the take-out sushi section of a grocery store or whole foods store. The flavor of the beans is slightly sweet and nutty—a cross between fresh green peas and lima beans. Fresh soybeans are high in protein, vitamin C, thiamine, and vitamin A. They can be served as a side dish (sprinkled with sea salt or a dash of soy sauce) or in salads, soups, stir-fries, and pasta dishes, or used as a substitute for green peas in recipes.

Dry whole soybeans: Rich in polyunsaturated oils, soybeans are the only legume that is a complete protein. Look for smooth beans with an even, creamy white color and no surface blemishes, such as holes or cracks. Dry whole soybeans have a very long cooking time, over 3 hours, and they tend to produce a lot of foam during cooking. For convenience, use canned soybeans, usually available in the bean aisle or health food section of grocery stores. Cooked beans can be used in the following ways: coarsely mashed for a substitute for ground meat in chilis, stews, and Mexican dishes (such as taco filling); ground for soy burgers or veggie patties; processed until smooth for a hummus-type dip; or left whole for bean salads, stir-fries, soups, and other bean dishes.

Soy flakes: Soy flakes are made from soybeans that have been dry-roasted, split, and tilled in a roller mill, then dehydrated. Soy flakes do not require presoaking, but they do take 30 to 40 minutes to cook. Soy flakes can be added to grains (such as brown rice or pearl barley), soups, stews, chilis, stuffings, and vegetable burgers.

Soy granules: Soy granules are made from cooked, defatted, and dehydrated soybeans. They do not need to be soaked or precooked before being added to hot cereals, casseroles, soups, or stews. They can be added to baked goods in place of nuts.

Soy grits: Soy grits are made from whole dry soybeans that are sometimes lightly toasted and then cracked into several pieces. They do not require presoaking and take about 40 minutes to cook (follow package directions, as cooking times vary). Cooked soy grits can be combined with other cooked or prepared grains such as rice, barley, quinoa, or bulgur, or added to pilafs, stuffings, and stews.

Soy powder: Soy powder is ground, cooked, dehydrated soybeans. It is similar to soy flour but contains less hull material, and, unlike the flour, it dissolves in liquid. Soy powder can be added to shakes or blender drinks for extra protein, or to baked goods, pancakes, and other breakfast food batters. (Soy flour is discussed on page 251.)

Texturized vegetable protein (TVP): TVP is a processed soy food made from high-protein defatted soy flour that is exposed to heat and pressure to form granules or small fibrous chunks. It is the main ingredient in meat-analog products such as soy burgers, sausages, bacon, and bacon bits. Keep in mind that while these soy products are high in protein, many also contain high amounts of fat. Packaged TVP sold in whole and health food stores can be reconstituted and added to tacos, burritos, bean stews, and Sloppy Joes.[6]

Sesame Tofu with Asian Greens

Heart-Health Benefits: Calcium, vitamin A, and folic acid; cholesterol free

---

This salad is a perfect lunch or a light dinner. Try to pick up as many ingredients as possible from a salad bar, such as the sliced or shredded cucumber, radishes, carrots, and fresh bean sprouts. If you want a simpler dressing using only garlic, soy sauce, and canola oil, see the Variation below.

■ *Serves 2* ■

Dressing

$1/2$ teaspoon miso (preferably brown rice miso)

2 teaspoons hot water

1 teaspoons soy sauce

1 tablespoon canola oil

Tiny amount of wasabi paste, to taste

4 cups Asian salad greens (such as a mix of baby spinach, mizuna, red and green chard, and red mustard greens) or other delicate greens, washed and dried

$1/2$ cup quartered and thinly sliced unpeeled cucumber

$1/2$ cup halved and sliced radishes, $1/2$ cup shredded carrots, $1/2$ cup thinly sliced celery, $1/2$ cup fresh bean sprouts, rinsed, or a combination

7 ounces extra-firm tofu (regular or lite), cut into $1/2$-inch cubes

2 tablespoons sesame seeds

Canola oil cooking spray or 1 tablespoon canola oil

$1/4$ teaspoon toasted sesame oil for sautéing the tofu

1. Combine the dressing ingredients in a small bowl and mix well; set aside.
2. Arrange the salad greens on two serving plates. Top with the cucumbers and radishes, and set aside.
3. Combine the tofu and sesame seeds in a small bowl and mix until the tofu cubes are well coated. Heat a medium nonstick skillet over medium-high heat, then spray with cooking spray or add the canola oil and sesame oil. Add the tofu and cook for 1 minute, or until the tofu cubes are nicely browned on one side, then turn the tofu pieces and cook the other sides for a total of about 3 minutes. Add 2 teaspoons of the dressing to the skillet, shake the skillet, and remove from the heat.
4. Drizzle the remaining dressing over the salads, top with the tofu and juices from the skillet, and serve immediately.

▶ **Variation:** For a simpler dressing, combine ½ teaspoon minced garlic, 2 teaspoons lite soy sauce, and 1 tablespoon canola oil in a small bowl and mix to blend.

Approximate Nutritional Information: Serving size: one-half sesame tofu with Asian greens (no dressing); Calories: 86 cals, 4%; Protein: 8 g, 17%; Total fat: 4 g, 6%; Saturated fat: 0.5 g, 3%; Cholesterol: 0 mg, 0%; Carbohydrates: 6 g, 2%; Fiber: 2 g, 9%; Sodium: 27 mg, 1%; Calcium: 198 mg, 20%; Vitamin A: 1,044 IU, 21%; Folic acid: 113 mcg, 28%; Vitamin K: 95 mcg, 119%; Diabetic Exchange Values: 1 Vegetable, 1 Lean Meat

Percentage of calories from fat: 38%. **Note:** It is more important to focus on the total fat value of this low-calorie recipe which is 4 grams, or 6% Daily Value, per serving, than on the percentage of calories from fat.

Approximate Nutritional Information: Serving size: one-quarter dressing; Calories: 65 cals, 3%; Protein: 0.3 g, 1%; Total fat: 6.8 g, 11%; Saturated fat: 0.4 g, 2%; Cholesterol: 0 mg, 0%; Carbohydrates: 0 g, 0%; Fiber: 0 g, 0%; Sodium: 224 mg, 9%; Vitamin K: 9 mcg, 11%; Diabetic Exchange Values: 1$^1/_2$ Fat

Percentage of calories from fat: 94%. **Note:** It is more important to focus on the total fat value of this dressing recipe which is 7 grams, or 11% Daily Value, per serving, than on the percentage of calories from fat.

Uses for Tofu

▶ Add firm tofu to curries.

▶ Use firm tofu for tofu burgers (see recipe for Old Bay Tofu Cakes on page 137).

▶ Add sautéed marinated firm tofu to noodle dishes.

▶ Add marinated firm tofu to stir-fries (see recipe on page 144).

▶ Use crumbled firm tofu in pasta sauces or to stuff pasta shells.

▶ Use marinated firm tofu in fajitas, burritos, tacos, and other Mexican dishes.

▶ Use grilled firm tofu to make vegetable and tofu sandwiches or roll-ups.

▶ Add crumbled or cubed firm tofu to chili (see recipe on page 138).

▶ Add crumbled or cubed firm tofu to casseroles and vegetable dishes (see recipe on page 130).

▶ Add soft or thinly sliced firm tofu to lasagna (see recipe on page 142).

▶ Top green salads with pieces of sautéed or grilled marinated firm tofu.

▶ Scramble crumbled tofu instead of eggs and top it with sautéed vegetables

▶ Add cubed firm tofu to miso soup and other soups (see recipe on page 54).

▶ Use silken tofu in salad dressings, mayonnaise, tartar sauce, and dips (see recipe on page 75).

▶ Use silken tofu in pureed vegetable soups and chowders instead of cream or milk.

▶ Use silken tofu in macaroni and cheese instead of cream or milk.

▶ Use silken tofu in milk shakes, smoothies, and other blender drinks (see recipe on page 36).

▶ Use silken or soft tofu in pie fillings, sorbets, cheesecakes, and mousse.

▶ Use silken tofu in batters that call for yogurt or sour cream.

Old Bay Tofu Cakes with Cocktail Sauce

Heart-Health Benefits: Protein and magnesium

Don't be surprised if these tofu cakes become a dinner staple. The Old Bay Seasoning provides the perfect kick, especially when paired with cocktail sauce. Other sauces to try with these tofu cakes include Sun-Dried Tomato Sauce, page 152, and Basil Sauce, page 156.

■ *Serves 4 (makes about 7 tofu cakes)* ■

One 14-ounce package lite extra-firm tofu, drained, finely crumbled (use your hands or a fork), and blotted dry with paper towels

1/2 cup plain bread crumbs

4 large egg whites

2 teaspoons Old Bay Seasoning

1/4 cup grated Parmesan cheese

1/4 cup chopped fresh cilantro, basil, or dill

1/4 cup diced jarred roasted red bell peppers or finely diced fresh red bell pepper

Canola oil cooking spray or 1 tablespoon canola oil

Cocktail sauce, for serving

1. To make the tofu cakes, combine all of the ingredients except the canola oil and cocktail sauce in a bowl and mix until well blended. Using a ⅓-cup measuring cup, scoop out portions of the tofu mixture and place on two large plates. Form each portion into a patty. (Note: The patties can be shaped, then covered and refrigerated for up to 24 hours.)
2. Heat a large nonstick skillet over medium-high heat. Spray with cooking spray or add the canola oil. Add the tofu cakes, in batches, and cook for about 3 to 4 minutes on each side, or until golden brown and heated through. If they are browning too quickly, reduce the heat. Serve hot with cocktail sauce. (Note: These tofu cakes are best sautéed, not grilled, because an indoor grill tends to mush the cakes, and they can fall through the grating of an outdoor grill.)

Approximate Nutritional Information: Serving size: one-quarter Old Bay tofu cakes with 2 tablespoons cocktail sauce; Calories: 182 cals, 9%; Protein: 17 g, 34%; Total fat: 7.8 g, 12%; Saturated fat: 1.8 g, 9%; Cholesterol: 4.4 mg, 1%; Carbohydrates: 13 g, 4%; Fiber: 1 g, 5%; Sodium: 648 mg, 27%; Magnesium: 80 mg, 20%; Vitamin K: 0 mcg, 0%; Diabetic Exchange Values: 1 Starch, 2 Lean Meat

Percentage of calories from fat: 37%. **Note:** This percentage is a bit high because of the Parmesan cheese, which can be omitted if you are on a fat-restricted diet.

Bean, Mushroom, and Tofu Chili

Heart-Health Benefits: Protein, iron, vitamins A, B vitamins, folic acid, magnesium, and fiber; cholesterol free

This chili is so tasty you won't miss the meat. If you are short on time, packaged chili mixes work well. Tempeh can be substituted for the tofu, and canned soybeans can be used instead of the black beans or red kidney beans. Shiitake mushrooms are the tastiest. Reduced-fat cheddar cheese, fat-free sour cream, taco sauce, and shredded lettuce are all great toppings. This chili is also fun served in soft or hard taco shells or with tortilla chips—kids especially like it this way.

■ *Serves 6 (makes about 7 cups)* ■

1 tablespoon canola oil

1 onion, finely chopped

1 garlic clove, minced

1 tablespoon plus 1 teaspoon chili powder

2 teaspoons ground cumin

1 teaspoon dried oregano

8 ounces mushrooms (any kind), stems trimmed, washed, halved, and thinly sliced

One 15-ounce can black beans, rinsed and drained

One 15-ounce can red kidney beans, rinsed and drained

One 14.5-ounce can diced tomatoes (do not drain)

1 cup fat-free low-sodium stock or water

One 15-ounce package extra-firm tofu, drained and cut into ¹/₂-inch cubes

A sprinkle or two of quick-dissolving flour, such as Wondra (optional)

¹/₂ cup chopped fresh cilantro, for garnish (optional)

1. Heat the canola oil in a 6-quart saucepan over medium-high heat. Add the onion and sauté for 1 minute. Add the garlic, chili powder, cumin, and oregano and sauté for 30 seconds. Add the mushrooms and sauté for 3 minutes, stirring occasionally.
2. Add the beans, diced tomatoes, and stock and bring to a boil. Reduce the heat to a gentle simmer and cook for 15 minutes.
3. Add the tofu and simmer for 10 minutes more, stirring occasionally. If the chili is not thick enough, add the quick-dissolving flour and cook for 2 minutes longer. Adjust the seasoning, garnish with the cilantro, if using, and serve immediately. Pass any extra toppings at the table.

▶ **Storage Tip:** This chili keeps for 5 days refrigerated, and it can be frozen for up to 1 month. Freeze in single-meal–size portions in zip-top freezer bags or plastic containers. Reheat in a microwave oven or on the stove.

Approximate Nutritional Information: Serving size: one-sixth bean, mushroom, and tofu chili; Calories: 249 cals, 12%; Protein: 18 g, 35%; Total fat: 6.5 g, 10%; Saturated fat: 0.7 g, 4%; Cholesterol: 0 mg, 0%; Carbohydrates: 34 g, 11%; Fiber: 11 g, 45%; Sodium: 149 mg, 6%; Iron: 5 mg, 27%; Vitamin A: 1,090 IU, 22%; Thiamin: .3 mg, 22%; Folic acid: 180 mcg, 45%; Magnesium: 101 mg, 25%; Vitamin K: 9 mcg, 11%; Diabetic Exchange Values: 2 Starch, 2 Lean Meat

Percentage of calories from fat: 22%

Mary Abernethy's Tofu and Vegetable Couscous with Harissa Sauce

Heart-Health Benefits: Protein, iron, vitamins A and C, B vitamins, folic acid, magnesium, and fiber; cholesterol free

Extra-firm tofu can be used in place of the tempeh in this delicious vegetable couscous. The fresh herbs give it a great kick, and a couple of drops of chili-based harissa sauce add a wonderfully spicy dimension. This stew is even better the second day.

■ *Serves 6* ■

2 tablespoons canola oil or olive oil

1 onion, finely diced

2 garlic cloves, minced

$^1/_2$ teaspoon caraway seeds

$^1/_2$ teaspoon cumin seeds

1 cup sliced peeled baby carrots

2 cups diced zucchini

1 cup diced peeled potatoes

$1^1/_2$ cups fat-free low-sodium stock

1 cup low-sodium tomato juice

$1^1/_2$ cups quartered canned artichoke hearts (in brine)

$1^1/_2$ cups canned chickpeas, rinsed and drained

One 15-ounce package extra-firm tofu, drained and cut into $^1/_2$-inch cubes

$^1/_4$ cup chopped fresh parsley

$^1/_4$ cup chopped fresh cilantro

Salt and freshly ground pepper, to taste

Harissa sauce (recipe follows), for serving

Cooked whole wheat couscous, for the table

1. In a large nonstick saucepan, heat the canola oil over medium-high heat. Add the onion and sauté for 2 minutes. Add the garlic, caraway seeds, cumin seeds, carrots, zucchini, and potatoes and sauté, stirring constantly, for 3 minutes.
2. Add the stock and tomato juice and bring to a boil, then reduce the heat and simmer, uncovered, for 15 minutes, or until the carrots and potatoes are tender.
3. Add the artichoke hearts, chickpeas, and tofu and continue to simmer for 5 minutes, or until heated through.
4. Stir in the parsley and cilantro, adjust the seasoning, and serve immediately, with the harissa sauce and couscous.

▶ **Substitution:** Use 3 cups (about 16 ounces) tempeh cut into ½-inch dice instead of the tofu.

Approximate Nutritional Information: Serving size: one-sixth tofu and vegetable couscous (no harissa sauce): Calories: 268 cals, 13%; Protein: 15 g, 31%; Total fat: 10.3 g, 16%; Saturated fat: 1.6 g, 8%; Cholesterol: 0 mg, 0%; Carbohydrates: 33 g, 11%; Fiber: 8 g, 30%; Sodium: 212 mg, 9%; Iron: 4 mg, 21%; Vitamin A: 3,190 IU, 64%; Vitamin C: 28 mg, 47%; Vitamin B_6: 0.5 mg, 23%; Folic acid: 137 mcg, 34%; Magnesium: 102 mg, 25%; Vitamin K: 58 mcg, 72%; Diabetic Exchange Values: 2 Starch, 1 Medium-Fat Meat, 1 Fat

Percentage of calories from fat: 33%

Harissa Sauce

■ *Makes ¼ cup* ■

¼ cup canola oil   2 teaspoons paprika

2 teaspoons chili powder

Combine all of the ingredients in a small saucepan and cook over low heat for about 2 minutes, or just until the spices are fragrant. Be careful not to burn the spices, which can happen easily. Immediately transfer the sauce to a small serving bowl.

Approximate Nutritional Information: Serving size: 2 teaspoons harissa sauce; Calories: 42 cals, 2%; Protein: 0 g, 0%; Total fat: 4.6 g, 7%; Saturated fat: 0.3 g, 2%; Cholesterol: 0 mg, 0%; Carbohydrates: 0 g, 0%; Fiber: 0 g, 0%; Sodium: 0 mg, 0%; Vitamin K: 6 mcg, 8%; Diabetic Exchange Values: 1 Fat

Percentage of calories from fat: 95%. **Note:** It is more important to focus on the total fat value of this harissa dressing which is 5 grams, or 7% Daily Value, per serving, than on the percentage of calories from fat.

SOLUBLE FIBER REDUCES LDL CHOLESTEROL

A RECENT STUDY showed that diets high in fiber from barley, oat bran, beans, and psyllium are modestly effective in reducing LDL (bad) cholesterol levels, compared with diets high in insoluble fiber or fiber primarily from fruits and vegetables.[7] Both soluble and insoluble fiber provide benefits to the digestive system by helping to maintain regularity. The main difference between the two is that soluble fiber forms a gel when mixed with liquid, while insoluble fiber does not. Insoluble fiber passes through the digestive tract largely intact.

In 1999, the Food and Drug Administration allowed manufacturers to make the health claim that 3 grams of soluble fiber from whole oats or psyllium seed husk per day, when included as part of a diet low in saturated fat and cholesterol, may reduce the risk of heart disease. While this claim specifically mentions only whole oats and psyllium seed husk, the same risk reduction benefits probably apply to barley, beans, and oat bran. Bottom line: Eat more soluble fiber![8,9]

Mushroom, Zucchini, Spinach, and Tofu Lasagna

Heart-Health Benefits: Protein, calcium, and vitamins A, C, and K

To save time, this recipe calls for high-quality jarred tomato sauce, presliced mushrooms, prewashed bagged baby spinach (or frozen spinach), and no-boil lasagna noodles. Muir Glen Organic diced tomatoes are the best.

■ *Serves 12* ■

One 24-ounce jar high-quality all-purpose tomato sauce, such as Rao's Homemade All Natural Premium Quality Marinara Sauce

One 14.5 ounce can diced tomatoes (do not drain)

1/2 cup thinly sliced fresh basil leaves

1 teaspoon dried oregano

1/2 cup water

Vegetables

1 tablespoon canola oil

1 small onion, finely diced

One 8-ounce package sliced baby bella mushrooms or shiitake mushrooms, stems trimmed (discarded if using shiitakes), washed, and thinly sliced

salt and freshly ground pepper, to taste

1 medium zucchini, washed, quartered lengthwise, and finely sliced

8 ounce package baby spinach leaves, washed, or 8 ounces frozen chopped spinach, thawed and well drained

One box no-boil (or oven-ready) lasagna noodles to fill a 13 x 9 x 2-inch pan

One 15-ounce package extra-firm tofu (regular or lite), drained, blotted dry with paper towels, and crumbled

2 1/2 cups shredded part-skim low-moisture mozzarella cheese

1. Combine the tomato sauce, diced tomatoes, basil, oregano, and water in a bowl and mix; set aside.
2. To cook the vegetables, heat the canola oil in a large nonstick skillet over medium-high heat. Add the onion and sauté for 1 minute, then add the mushrooms, season with salt and pepper, and sauté for 4 minutes. Transfer the onion and mushrooms to a large bowl and set aside. Return the skillet to medium-high heat, add the zucchini, season with salt and pepper, and sauté for 4 minutes, or until wilted. If the zucchini sticks to the pan, add 2 tablespoons water. Transfer the zucchini to the bowl containing the mushrooms. Return the skillet to medium-high heat, add 2 tablespoons water and the baby spinach, and sauté until just wilted, about 3 minutes. (If using frozen spinach, add the drained spinach directly to the mushrooms.) Add the spinach to the mushrooms and set aside.
3. Adjust an oven rack to the middle position and preheat the oven to 375 degrees F.
4. To assemble the lasagna, spread 1 cup sauce over the bottom of an ungreased

13 x 9 x 2-inch pan. Place 3 or 4 no-boil lasagna noodles over the sauce (follow the instructions on your lasagna box, as different brands require different preparation methods). Spread about half of the vegetables (including the juices) evenly over the noodles, followed by half of the crumbled tofu, 1¼ cups of the sauce, and 1 cup of the mozzarella cheese. Repeat with another layer of noodles, vegetables, tofu, sauce, and cheese. Add another layer of noodles, then cover with the remaining 1½ cups sauce and sprinkle with the remaining ½ cup mozzarella cheese.

5. Cover the lasagna with foil and bake for about 1 hour, or until all of the layers of noodles feel soft when pierced with a knife. Remove the foil and bake for 5 minutes longer to allow the top to firm up. Remove from the oven and let cool for 10 minutes before slicing.

▶ **Storage Tip:** Any leftover cooked lasagna can be frozen. Reheat it in a microwave oven or conventional oven.

Approximate Nutritional Information: Serving size: one-twelfth mushroom, zucchini, spinach, and tofu lasagna; Calories: 180 cals, 9%; Protein: 13 g, 26%; Total fat: 6.7 g, 10%; Saturated fat: 2.3 g, 12%; Cholesterol: 9.3 mg, 3%; Carbohydrates: 20 g, 7%; Fiber: 4 g, 16%; Sodium: 471 mg, 20%; Calcium: 229 mg, 23%; Vitamin A: 1,731 IU, 35%; Vitamin C: 17 mg, 28%; Vitamin K: 82 mcg, 103%; Diabetic Exchange Values: 1 Starch, 1 Vegetable, 1 Medium-Fat Meat

Percentage of calories from fat: 31%

HIGH CALCIUM INTAKE FROM DAIRY SOURCES BOOSTS WEIGHT LOSS

RECENT STUDIES SHOW that dietary calcium from dairy products—not calcium supplements—plays a key role in a healthy metabolism and in the likelihood of loosing weight. Over the past four years, evidence has emerged in support of the "anti-obesity" effect of dietary calcium and dairy products. Dairy sources of calcium show greater effects than supplements, which are most likely attributable to the additional bioactive compounds in dairy sources, which act together with calcium to reduce body fat. So, if you are trying to lose weight, including three to four servings of low-fat or fat-free dairy products (equal to 1,200 to 1,300 mg of calcium) in your daily diet may help take the pounds off.[10,11]

Tofu Vegetable Stir-Fry

Heart-Health Benefits: Protein, vitamins A and C, and folic acid; cholesterol free

t is essential to have all of the ingredients for this stir-fry prepped before you begin, as the cooking goes very quickly. A mini food processor is an easy way to mince the garlic and ginger. Chicken, shrimp, or scallops can be used in place of the tofu. Use any of your favorite vegetables, for a total of 6 or 7 cups (1 to 1¼ pounds). Try to cut all of the vegetables approximately the same size for even cooking.

■ *Serves 4* ■

Marinade

2 tablespoons lite soy sauce

2 tablespoons hoisin sauce

2 tablespoons water

1 garlic clove, minced

1 tablespoon minced fresh ginger

15 ounces extra-firm tofu, drained and cut into ½-inch cubes

Stir-Fry Sauce

1 tablespoon hoisin sauce

3 tablespoons water

2 tablespoons lite soy sauce

1 teaspoon cornstarch

1 teaspoon brown sugar

1 tablespoon canola oil

A few drops of toasted sesame oil

1 tablespoon minced fresh ginger

1 garlic clove, minced

1 cup thinly sliced carrots

2½ cups broccoli florets

1 cup sliced zucchini or yellow squash

½ red bell pepper, washed, cored, seeded, and thinly sliced

3 scallions, trimmed and thinly sliced

⅓ cup cashew nuts, coarsely chopped (optional)

¼ cup chopped fresh cilantro

1. To make the marinade, combine all of the ingredients in a medium bowl and mix. Add the tofu, cover, and refrigerate for at least 15 minutes, or up to 12 hours.
2. To make the stir-fry sauce, combine all of the ingredients in a small bowl and mix until the cornstarch is completely dissolved; set aside.
3. To stir-fry, heat the canola oil and sesame oil in a very large nonstick skillet or large nonstick wok over medium-high to high heat. Add the ginger and garlic and sauté for 30 seconds. Add the carrots, broccoli florets, zucchini, and red bell pepper and sauté, stirring occasionally, for 3 minutes. Add 3 tablespoons water and continue to cook and stir for 2 minutes, or until the vegetables are crisp-tender; do not overcook. Transfer the vegetables to a large serving bowl and cover with foil to keep warm. (Do not rinse the skillet.)

4. Reheat the skillet over medium-high heat. Add the tofu, with its marinade, and the stir-fry sauce, stir, and cook for 3 minutes. Add the scallions and cook 1 minute more.
5. Add the contents of the skillet to the vegetables and gently mix. Adjust the seasoning, garnish with the cashew nuts, if using, and cilantro, and serve immediately.

▶ **Advance Preparation:** The vegetables can be prepared up to 3 days in advance and refrigerated. The stir-fry sauce can be made 1 day in advance, covered, and refrigerated.

▶ **Timesaving Tip:** Convenient fresh vegetable stir-fry packs are available in some grocery stores. They usually come in 12-ounce bags and can be supplemented with your favorite vegetables. Sixteen-ounce bags of frozen stir-fry vegetables are also available in many grocery stores. Follow the package directions for sautéing.

Approximate Nutritional Information: Serving size: one-quarter tofu vegetable stir-fry (no cashew nuts); Calories: 217 cals, 11%; Protein: 15g, 30%; Total fat: 10.8 g, 17%; Saturated fat: 1.3 g, 7%; Cholesterol: 0 mg, 0%; Carbohydrates: 20 g, 7%; Fiber: 3 g, 12%; Sodium: 846 mg, 35%; Vitamin A: 6,041 IU, 121%; Vitamin C: 88 mg, 147%; Folic acid: 93 mcg, 23%; Vitamin K: 104 mcg, 131%; Diabetic Exchange Values: 1 Starch, 1 Vegetable, 1 Medium-Fat Meat, 1 Fat

Percentage of calories from fat: 41%. **Note:** It is more important to focus on the total fat value of this low-calorie recipe which is 11 grams, or 17% Daily Value, per serving, than on the percentage of calories from fat.

TIPS FOR DEALING WITH LACTOSE INTOLERANCE

DAIRY PRODUCTS CONTAIN two essential minerals that are good for your heart—calcium and magnesium. High levels of calcium protect against bone loss, high blood pressure, and colon cancer. Magnesium helps keep blood pressure at an optimal level. If you consider yourself lactose intolerant, the following tips might help you get low-fat and nonfat dairy products into your diet.

▶ Try fat-free yogurt and fermented dairy products such as kefir. Start with 1/4 cup a day.
▶ Try hard cheeses (such as low-fat cheddar, Swiss, or Parmesan), which are lower in lactose than softer ones.
▶ Try lactose-free fat-free milk; start slowly.
▶ Take lactase tablets before drinking milk.
▶ Try fat-free frozen yogurt instead of ice cream.
▶ Try soy products (such as soy milk, yogurt, sour cream, or cheese), which are all lactose free.

Preventing Osteoporosis

IN ADDITION TO controlling blood pressure (see page 65) and helping to shed unwanted pounds (see page 143), a high intake of calcium helps prevent a crippling disease called osteoporosis. Eight million women and two million men suffer from osteoporosis, and millions more are on the verge of developing this widespread, underdiagnosed disease. According to the Osteoporosis and Related Bone Diseases National Resource Center at the National Institutes of Health (NIH), one out of every two women and one in eight men over fifty years of age will have an osteoporosis-related fracture in their lifetimes.[12]

Osteoporosis is a disease in which bones become thin, brittle, and easily broken or fractured due to a decrease in bone density and strength. During childhood, bones grow rapidly in length and density. Bones reach a maximum length in the teen years, but their density continues to develop until about age thirty. After thirty, bones slowly begin lose their density and strength.[13]

Men have larger, stronger bones than women, which explains, in part, why osteoporosis affects more women than men. Hormonal changes related to menopause are another reason why women are more susceptible to developing osteoporosis.

Ways to Prevent Osteoporosis

▶ Awareness is key. If you notice a loss of height, change in posture, or sudden back pain, it is important to inform your doctor. Depending on your age and family history, a Bone Mineral Density (BMD) Test may be ordered, to determine your bone mass.

▶ Change unhealthy habits, such as smoking, excessive alcohol intake, and inactivity.

▶ Ensure a calcium intake of 1,000 milligrams per day to age 50, and 1,200 milligrams per day over the age of 51.

▶ Ensure adequate vitamin D intake, at least 400 IU, but not more than 800 IU, per day. Vitamin D helps the body absorb calcium. Normally, our bodies make enough vitamin D from about 10 minutes of daily exposure to sunlight.

▶ Engage in a regular regimen of weight-bearing exercises, where bone and muscles work against gravity, such as walking, jogging, racquet sports, stair climbing, team sports, lifting weights, and/or using resistance machines. *Health Note:* If you have already been diagnosed with osteoporosis, any exercise program should be evaluated for safety by your doctor before you begin.

Attention Parents: Building strong bones in girls and boys during childhood and adolescence is the best defense against developing osteoporosis later in life. See How Much Calcium Do You Need?, page 68, for information on adequate calcium intake at any age. And regular exercise is just as important for children as it is for adults.

FIVE

FISH AND SHELLFISH

HEART-HEALTH TIPS AT A GLANCE

▶ Fish and shellfish are excellent sources of protein, with very little fat and saturated fat. The American Heart Association recommends eating fish at least two times a week (see Eat Seafood Twice a Week, page 153).

▶ Certain fish, such as salmon, tuna, halibut, herring, and mackerel, are excellent sources of heart-healthy omega-3 fatty acids (see What Are Omega-3 Fatty Acids and Why Are They Good For You?, page 150).

▶ While it is true that shellfish contain high levels of cholesterol, their low levels of fat, particularly saturated fat, make them a good source of protein and omega-3 fatty acids (see What about Shellfish?, page 161).

▶ How fish and shellfish are cooked is important to heart health. Avoid batter-coated and deep-fried fish and shellfish in restaurants, fast food establishments, or frozen dinners. Baking, broiling, grilling, steaming, and sautéing are the healthiest way to cook fish and shellfish. Artery-clogging butter or cream sauces can turn a healthy, low-fat fish into a high-fat nightmare; instead, a squirt of fresh lemon or lime juice and some fresh herbs add great flavor, particularly if you don't have the time to assemble a healthy sauce or salsa.

▶ Always buy the freshest fish you can find. Ask your fishmonger for advice, and remember that sometimes fish on sale is past its prime—which is why it is on sale (see How to Buy and Cook Fish and Shellfish, page 160).

▶ If the wild salmon versus farm-raised salmon debate has you confused, the information in Choose Wild Salmon over Farm-Raised, page 166, may help clarify things. Bottom line: Whenever possible, choose wild salmon, but don't eliminate salmon from your diet if you cannot find wild salmon.

▶ If you are concerned about potentially harmful mercury levels in fish, see Mercury Levels and Fish Consumption: Warnings for Women and Children, page 159, for the latest guidelines.

▶ Before you reach for your next frozen dinner, read Smart Choice Frozen Dinners, page 176, and Deep-Fried Dangers, page 173, to make the healthiest selection possible.

▶ Mix and match the sauces, dry rubs, and marinades in this chapter with lean white or red meats or tofu.

Dinner for One Baked in Foil: Haddock with Baby Spinach, Red Bell Peppers, and Basil Pesto

Heart-Health Benefits: Protein, calcium, iron, vitamins A, C and E, B vitamins, folic acid, magnesium, and fiber

*F*ish **baked in** foil is a nutritious, tasty, and almost effortless way to prepare any fillet. You can make the foil pack in the morning and pop it in the oven when you get home from work.

■ *Serves 1* ■

Canola oil cooking spray or canola oil

6 ounces skinless haddock, sea bass, or salmon
   (preferably wild) fillet, any pinbones removed

1¹/₂ tablespoons store-bought basil pesto sauce

2¹/₂ cups lightly packed baby spinach leaves,
   washed

¹/₂ cup thinly sliced red bell pepper

2 tablespoons grated Parmesan cheese

Salt and freshly ground pepper, to taste

1. Preheat the oven to 450 degrees F.
2. Cut two 18 x 12-inch rectangles of aluminum foil. Spray the center of one of the rectangles with cooking spray or lightly grease with canola oil, then arrange the fish in the center and evenly spread the pesto sauce over the fish. Pile the spinach leaves and red bell peppers on top of the fish, sprinkle with the Parmesan cheese, and season with salt and pepper. Spray the center of the other piece of foil with canola oil cooking spray, or lightly grease it then place it on top of the mound of spinach and tightly seal the pack by rolling and crimping the four edges.
3. Place the foil pack on a baking sheet and bake for 15 minutes. Remove the foil pack, and using a sharp knife or scissors, carefully open it—be careful not to burn yourself with the steam. Transfer the fish to a plate and enjoy.

▶ **Advance Preparation:** The foil pack can be made up to 8 hours in advance and kept refrigerated.

Approximate Nutritional Information: Serving size: 1 serving haddock with baby spinach, red bell peppers, and basil pesto; Calories: 319 cals, 16%; Protein: 46 g, 91%; Total fat: 5.8 g, 9%; Saturated fat: 2.0 g, 10%; Cholesterol: 106 mg, 35%; Carbohydrates: 23 g, 8%; Fiber: 12 g, 49%; Sodium: 1,155 mg, 48%; Calcium: 960 mg, 96%; Iron: 8 mg, 46%; Vitamin A: 39,899 IU, 798%; Vitamin C: 633 mg, 1,054%; Vitamin E: 11 IU, 38%; Thiamin: 0.3 mg, 24%; Riboflavin: 0.5 mg, 31%; Niacin: 10 mg, 49%; Vitamin B_6: 1 mg, 65%; Vitamin B_{12}: 2 mcg, 38%; Folic acid: 631 mcg, 158%; Magnesium: 120 mg, 30%; Vitamin K: 4 mcg, 5%; Diabetic Exchange Values: 1 Starch, 1 Vegetable, 5 Very Lean Meat, 1 Fat

Percentage of calories from fat: 16%

What Are Omega-3 Fatty Acids and Why Are They Good for You?

OMEGA-3 FATTY ACIDS (sometimes written as n-3 or w-3) are a form of polyunsaturated fat. The omega-3 fatty acids include:

▶ Alpha-linolenic acid (ALA)
▶ Eicosapentaenoic acid (EPA) and
▶ Docosahexaenoic acid (DHA)

Of the three, ALA is the only essential omega-3 fatty acid, meaning that the body cannot make this fatty acid on its own. ALA must be obtained from plant sources, including flaxseed, pumpkin seeds, walnuts, hemp seeds, soybeans, canola oil, ground linseeds, wheat and barley grass, grains, legumes, and some dark green leafy vegetables. EPA and DHA omega-3 fatty acids are synthesized in the body, and therefore are not essential. Good sources of EPA and DHA include coldwater fish, such as salmon, tuna, halibut, herring, and mackerel. The body can convert ALA to EPA and DHA, but inefficiently.[1]

According to the Agency for Healthcare Research and Quality, a government agency of the Department of Health and Human Services, omega-3s ingested by eating fish or by taking a fish oil supplement may reduce heart attacks as well as other problems related to heart and blood vessel disease in people who already have such conditions. In 2004, the U.S. Food and Drug Administration announced a health claim that supportive—but not conclusive—research has shown that consumption of EPA and DHA omega-3 fatty acids may reduce the risk of coronary disease. [2]

Although omega-3 fatty acids do not alter total cholesterol, HDL cholesterol, or LDL cholesterol, evidence suggests that they can reduce levels of triglycerides, a fat in the blood that may contribute to heart disease. ALA omega-3s appear to have similar benefits, but to a much lesser extent than food sources and fish oil that supply EPA and DHA. However, the American Heart Association recommends eating tofu and other forms of soybeans, walnuts and walnut oil, ground flaxseed and flaxseed oil, and canola oil despite the fact that the exact level of the conversion of the ALA in these foods to EPA and DHA remains unknown.

BENEFITS OF OMEGA-3 FATTY ACIDS[3]

▶ Reduce the risk of arrhythmias (irregular heartbeats) that can lead to sudden cardiac death
▶ Decrease triglyceride levels
▶ Decrease the growth rate of atherosclerotic plaque
▶ Slightly lower high blood pressure

Roasted Cod with Cherry Tomatoes, Black Olives, and Fresh Basil

---

Heart-Health Benefits: Protein, vitamin C, and B vitamins

This quick and easy Mediterranean-style sauce is a wonderful accompaniment to any fish from meaty swordfish to delicate cod. The hardest part of the dish is the timing. The cod takes about ten minutes to cook, and the sauce takes only three minutes. So, have everything ready, and make the sauce while the cod finishes cooking. When the fish comes out of the oven, transfer it to a serving platter and pour the sauce over it. Serve with brown rice and a green salad.

■ *Serves 4* ■

2 tablespoons olive oil

1¼ pounds cod fillet

Salt and freshly ground pepper, to taste

1 garlic clove, minced

¾ cup pitted brine-cured black olives (such as Kalamata), coarsely chopped

3 cups (about 15 ounces) cherry tomatoes, halved

1 tablespoon freshly squeezed lemon juice, or to taste

½ cup thinly sliced fresh basil leaves

1. Preheat the oven to 450 degrees F. Have all of your sauce ingredients ready to go.
2. Line a baking sheet with foil. Place 1 tablespoon of the olive oil on the foil, then rub both sides of the cod fillet in the oil. Season the cod with salt and pepper. Place the cod in the oven and cook for 7 to 10 minutes, depending on the thickness of the fish.
3. While the cod is cooking, heat the remaining 1 tablespoon olive oil in a large nonstick skillet over medium-high heat. Add the garlic and sauté for 30 seconds. Add the olives, cherry tomatoes, and lemon juice and cook for 2 minutes, or just until the cherry tomatoes are soft and their skin begins to wrinkle. Remove from the heat, adjust the seasoning, and set aside.
4. Transfer the cooked fish to a serving platter. Pour the sauce over the fish and garnish with the basil. Serve immediately.

Approximate Nutritional Information: Serving size: one-quarter roasted cod with cherry tomatoes, black olives, and fresh basil; Calories: 186 cals, 9%; Protein: 26 g, 53%; Total fat: 6.1 g, 9%; Saturated fat: 0.8 g, 4%; Cholesterol: 61 mg, 20%; Carbohydrates: 6 g, 2%; Fiber: 2 g, 7%; Sodium: 347 mg, 14%; Vitamin C: 24 mg, 41%; Vitamin B_6: 0.4 mg, 23%; Vitamin B_{12}: 1 mcg, 21%; Vitamin K: 20 mcg, 25%; Diabetic Exchange Values: 1 Vegetable, 3 Lean Meat

Percentage of calories from fat: 30%

Broiled Marinated Halibut Steaks with Sun-Dried Tomato Sauce

Heart-Health Benefits: Protein, vitamin D, B vitamins, and magnesium

---

*Y*ou'll find yourself eating this sauce with everything from pasta to grilled chicken. The lemon-oregano marinade is also great for flavoring other fish, shellfish, chicken, or pork.

■ *Serves 4* ■

Lemon-Oregano Marinade

  ⅓ cup freshly squeezed lemon juice

  1 tablespoon dried oregano

  2 tablespoons minced shallots or 2 garlic
    cloves, minced

  1 tablespoon olive oil or canola oil

  1 tablespoon Dijon mustard

1¼ to 1½ pounds halibut steaks, skin on (see
    Cooking Note on page 153)

Sun-Dried Tomato Sauce (makes about ½ cup)

  ½ cup sun-dried tomatoes in oil, preferably
    without any added seasonings

  ½ vine-ripened tomato

  1½ teaspoons light mayonnaise

  1½ tablespoons nonfat plain yogurt or fat-
    free sour cream

  1 tablespoon water

  Salt and freshly ground pepper, to taste

Canola oil cooking spray or canola oil, for
    greasing the baking sheet

Salt and freshly ground pepper, to taste

¼ cup thinly sliced fresh basil leaves, for garnish
    (optional)

Lemon wedges, for serving (optional)

1. Combine the marinade ingredients in a bowl and mix. Add the halibut, turn to coat fish and marinate in the refrigerator for at least 3 hours, or up to 12 hours (the longer, the better).

2. Combine the sauce ingredients in the bowl of a food processor and process until fairly smooth. Adjust the seasoning, and transfer to a serving bowl. This sauce will be served at room temperature, so set it aside if serving within 1 hour; otherwise refrigerate and bring it to room temperature before serving. (The sauce can be made 2 days ahead and kept refrigerated.)

3. To cook the halibut, preheat the broiler. Line a baking sheet with foil and spray with cooking spray or lightly grease with canola oil. Place the fish on the foil and season with salt and pepper. Flip the fish and season the other side. Broil for 5 minutes on one side, then flip and broil for 7 minutes more, or until the fish is cooked through. The cooking time will depend on the strength of the broiler and the thickness of the fish. (Note: When broiling anything, watch the oven carefully to avoid fires.)

4. Transfer the halibut to a serving platter and remove the skin. Garnish with the basil and arrange the lemon wedges around the platter. Serve immediately, with the sun-dried tomato sauce on the side.

▶ **Cooking Note:** Ask your fishmonger for Atlantic halibut, which has 2 grams of fat per 3-ounce serving of raw fish, versus Greenland halibut, which has 12 grams of fat per the same amount of raw fish. Also, ask for a full steak, with four sections, versus the belly cut or boneless steak.

Approximate Nutritional Information: Serving size: one-quarter broiled marinated halibut; Calories: 156 cals, 8%; Protein: 29 g, 59%; Total fat: 3.2 g, 5%; Saturated fat: 0.4 g, 2%; Cholesterol: 45 mg, 15%; Carbohydrates: 0 g, 0%; Fiber: 0 g, 0%; Sodium: 77 mg, 3%; Vitamin D: 851 IU, 213%; Niacin: 8 mg, 41%; Vitamin B_6: 0.4 mg, 24%; Vitamin B_{12}: 2 mcg, 28%; Magnesium: 118 mg, 29%; Diabetic Exchange Values: 4 Very Lean Meat, 1 Fat

Percentage of calories from fat: 20%

Approximate Nutritional Information: Serving size: 2 tablespoons sun-dried tomato sauce; Calories: 16 cals, 1%; Protein: 0.6 g, 1%; Total fat: 0.4 g, 1%; Saturated fat: 0 g, 0%; Cholesterol: 0 mg, 0%; Carbohydrates: 3 g, 1%; Fiber: 0.5 g, 2%; Sodium: 153 mg, 6%; Vitamin K: 3 mcg, 4%; Diabetic Exchange Values: FREE

Percentage of calories from fat: 22%

Approximate Nutritional Information: Serving size: one-quarter lemon-oregano marinade; 44 cals, 2%; Protein: 0.9 g, 2%; Total fat: 3.3 g, 5%; Saturated fat: 0.4 g, 2%; Cholesterol: 0 mg, 0%; Carbohydrates: 4 g, 1%; Fiber: 0.4 g, 2%; Sodium: 91 mg, 4%; Vitamin K: 2 mcg, 3%; Diabetic Exchange Values: 1 Fat

Percentage of calories from fat: 59%. **Note:** The fat value of this marinade is not important, since it will be discarded before broiling the fish.

EAT SEAFOOD TWICE A WEEK

THE AMERICAN HEART Association (AHA) recommends eating fish, particularly fatty fish high in EPA and DHA omega-3 fatty acids, at least two times a week. Fish is a good source of protein and does not have the high saturated fat that fatty meats and meat products do.[4]

Broiled Swordfish with Artichoke Heart–Green Olive Tapenade

Heart-Health Benefits: Protein and B vitamins

Don't be surprised if you find yourself eating this artichoke tapenade straight out of the bowl of the food processor. Add couscous, tabbouleh, quinoa, or any other whole grain and a big green salad to make a perfect meal. The swordfish is also fabulous on the grill (see Cooking Tip on page 155).

■ *Serves 4* ■

1 recipe Lemon-Oregano Marinade (page 152)

1¼ pounds swordfish steaks (about 1¼ inches thick)

Artichoke Heart–Green Olive Tapenade (makes about ¾ cup)

¾ cup canned artichoke hearts in brine, (about 4 hearts) drained

10 pitted green olives (not with pimentos)

2 tablespoons freshly squeezed lemon juice, or to taste

2 tablespoons olive oil or canola oil

1 garlic clove

1 teaspoon ground coriander

Salt and freshly ground pepper, to taste

¼ cup lightly packed fresh cilantro leaves

Canola oil cooking spray or canola oil, for greasing the baking sheet

Salt and freshly ground pepper, to taste

1. Pour the marinade into a shallow dish. Add the swordfish and marinate, refrigerated, for at least 30 minutes, or up to 24 hours.
2. For the tapenade, combine all of the ingredients except the cilantro leaves in the bowl of a food processor and process until almost smooth. Add the cilantro and pulse a few times, until the cilantro leaves are chopped but not pureed. If the tapenade is too thick, add 1 tablespoon of water and pulse a couple more times. Adjust seasoning and transfer to a serving bowl. This sauce will be served at room temperature, so set it aside if serving within 1 hour; otherwise, refrigerate and bring it to room temperature before serving. (The tapenade can be made up to 2 days in advance and kept refrigerated.)
3. To broil the fish, preheat the broiler. Line a baking sheet with foil and spray with cooking spray or grease with canola oil. Place the fish on the foil and season with salt and pepper. Flip the fish and season the other side. Broil the fish for 4 minutes on one side, then flip and broil for 3 to 4 minutes more, or until the fish is cooked through. The cooking time will depend on the strength of the broiler and the thickness of the fish. (Note: When broiling anything, watch the oven carefully to avoid fires.)

4. Transfer the swordfish to a serving platter. Serve immediately, with the tapenade on the side.

▶ **Cooking Tip:** The swordfish steaks can be cooked on an outdoor grill for about 7 minutes total grilling time, or on an indoor grill for about 5 minutes total grilling time. They can also be pan fried for about 3 minutes on each side.

Approximate Nutritional Information: Serving size: one-quarter broiled swordfish: Calories: 172 cals, 9%; Protein: 28 g, 56%; Total fat: 5.6 g, 9%; Saturated fat: 1.5 g, 8%; Cholesterol: 55 mg, 18%; Carbohydrates: 0 g, 0%; Fiber: 0 g, 0%; Sodium: 273 mg, 11%; Niacin: 14 mg, 69%; Vitamin B$_6$: 0.4 mg, 23%; Vitamin B$_{12}$: 2 mcg, 41%; Diabetic Exchange Values: 4 Very Lean Meat, 1 Fat

Percentage of calories from fat: 31%

Approximate Nutritional Information: Serving size: 2 tablespoons artichoke heart–green olive tapenade; Calories: 69 cals, 3%; Protein: 2 g, 3%; Total fat: 5.0 g, 8%; Saturated fat: 0.6 g, 3%; Cholesterol: 0 mg, 0%; Carbohydrates: 5 g, 2%; Fiber: 0.9 g, 4%; Sodium: 207 mg, 9%; Vitamin K: 24 mcg, 29%; Diabetic Exchange Values: 1 Fat

Percentage of calories from fat: 63%. **Note:** It is more important to focus on the total fat value of this low-calorie recipe which is 5 grams, or 8% Daily Value, per serving, than on the percentage of calories from fat.

Approximate Nutritional Information: Serving size: one-quarter lemon-oregano marinade: 44 cals, 2%; Protein: 0.9 g, 2%; Total fat: 3.3 g, 5%; Saturated fat: 0.4 g, 2%; Cholesterol: 0 mg, 0%; Carbohydrates: 4 g, 1%; Fiber: 0.4 g, 2%; Sodium: 91 mg, 4%; Vitamin K: 2 mcg, 3%; Diabetic Exchange Values: 1 Fat

Percentage of calories from fat: 63%. **Note:** The fat value of this marinade is not important since it will be discarded before broiling the fish.

HOW MUCH OMEGA-3 SHOULD YOU CONSUME?

THE IDEAL AMOUNT is not clear. Evidence from prevention studies suggests that taking eicosapentaenoic acid (EPA) and docosahexaenoic acid (DHA) ranging from 0.5 to 1.8 grams per day, (either in the form of fatty fish or supplements), significantly reduced deaths from heart disease and all causes (see Omega-3 Sources, page 158, for a list of fish high in omega-3 fatty acids). For those who cannot consume fish or fish oil, an intake of 1.5 to 3 grams per day of alpha-linolenic fatty acid seems beneficial. Patients taking more than 3 grams of omega-3 fatty acids from supplements should do so only under a physician's care (see Omega-3 Supplement Warning, page 157). Further guidelines can be found on page 157.

Christian Zagler's Poached Salmon with Fresh Basil Sauce

Heart-Health Benefits: Protein and B vitamins

---

*P*oached salmon with fresh basil sauce is a light, easy dinner that can be made in advance. The basil sauce is equally good with cooked shellfish or white or red meat.

■ *Serves 4* ■

Basil Sauce (makes about ¹/₂ cup)
  1 cup lightly packed fresh basil leaves
  2 tablespoons light mayonnaise
  3 tablespoons nonfat plain yogurt or fat-free
    sour cream
  Salt and freshly ground pepper, to taste

4 cups water, or as needed
2 bay leaves
5 black peppercorns
Juice of ¹/₂ lemon
1¹/₄ pounds salmon fillet (preferably wild), skin on
Lemon wedges, for serving

1. For the basil sauce, combine all of the ingredients in the bowl of a food processor and process until smooth, then transfer to a serving bowl. This sauce will be served at room temperature, so set it aside if serving within 1 hour; otherwise, refrigerate and bring it to room temperature before serving.
2. To poach the salmon, combine the water, bay leaves, peppercorns, and lemon juice in a medium saucepan or deep skillet and bring to a boil. Reduce the heat to a simmer and add the salmon fillet (skin side up). The poaching liquid should completely cover the salmon, so add more water if necessary. Cook for 15 to 20 minutes, or until cooked through.
3. Transfer the salmon to a serving platter, and when it is cool enough to handle, remove the skin. Serve immediately, or at room temperature, with the basil sauce and lemon wedges on the side.

▶ **Advance Preparation:** The basil sauce can be made up to 2 days in advance. The poached salmon can be made up to 8 hours ahead and refrigerated. Serve chilled or at room temperature.

Approximate Nutritional Information: Serving size: one-quarter poached salmon; Calories: 204 cals, 10%; Protein: 28 g, 56%; Total fat: 8.9 g, 14%; Saturated fat: 1.3 g, 7%; Cholesterol: 78 mg, 26%; Carbohydrates: 0 g, 0%; Fiber: 0 g, 0%; Sodium: 62 mg, 3%; Thiamin: 0.3 mg, 22%; Riboflavin: 0.5 mg, 32%; Niacin: 11 mg, 56%, Vitamin B$_6$: 1 mg, 58%; Vitamin B$_{12}$: 5 mcg, 75%; Diabetic Exchange Values: 4 Very Lean Meat, 2 Fat

Percentage of calories from fat: 41%. **Note:** It is important to remember that salmon contains heart-healthy omega-3 fatty acids which accounts, in part, for this high percentage.

Approximate Nutritional Information: Serving size: 2 tablespoon fresh basil sauce; Calories: 17 cals, 1%; Protein: 0.4 g, 1%; Total fat: 1.2 g, 2%; Saturated fat: 0.2 g, 1%; Cholesterol: 0 mg, 0%; Carbohydrates: 0 g, 0%; Fiber: 0.2 g, 1%; Sodium: 100 mg, 4%; Vitamin K: 27 mcg, 34%; Diabetic Exchange Values: FREE

Percentage of calories from fat: 64%. **Note:** It is more important to focus on the total fat value of this low-calorie recipe, which is 1 gram, or 2% Daily Value, per serving than on the percentage of calories from fat.

American Heart Association Recommendations for Omega-3 Fatty Acid Intake

▶ People without documented coronary heart disease (CHD): Eat a variety of fatty fish, at least twice a week. Include oils and foods rich in alpha-linolenic acid (such as flaxseed oil, canola oil, soybean oil, ground flaxseed, and walnuts).

▶ People with documented CHD: Consume about 1 gram of EPA and DHA per day, preferably from fatty fish. EPA and DHA supplements could be considered with a physician.

▶ Patients who need to lower triglycerides: 2 to 4 grams of EPA and DHA per day provided as capsules under a physician's care.[5]

OMEGA-3 SUPPLEMENT WARNING

INCREASING OMEGA-3 fatty acids through food is always preferable to taking supplements. However, people with coronary artery disease and those with high triglycerides may not be able to get enough omega-3 by diet alone. These people may want to talk to their doctors about taking a supplement. The FDA recommends that consumers not exceed more than a total of 3 grams per day of EPA and DHA omega-3 fatty acids, with no more than 2 grams per day from a dietary supplement. Anyone taking more than 3 grams of omega-3 fatty acids from supplements should do so only under a physician's care. High intakes could cause excessive bleeding. This is especially important for people who take prescription blood pressure medications and/or anticoagulants and for people who take aspirin on a regular basis.[6]

Omega-3 Sources

Amounts of EPA and DHA in Fish and Fish Oils and the Amount of Fish and Shellfish Required to Provide about 1 Gram of EPA and DHA per Day[1]

SOURCE	EPA AND DHA CONTENT*	DAILY AMOUNT REQUIRED FOR ABOUT 1 GRAM OF EPA AND DHA**
Fish and Shellfish		
Tuna, light, canned in water, drained	0.26	12
Tuna, white, canned in water, drained	0.73	4
Tuna, fresh	0.24–1.28	2.5–12
Sardines	0.98–1.7	2–3
Salmon, chum	0.68	4.5
Salmon, sockeye	0.68	4.5
Salmon, pink	1.09	2.5
Salmon, Chinook	1.48	2
Salmon, Atlantic, farmed	1.09–1.83	1.5–2.5
Salmon, Atlantic, wild	0.9–1.56	2–3.5
Mackerel	0.34–1.57	2–8.5
Herring, Pacific	1.81	1.5
Herring, Atlantic	1.71	2
Trout, rainbow, farmed	0.98	3
Trout, rainbow, wild	0.84	3.5
Halibut	0.4–1	3–7.5
Cod, Pacific	0.13	23
Cod, Atlantic	0.24	12.5
Haddock	0.2	15
Catfish, farmed	0.15	20
Catfish, wild	0.2	15
Flounder/sole	0.42	7
Oyster, Pacific	1.17	2.5
Oyster, eastern	0.47	6.5
Oyster, farmed	0.37	8
Lobster	0.07–0.41	7.5–42.5
Crab, Alaskan king	0.35	8.5
Shrimp	0.27	11
Clam	0.24	12.5
Scallop	0.17	17.5
Capsules		
Cod liver oil	0.19	5***
Standard fish body oil	0.3	3
Omega-3 fatty acid Concentrate	0.50	2

*The EPA and DHA content of fish is per 3 ounce serving (edible portion), and per grams per gram of oil.

**The amount required to provide about 1 gram of EPA and DHA per day is measured in ounces of fish per day, or grams per gram of oil per day.

***This amount of cod liver oil would provide approximately the Recommended Dietary Allowance of vitamins A and D.

Source Notes

Data from the USDA Nutrient Data Laboratory, available at: www.nalusda.gov/fnic/foodcomp/; accessed October 3, 2002. The amounts of fish given above are very rough estimates because oil content can vary markedly (>300%), depending on species, season, diet, and packaging and cooking methods.

Alpha-Linolenic Acid Content of Selected Vegetable Oils, Nuts, and Seeds

SOURCE	ALPHA-LINOLENIC ACID CONTENT (GRAMS PER TABLESPOON)
Olive oil	0.1
Walnuts, English	0.7
Soybean oil	0.9
Canola oil	1.3
Walnut oil	1.4
Flaxseeds	2.2
Flaxseed oil	8.5

Source Note
Data from the USDA Nutrient Data Laboratory, available at: www.nalusda.gov/fnic/foodcomp/; accessed October 3, 2002.

MERCURY LEVELS AND FISH CONSUMPTION: WARNINGS FOR WOMEN AND CHILDREN

NEARLY ALL FISH and shellfish contain traces of mercury, and for most people this mercury is not a health concern. However, some fish and shellfish contain high levels of mercury that can pose a threat to children, pregnant women, and women who are planning to become pregnant. The Food and Drug Administration (FDA) and the Environmental Protection Agency (EPA) advise women who might become pregnant, pregnant women, nursing mothers, and young children to follow these guidelines.

▶ Do not eat shark, swordfish, king mackerel, or tilefish, which contain high levels of mercury.
▶ Eat up to 12 ounces (2 average servings) a week of a variety of fish and shellfish that are lower in mercury.
▶ Five of the most popular fish that are low in mercury are shrimp, canned light tuna, salmon, pollock, and catfish.
▶ Another popular fish, albacore ("white") tuna, has more mercury than canned light tuna. So, eat no more than 6 ounces (one average serving) of albacore tuna per week.
▶ Check local advisories about the safety of fish caught by family and friends in your local lakes, rivers, and coastal areas. If advice is unavailable, eat no more than 6 ounces (one average serving) per week of fish caught from local waters, and do not consume any other fish that week.

Answers to Frequently Asked Questions about Mercury in Fish and Shellfish

What Are mercury and methylmercury?

Mercury occurs naturally in the environment and can also be released into the air through industrial pollution. Mercury falls from the air and can accumulate in streams and oceans, where it turned into methylmercury. It is this type of mercury that can be harmful to an unborn baby and young child. Fish absorb the methylmercury as they feed in these waters and it builds up in them. It builds up more in some types of fish and shellfish than others depending on what the fish eat, which is why the levels vary.

Should women who could have children but who are not pregnant be concerned about methylmercury?

If a woman regularly eats fish that are high in methylmercury, it can accumulate in her bloodstream over time. Methylmercury is removed from the body naturally, but it may take over a year for levels to drop significantly. Thus it may be present in a woman before she becomes pregnant.

Is there methylmercury in all fish and shellfish?

Nearly all fish and shellfish contain traces of methylmercury. However, larger fish that have lived longer have the highest levels of methylmercury because they've had more time to accumulate it. These large fish (e.g., swordfish, shark, king mackerel, and tilefish) pose the greatest risk. Other types of fish maybe eaten in the amounts recommended by the FDA and EPA.

What about fish sticks and fast-food sandwiches?

Fish sticks and fast-food sandwiches are commonly made from fish that are low in mercury.

What about tuna steaks?

Because tuna steaks generally contain higher levels of mercury than canned light tuna, when choosing your two meals of fish and shellfish, eat no more than 6 ounces (one average serving) of tuna steak per week.

What if one eats more than the recommended amount of fish and shellfish in a week?

One week's consumption of fish will not change the level of methylmercury in the body much. If you eat a lot of fish one week, cut back for the next week or two. Just make sure to *average* the recommended amount per week.[8]

How to Buy and Cook Fish and Shellfish

Tips for Buying Fresh Fish Fillets and Steaks
- ▶ Look for firm, shiny flesh that gives slightly when pressed. The flesh should not be mushy, and it should not separate easily.
- ▶ If the head is on, the fish's eyes should be clear and should bulge a bit. Avoid fish with dull, cloudy, sunken, or bloody eyes.
- ▶ The gills should be bright pink or red, not brown or gray.
- ▶ The fish should have a pleasant ocean-fresh smell, not a fishy or ammonia-like odor.
- ▶ Scales (if any) should be shiny and should cling tightly to the flesh.
- ▶ Steaks and fillets should be moist, not slimy or dry, and the color should be uniformly bright, not dull.

Tips for Buying Crabs, Lobsters, and Shrimp
- ▶ The legs should be lively when touched unless the crustacean is soft-shelled (such as soft-shell crabs) or shrimp which is not sold live.
- ▶ The tail of a live lobster should curl under when the lobster is lifted up; it should not hang limp.
- ▶ Shellfish should feel heavy, not light or dry.
- ▶ Raw shrimp should have translucent shells with a grayish green, pinkish tan, or pink tint. They should be moist and firm, not mealy.

Tips for Buying Live Clams, Mussels, Oysters, Scallops, and Other Mollusks
- ▶ Shells should be tightly closed. If any are open, they should shut immediately if gently tapped. Avoid or discard gaping shells that do not close when tapped.
- ▶ Shells should be moist and intact, not cracked, dry, or chipped.
- ▶ Mollusks should have a clean ocean-fresh scent, not a fishy odor.

Tips For Buying Shucked Clams, Mussels, Oysters, Scallops, and Other Mollusks
- ▶ Meat should be plump, not shriveled, dark, or dry.
- ▶ Meat should be free of shell particles and sand.
- ▶ Any liquid should be clear, not cloudy or opaque, and it should be less than 10 percent of the volume.
- ▶ Mollusks should have a clean ocean-fresh scent, not a fishy odor.

Tips for Buying Frozen Fish and Shellfish
- ▶ Flesh should be frozen solid.
- ▶ Fish should be in a tight moisture-proof package.
- ▶ Fish should not have any freezer burn or ice crystals.
- ▶ When thawed, fish should pass the same tests as outlined for fresh fish and shellfish above.
- ▶ Frozen fish or shellfish should remain frozen until it is thawed for cooking. Do not refreeze.

Tips for Cooking Fresh Fish

▶ Marinades and dry rubs add tremendous taste to fish, and the choices are endless. Play around to find your favorites.

▶ Keep marinating fish refrigerated; do not leave it at room temperature.

▶ Do not use the plate or platter that held the raw fish to serve the cooked fish. Discard any marinades or sauces that came in contact with the raw fish. Do not serve them as sauce, unless you boil them for a few minutes, and do not recycle them.

▶ The healthiest and tastiest ways to cook fish are grilling, broiling, poaching, steaming, sautéing, and baking. Avoid deep-frying.

▶ The 10-Minute-Per-Inch Rule for Fish: Measure fish at its thickest point (if stuffed or rolled, measure after preparing). If baking (at a high temperature), grilling, broiling, poaching, steaming, or sautéing, cook the fish for about 10 minutes per inch of thickness. Add 5 minutes of cooking time to the total cooking for fish wrapped in foil or covered with a sauce. Double the cooking time for frozen fish that has not been thawed prior to cooking.

▶ Fish is done when the flesh turns from translucent to opaque. It should flake easily with a fork or knife, and a thermometer inserted into the thickest part should read 140 degrees F.[9]

What about Shellfish?

SHELLFISH IS AN excellent low-fat source of protein, with a moderate amount of cholesterol. Shrimp and crab have the highest levels of cholesterol, scallops and mussels have the lowest. Most shellfish have less than 1 gram of saturated fat per serving, and many varieties have almost none. Butter and other sauces of course, as well as deep-frying, can make shellfish less healthy.

SHELLFISH	SATURATED FAT (GRAMS)	CHOLESTEROL (GRAMS)
Shrimp	0.2	166
Crab (3 ounces) baked	1	80
King crab (1 leg)	0.1	71
Lobster (3 ounces)	0.1	61
Oysters (6 medium)	0.5	58
Clams (19 small)	0.2	57
Mussels (4–5)	0.7	48
Sea Scallops (3–4)	0.6	34

Sautéed Shrimp with Zucchini and Tomatoes on Pasta

Heart-Health Benefits: Protein, iron, vitamins A and C, B vitamins, folic acid and magnesium

A **quick and easy** pasta dish that can be made with high-quality canned diced tomatoes (such as Glen Muir) or with 2 cups of diced vine-ripened tomatoes. Chicken, tofu, or scallops can be substituted for the shrimp.

■ *Serves 4* ■

12 ounces whole wheat thin spaghetti

1 tablespoon plus 2 teaspoons olive oil

3 cups diced zucchini

Salt and freshly ground pepper, to taste

1 cup thinly sliced scallions

1 small garlic clove, minced

1 to 1¼ pounds medium shrimp, peeled and deveined

One 14.5-ounce can diced tomatoes (do not drain) or 2 cups diced ripe tomatoes

2 teaspoons grated lime or lemon zest

2 tablespoons freshly squeezed lime or lemon juice, or to taste

½ cup thinly sliced fresh basil leaves or chopped fresh cilantro

1. Cook the pasta according to the package directions; drain. Place it back in the pot, stir in 2 teaspoons of the olive oil (to prevent sticking), cover, and set aside in a warm place.
2. Meanwhile, heat 1½ teaspoons of the olive oil in a large nonstick skillet over medium-high heat. Add the zucchini, season with salt and pepper, and sauté, stirring occasionally, for 2 minutes, or just until crisp-tender; do not overcook. Add the zucchini to the pasta, and re-cover the pot. (Do not rinse the skillet.)
3. Return the skillet to medium-high heat and add the remaining 1½ teaspoons olive oil. Add the scallions, garlic, and shrimp and sauté for 3 minutes, stirring occasionally, or until the shrimp are cooked. Gently stir in the diced tomatoes, lime zest, and lime juice and sauté for 1 minute longer.
4. Add the shrimp mixture and sauce to the pasta. Add the basil and gently stir until all of the ingredients are well combined. Adjust the seasoning and serve immediately.

▶ **Timesaving Tip:** Buy frozen shrimp that is already peeled and deveined.

Approximate Nutritional Information: Serving size: one-quarter sautéed shrimp with zucchini and tomatoes on pasta; Calories: 526 cals, 26%; Protein: 43 g, 87%; Total fat: 9.0 g, 14%; Saturated fat: 1.4 g, 7%; Cholesterol: 215 mg, 72%; Carbohydrates: 73 g, 24%; Fiber: 2 g, 9%; Sodium: 376 mg, 16%; Iron: 7 mg, 41%; Vitamin A: 1,380 IU, 28%; Vitamin C: 33 mg, 54%; Vitamin D: 215 IU, 54%; Thiamin: 0.5 mg, 36%; Riboflavin: 0.3 mg, 19%; Niacin: 9 mg, 45%; Vitamin B$_6$: 0.6 mg, 30%; Vitamin B$_{12}$: 2 mcg, 27%; Folic acid: 99 mcg, 25%; Magnesium: 204 mg, 51%; Vitamin K: 37 mcg, 46%; Diabetic Exchange Values: 4 Starch, 2 Vegetable, 4 Very-Lean Meat, 2 Fat

Percentage of calories from fat: 15%

Sautéed Scallops with Capers and Red Bell Peppers with Pasta

Heart-Health Benefits: Protein, vitamins A, C, and E, B vitamins, folic acid, and magnesium

---

A delicious and sophisticated dish that is surprisingly easy to make.

■ *Serves 4* ■

10 ounces whole wheat thin spaghetti

5 tablespoons canola oil

1 cup finely diced celery

3 tablespoons capers

1/4 cup finely diced red bell peppers

2 tablespoons freshly squeezed lemon juice

1 1/4 pounds sea scallops, rinsed and patted dry with paper towels

Salt and freshly ground pepper, to taste

Canola oil cooking spray or canola oil

1/2 cup chopped fresh cilantro

1. Cook the pasta according to the package directions; drain. Place it back in the pot, stir in 1 tablespoon of the canola oil (to prevent sticking), cover, and set aside in a warm place.
2. Meanwhile, heat a small saucepan over medium-high heat. Add the remaining 4 tablespoons (about 1/4 cup) canola oil, the celery, capers, red bell peppers, and lemon juice. Sauté for 2 minutes, then remove from the heat and add the sauce to the pasta. Re-cover the pot and set aside.
3. To sauté the scallops, season them on both sides with salt and pepper. Heat a large nonstick skillet over medium-high heat. Spray with cooking spray or lightly grease with canola oil, then add the scallops and cook on one side for 2 minutes, or until golden brown. Flip the scallops and cook on the other side for 2 to 3 minutes, or until golden brown and completely cooked.
4. Add the scallops and any juices to the pasta. Add the cilantro and gently stir until all of the ingredients are well combined. Adjust the seasoning and serve immediately.

Approximate Nutritional Information: Serving size: one-quarter sautéed scallops with capers and red bell peppers with pasta: Calories: 555 cals, 28%; Protein: 33g, 67%; Total fat: 19.5 g, 30%; Saturated fat: 1.3 g, 7%; Cholesterol: 47 mg, 16%; Carbohydrates: 59 g, 20%; Fiber: 3 g, 10%; Sodium: 449 mg, 19%; Vitamin A: 1,388 IU, 28%; Vitamin C: 48 mg, 80%; Vitamin E: 8 IU, 27%; Thiamin 0.7 mg, 47%; Riboflavin: 0.4 mg, 28%; Niacin: 6 mg, 29%; Vitamin B 12: 2 mcg, 36%; Folic acid: 195 mcg, 49%; Magnesium: 90 mg, 22%; Vitamin K: 32 mcg, 40%; Diabetic Exchange Values: 3 Starch, 3 Vegetable, 3 Medium-Fat Meat, 1 Fat

Percentage of calories from fat: 32%

Grilled Curry-Rubbed Salmon with Papaya Salsa

Heart-Health Benefits: Protein, vitamins A and C, and B vitamins

A **fast and simple** weekday dinner fancy enough for weekend friends. The papaya can be substituted with your favorite fruit—plums, peaches, or mangoes are delicious—and fresh herbs. Polenta, brown rice, or quinoa makes a great side dish.

■ *Serves 4* ■

Papaya Salsa

- 1 cup peeled, seeded, and finely diced papaya
- ¹/₃ cup finely diced red bell pepper
- ¹/₂ cup quartered cherry tomatoes
- ¹/₄ cup finely diced red onion
- 2 to 3 tablespoons chopped fresh cilantro or mint leaves, to taste
- One 8-ounce can Mandarin oranges in light syrup, drained and sliced widthwise

- 1 tablespoon freshly squeezed lime juice or seasoned rice vinegar, or to taste

- 1¹/₄ pounds salmon fillet or salmon steaks (preferably wild), skin on
- 1 tablespoon curry powder, or to taste
- Canola oil cooking spray
- Salt and freshly ground pepper, to taste

1. To make the papaya salsa, mix all of the ingredients in a bowl. Cover and refrigerate until ready to serve. (Note: The salsa is best if allowed to sit for 30 minutes before serving for the flavors to develop; it can be made up to 3 hours in advance.)
2. Preheat a grill (indoor or outdoor) to high. Rub the salmon with a light coating of curry powder, then generously spray with cooking spray and season with salt. Grill the salmon for a total cooking time of about 7 to 10 minutes (turning once) on an outdoor grill, about 5 minutes on an indoor grill. The cooking time will depend on the thickness of the salmon.
3. Transfer the salmon to a serving platter. Serve immediately, with the papaya salsa on the side.

Approximate Nutritional Information: Serving size: one-quarter curry-rubbed grilled salmon; Calories: 205 cals, 10%; Protein: 28 g, 56%; Total fat: 9.1 g, 14%; Saturated fat: 1.4 g, 7%; Cholesterol: 78 mg, 26%; Carbohydrates: 0 g, 0%; Fiber: 0.3 g, 1%; Sodium: 63 mg, 3%; Thiamin: 0.3 mg, 22%; Riboflavin: 0.5 mg, 32%; Niacin: 11 mg, 56%; Vitamin B_6: 1 mg, 59%; Vitamin B_{12}: 5 mcg, 75%; Vitamin K: 0.9 mcg, 1%; Diabetic Exchange Values: 4 Very Lean Meat, 2 Fat

Percentage of calories from fat: 42%. **Note:** It is more important to focus on the total fat of this low-calorie high-omega-3 recipe which is 9 grams, or 14% of Daily Value, focus on the percentage of calorie's from fat.

Approximate Nutritional Information: Serving size: one-quarter papaya salsa; Calories: 53 cals, 3%; Protein: 1 g, 3%; Total fat: 0 g, 0%; Saturated fat: 0 g, 0%; Cholesterol: 0 mg, 0%; Carbohydrates: 13 g, 4%; Fiber: 2 g, 8%; Sodium: 10 mg, 0%; Vitamin A: 1,786 IU, 36%; Vitamin C: 77 mg, 129%; Vitamin K: 4 mcg, 5%; Diabetic Exchange Values: 1 Fruit

Percentage of calories from fat: 4%

Choose Wild Salmon over Farm-Raised

THERE IS NO doubt that salmon, a fatty, cold-water fish that is high in omega-3 fatty acids, is good for your heart. There is some debate, however, over the levels of PCBs (polychlorinated biphenyls) and other toxins found in farm-raised salmon, and how much is safe to eat. High levels of PCBs may pose a risk of cancer, but your risk for heart disease is probably far greater. Confusing? You bet! Perhaps these questions and answers can shed some light.

What are PCBs and how do they get into the fish?

PCBs are organic pollutants that have been shown to cause cancer in animals. The toxins come from plastics, waste incinerators, leaky transformers, and insecticide residues. Farmed salmon get concentrated levels of PCBs from their food, which is a mixture of ground-up fish and oils. Wild salmon get some PCBs too; however, their diet is more varied so the PCB levels are lower. Fortunately, fish food is constantly being improved and tested, so the toxin levels are decreasing.

How does one know if salmon is farm-raised or wild?

If this information is not provided in the fish case or on the packaging of the fish (which it should be), ask the fishmonger. Names such as "Atlantic salmon" or "Icelandic salmon" may sound like wild, but these are usually farm-raised. Depending on where you live, the price of salmon can also be an indicator: Higher prices usually mean the salmon is wild. Also, wild salmon is generally available fresh on the East Coast of the United States only from May until the end of August. Alaska and the West Coast enjoy a year-round supply of wild salmon at a reasonable cost. Wherever you live, wild salmon can be purchased frozen (year-round) from the mail-order companies listed in Sources, page 268–69.

Where do wild salmon come from and are they endangered?

Many wild salmon runs are threatened, endangered, or even extinct, but many are still healthy. As a general rule, wild stocks in Alaska are faring far better than those of California and the Pacific Northwest. As for Atlantic salmon, there are virtually no harvestable runs left in the United States.[11]

The life cycles of wild salmon are threatened by the building and draining of dams, urban development, pollution, El Niño events, and the integration of farm-raised salmon with wild salmon. There are five different species of Pacific wild salmon: Chinook (also called king or spring), chum (or keta), coho, sockeye, and pink. Wild salmon are anadromous, meaning that they spawn in fresh water and spend much of their life at sea, in salt water. To learn more about the fascinating life cycle of wild salmon, see Sources, page 269.

How much farm-raised salmon is safe to eat?

There are no official guidelines on the amount of farm-raised salmon that is safe to eat. As a matter of common sense, if you tend to consume a lot of salmon, try to buy wild salmon whenever it is available and affordable. If wild salmon is not an option, though, do not completely eliminate salmon from your diet. Eat the amount of farm-raised salmon you feel comfortable with, and branch out and try other fish and shellfish that are high in heart-healthy omega-3 fatty acids, such as halibut, mackerel, lake trout, herring, sardines, scallops, and shrimp.

Should pregnant women and children limit their intake of farm-raised salmon?

Because of potential harmful effects from PCBs on fetuses and growing children, it is advisable for women who may become pregnant, pregnant women, nursing women, and young children to limit their consumption of farm-raised salmon. While there are no official guidelines, many health professionals believe that those in this group should limit their intake to once a month.

Is canned salmon from farm-raised salmon?

No, almost all of it comes from wild salmon.

Can I reduce the levels of PCBs in the farm-raised salmon that I eat?

Consumers can possibly reduce their exposure to PCBs by removing the skin and fat from fish before cooking it. However, because methylmercury is distributed throughout the muscle, skinning and trimming the fat does not significantly reduce mercury concentrations.[12]

Cajun Dry-Rubbed Tilapia with Spinach and Shiitake Mushrooms

Heart-Health Benefits: Protein, calcium, iron, vitamins A and C, B vitamins, folic acid, and magnesium

*M*ake this easy Cajun dry rub from scratch or use your favorite store-bought rub. These tilapia fillets can be broiled, baked, or panfried. Tilapia is too fragile for an outdoor grill, but an indoor grill is perfect.

■ *Serve 2* ■

Cajun Dry Rub (makes 1 tablespoon)
- 1 teaspoon chili powder
- $^1/_2$ teaspoon paprika
- $^1/_2$ teaspoon dried oregano
- $^1/_2$ teaspoon ground cumin
- $^1/_8$ teaspoon powdered garlic
- $^1/_8$ teaspoon red pepper flakes (optional)

- 12 ounces tilapia fillets
- $1^1/_2$ tablespoons canola oil
- 4 ounces shiitake mushrooms, stems discarded, washed, and thinly sliced
- Salt and freshly ground pepper, to taste
- $^1/_2$ teaspoon minced garlic
- One 8-ounce bag prewashed baby spinach
- Canola oil cooking spray, if using an indoor grill
- Lemon wedges, for the table

1. Combine all of the rub ingredients in a large bowl or zip-top bag and mix until well blended. Add the tilapia and coat with the dry rub. Let marinate, refrigerated, for at least 15 minutes, or up to 8 hours.
2. Heat $1^1/_2$ teaspoons of the canola oil in a large nonstick skillet over medium-high heat. Add the mushrooms, season with salt and pepper, and sauté for 5 minutes, or until wilted and golden brown. Transfer the mushrooms to a bowl, cover with foil, and set aside. (Do not rinse the skillet.)
3. Add $1^1/_2$ teaspoons of the canola oil to the skillet and heat over medium-high heat. Add the garlic and spinach, season with salt and pepper, and sauté for 2 minutes, or until the spinach is wilted. Transfer the spinach to the serving bowl containing the mushrooms, re-cover, and set aside. (Do not rinse the skillet.)
4. Add the remaining $1^1/_2$ teaspoons canola oil to the skillet and heat over medium-high heat. Season the tilapia fillets on both sides with salt, then add them to the skillet and cook for 3 to 4 minutes on each side, or until cooked through. Or, if using an indoor grill, preheat the grill to high. Spray both sides of the fish with cooking spray, and cook the fish for 1 to 2 minutes, or until cooked through.
5. To serve, stir the spinach and mushrooms together, then adjust the seasoning. Place some of the spinach mixture on each plate and top with a tilapia fillet. Serve with lemon wedges on the side.

Approximate Nutritional Information: Serving size: one-half Cajun dry-rubbed tilapia (see Nutrition Note below) with spinach and shiitake mushrooms; Calories: 225 cals, 11%; Protein: 37 g, 73%; Total fat: 5.5 g, 8%; Saturated fat: 0.5 g, 3%; Cholesterol: 97 mg, 32%; Carbohydrates: 8 g, 3%; Fiber: 4 g, 18%; Sodium: 154 mg, 6%; Calcium: 282 mg, 28%; Iron: 4 mg, 23%; Vitamin A: 10,603 IU, 212%; Vitamin C: 132 mg, 220%; Riboflavin: 0.4 mg, 24%; Niacin: 10 mg, 48%; Vitamin B_6: 0.8 mg, 41%; Vitamin B_{12}: 2 mcg, 34%; Folic acid: 189 mcg, 47%; Magnesium: 86 mg, 22%; Vitamin K: 6 mcg, 8%; Diabetic Exchange Values: 1 Vegetable, 5 Very Lean Meat, 1 Fat

Percentage of calories from fat: 22%

Nutrition Note: Haddock was used to determine this nutritional breakdown instead of tilapia because Nutritionist Pro software does not have a cholesterol value for tilapia.

FAKE SHELLFISH

HAVE YOU EVER wondered what that "fake shellfish" you see in salad bars, seafood salads, and Japanese roll-ups is made of? Most likely it is Alaskan pollock, which is ground, washed, strained, and mixed with salt, sugar, flavorings, egg whites, and starch. After it is cooked, the fish paste is shaped and colored to resemble crab, shrimp, or scallops. Fake shellfish has 75 percent less cholesterol than most shellfish, and it is very low in fat. The downside is that it has no heart-healthy omega-3 benefits and it is high in sodium, not to mention the bland flavor.

Sesame-Coated Yellowfin Tuna with Wasabi–Soy Sauce and Kim Chee Salsa

---

Heart-Health Benefits: Protein, vitamin C, and B vitamins

An **Asian twist** on tuna—swordfish works well, too. Make the salsa as spicy as you like, and substitute your favorite salad ingredients for those called for. If you are short on time, pick up some store-bought kim chee.

■ *Serves 4* ■

Kim Chee Salsa

- 4 cups finely chopped Napa cabbage or Chinese cabbage
- 1 garlic clove, minced
- ³/₄ cup thinly sliced scallion greens
- ¹/₄ cup grated carrots
- ¹/₄ cup grated cucumber
- 1 cup fresh bean sprouts, rinsed (optional)
- 1 teaspoon chili powder or red pepper flakes, or to taste
- 1 teaspoon toasted sesame oil, or to taste
- 2 teaspoons lite soy sauce, or to taste
- 1 teaspoon seasoned rice vinegar, or to taste

- 2 teaspoons crushed fresh ginger (use a garlic press to extract the juice, reserve 2 teaspoons of the pressed ginger pulp)

Wasabi-Soy Sauce

- 2 tablespoons lite soy sauce
- 1 teaspoon wasabi paste or to taste
- ¹/₂ cup sesame seeds
- 1¹/₄ pounds yellowfin tuna steaks (about 1¹/₄ inches thick)
- Salt and freshly ground pepper, to taste
- Canola oil cooking spray or canola oil

1. To make the kim chee salsa, bring a large saucepan of water to a boil. Add the cabbage and cook for 30 seconds, or just until wilted. Drain, rinse under cold running water, and drain again; gently squeeze to remove excess water, and place in a large bowl.
2. When the cabbage is completely cool, add the remaining salsa ingredients and stir gently. Set aside.
3. For the wasabi-soy sauce, mix the soy sauce and wasabi in a small bowl; set aside.
4. Spread the sesame seeds in a shallow baking dish or pie plate. Pat the tuna steaks dry with paper towels. Season the tuna with salt and pepper, then press both sides and the edges of each steak in the sesame seeds to coat; set aside.
5. Heat a large nonstick skillet over medium-high heat and spray with cooking spray or lightly grease with canola oil. Add the tuna steaks to the skillet and cook the first side for about 2 minutes, then carefully flip with a large spatula and cook the other side for about 2 minutes. The cooking time will depend on

the thickness of the steaks and how done you like them: Rare 1¼-inch tuna steaks (opaque around the edges and red in the middle) will take about 3 minutes, medium-rare (opaque around the edges and pink in the middle) will take about 4 minutes, and well-done (completely opaque throughout) will take about 6 minutes; try not to overcook the tuna (even if you like it well-done), as it tends to dry out the fish.

6. Transfer the tuna to a serving platter and serve with the wasabi-soy sauce and kim chee salsa on the side.

▶ **Cooking Tip:** Cooking the tuna steaks coated with sesame seeds on an indoor grill works really well. However, keep in mind that the tuna will cook twice as fast, so the total cooking time will only be about 2 minutes.

▶ **Advance Preparation:** The salsa can be made up to 1 day in advance and kept refrigerated.

Approximate Nutritional Information: Serving size: one-quarter sesame-coated sautéed yellowfin tuna; Calories: 155 cals, 8%; Protein: 33 g, 66%; Total fat: 1.4 g, 2%; Saturated fat: 0.3 g, 3%; Cholesterol: 64 mg, 21%; Carbohydrates: 0 g, 0%; Fiber: 0 g, 0%; Sodium: 52 mg, 2%; Thiamin: 0.6 mg, 41% Niacin: 14 mg, 70%; Vitamin B$_6$: 1 mg, 64%; Diabetic Exchange Values: 5 Very Lean Meat

Percentage of calories from fat: 9%

Approximate Nutritional Information: Serving size: one-quarter kim chee salsa; 38 cals, 2%; Protein: 2 g, 4%; Total fat: 1.6 g, 2%; Saturated fat: 0.2 g, 1%; Cholesterol: 0 mg, 0%; Carbohydrates: 5 g, 2%; Fiber: 2 g, 7%; Sodium: 116 mg, 5%; Vitamin C: 23 mg, 39%; Vitamin K: 37 mcg, 46%; Diabetic Exchange Values: 1 Vegetable

Percentage of calories from fat: 35%. **Note:** It is more important to focus on the total fat value of this low-calorie recipe, which is 2 grams, or 2% Daily Value, per serving than on the percentage of calories from fat.

Approximate Nutritional Information: Serving size: 2 teaspoons wasabi-soy sauce; 4 cals, 0%; Protein: 0.3 g, 0%; Total fat: 0 g, 0%; Saturated fat: 0 g, 0%; Cholesterol: 0 mg, 0%; Carbohydrates: 0 g, 0%; Fiber: 0 g, 0%; Sodium: 192 mg, 8%; Diabetic Exchange Values: FREE

Percentage of calories from fat: 0%

Shrimp and Bay Scallops with Corn, Zucchini, and Tomatoes

Heart-Health Benefits: Protein and vitamin C

A **scrumptious and beautiful** main course, especially during summer when light meals make use of the freshest produce available. Serve with a crusty whole wheat baguette or a hearty whole-grain country-style bread.

■ *Serves 4* ■

1 tablespoon canola oil or olive oil

8 ounces medium shrimp, peeled and deveined

8 ounces bay scallops, rinsed and patted dry

1 small garlic clove, minced

1 medium zucchini, washed, quartered lengthwise, and cut into ¹/₂-inch pieces

2 ears fresh corn (white or yellow), kernels cut off the ears, or 1¹/₂ cups frozen corn, thawed

1 cup halved cherry tomatoes

¹/₃ cup thinly sliced scallions

¹/₃ cup chopped fresh cilantro

1 tablespoon freshly squeezed lime juice, or to taste

Salt and freshly ground pepper, to taste

1. Heat 1 teaspoon of the canola oil in a large nonstick skillet over medium-high heat. Add the shrimp, season with salt and pepper, and sauté for 2 minutes, or just until done. Transfer the cooked shrimp to a large serving dish, cover with foil, and set aside. (Do not rinse the skillet.)
2. Heat another teaspoon of canola oil in the skillet over medium-high heat. Add the bay scallops, season, and cook for 2 minutes, or until cooked through. Transfer the cooked scallops to the serving dish, re-cover, and set aside. (Do not rinse the skillet.)
3. Heat the remaining 1 teaspoon canola oil in the skillet over medium-high heat. Add the garlic, zucchini, and corn, season, and sauté for 3 minutes, or just until the zucchini is crisp-tender. Transfer the vegetables to the serving dish, then add the cherry tomatoes, scallions, cilantro, and lime juice and mix gently. Adjust the seasoning and serve immediately, or cool and serve at room temperature.

Approximate Nutritional Information: Serving size: one-quarter shrimp and bay scallops with corn, zucchini, and tomatoes; Calories: 140 cals, 7%; Protein: 15g, 31%; Total fat: 4.6 g, 7%; Saturated fat: 0.3 g, 2%; Cholesterol: 69 mg, 23%; Carbohydrates: 10 g, 3%; Fiber: 2 g, 7%; Sodium: 328 mg, 14%; Vitamin C: 16 mg, 27%; Vitamin K: 7 mcg, 9%; Diabetic Exchange Values: 2 Vegetable, 2 Very Lean Meat, 1 Fat

Percentage of calories from fat: 29%

Deep-Fried Dangers

IT IS ALWAYS best to avoid deep-fried food no matter what it is or how tempting it may smell or look. For the sake of comparison, a roasted 3-ounce portion of chicken has about 3 grams of fat and 140 calories, while a deep-fried portion of the same size has about 11 grams of fat and 221 calories. Common deep-fried foods include French fries, onion rings, Tater Tots, batter-coated or breaded fish, oysters, shrimp, chicken nuggets, meats, mozzarella sticks, fried dough, and doughnuts. When dining out, always opt for grilled, broiled, baked, steamed, boiled, or sautéed dishes.

Attention Parents: Almost all of the fried frozen foods designed for kids, such as chicken nuggets, fish sticks, and TV dinners, contain partially hydrogenated oil. Bell & Evans is one brand of chicken nuggets and chicken tenders that does not.

Crab Cakes
with Tomatillo-Avocado Sauce

Heart-Health Benefits: Protein and B vitamins

Admittedly, crab cakes, especially those made with 100 percent jumbo lump crabmeat, are a luxury; but, when your budget allows, go for it! Other times, use half jumbo lump and half backfin crabmeat, which is cheaper. The tomatillo-avocado sauce is also a fabulous dip for baked tortilla chips or raw vegetables, and an interesting alternative to traditional guacamole. The recipes for the sauce and the crab cakes can be cut in half for a smaller yield.

■ *Serves 4 to 5* ■

Tomatillo-Avocado Sauce (makes about 2 cups)

- 4 small tomatillos, papery husks removed, washed, and coarsely chopped
- 1 tablespoon olive oil or canola oil
- 1 tablespoon seasoned rice vinegar
- 1 tablespoon freshly squeezed lime juice
- 1 small garlic clove, peeled
- 1/4 teaspoon ground cumin
- 1/2 cup loosely packed fresh cilantro leaves
- Salt and freshly ground pepper, to taste
- 1 small avocado, halved, pitted, and peeled

Crab Cakes (makes 7 crab cakes)

- 8 ounces jumbo lump crabmeat, picked over to remove any shells and cartilage
- 8 ounces backfin crabmeat, picked over to remove any shells and cartilage
- 1/2 cup plain bread crumbs
- 2 tablespoons thinly sliced scallions or fresh chives
- 1/4 cup chopped fresh dill, cilantro, or basil
- 2 teaspoons grated lemon zest (optional)
- 2 teaspoons Dijon mustard
- 3 large egg whites
- 2 tablespoons light mayonnaise
- 1 tablespoon canola oil

1. To make the tomatillo-avocado sauce, combine all of the ingredients except the avocado in the bowl of a food processor and pulse to a chunky consistency. Add the avocado and pulse a few more times. Transfer to a serving bowl, cover with plastic wrap pressed flush against the surface of the sauce, and refrigerate until ready to serve. (Note: This sauce can be made up to 1 day in advance.)
2. To make the crab cakes, combine all of the ingredients except the canola oil in a bowl. Mix gently until well incorporated. To form the crab cakes, use a 1/3-cup measuring cup to portion out each crab cake, then form each portion into a patty and place it on a large plate. Cover and refrigerate until ready to cook. (Note: These crab cakes can be made up to 8 hours in advance.)

3. Heat the canola oil in a large nonstick skillet over medium-high heat. Add 3 or 4 of the crab cakes (avoid overcrowding) and cook on one side for about 3 minutes, or until golden brown. Carefully flip and cook on the other side for about 3 minutes, or until golden brown and thoroughly cooked. (Note: You may need to adjust the heat if the crab cakes are browning too quickly.) Transfer the cooked crab cakes to a serving plate and cover loosely with foil to keep warm. Cook the remaining crab cakes, and transfer to the plate. Serve immediately with the tomatillo-avocado sauce.

▶ **Cooking Tip:** The crab cakes can be baked instead of sautéed, but they will not be a nice golden brown on the outside. Preheat the oven to 400 degrees F. Line a baking sheet with foil and spray with canola oil cooking spray. Bake for 15 minutes, or until the crab cakes are thoroughly cooked.

Approximate Nutritional Information: Serving size: 1 crab cake (no sauce); Calories: 99 cals, 5%; Protein: 15 g, 30%; Total fat: 2.7 g, 4%; Saturated fat: 0.4 g, 2%; Cholesterol: 66 mg, 22%; Carbohydrates: 3 g, 1%; Fiber: 0.1 g, 1%; Sodium: 287 mg, 12%; Vitamin B_{12}: 5 mcg, 79%; Vitamin K: 6 mcg, 8%; Diabetic Exchange Values: 2 Very Lean Meat, 1/2 Fat

Percentage of calories from fat: 25%

Approximate Nutritional Information: Serving size: 2 tablespoons tomatillo-avocado sauce; Calories: 33 cals, 2%; Protein: 0.4 g, 1%; Total fat: 2.8 g, 4%; Saturated fat: 0.2 g, 1%; Cholesterol: 0 mg, 0%; Carbohydrates: 2 g, 1%; Fiber: 0.9 g, 4%; Sodium: 3 mg, 0%; Vitamin K: 5 mcg, 6%; Diabetic Exchange Values: 1 Fat

Percentage of calories from fat: 73%. **Note:** It is more important to focus on the total fat value of this low-calorie recipe, which is 3 grams, or 4% Daily Value, per serving than on the percentage of calories from fat.

Smart Choice Frozen Dinners

NEW CHOICES OF frozen dinners appear on the market almost daily, and different brands cater to specific dietary needs. For instance, if you are trying to lose weight, Smart Ones, Lean Cuisine, Healthy Choice, Lean Gourmet, and Weight Watchers have less fat and fewer calories than other major brands. If you need to watch your sodium intake, reduced-sodium meals are available. If you just want a tasty, healthy meal, Amy's line of frozen foods is a great choice. Following are some tips to keep in mind as you browse the frozen food aisles.

▶ Look for dinners with the highest amount of protein (usually about 10 grams) and the least amount of fat per serving.
▶ Look for vegetarian frozen dinners, which are usually low in fat and cholesterol.
▶ Look for reduced-sodium dinners.
▶ Buy frozen dinners from a whole foods store. Their in-house brands tend to be less processed, though slightly more expensive.
▶ Look for dinners that are baked, not fried.
▶ Choose frozen dinners that do not contain trans fats or partially hydrogenated oil. Pizzas and other dinners with crusts or breading often contain trans fats.

Attention Parents: Be sure to read the nutritional information on frozen dinners designed for kids. Many of them are extremely high in fat and sodium, and most of them are deep-fried, not baked. Your kid(s) may prefer the fancy packaging or the other gimmicks, but don't succumb to their desires. A nutritious "adult-style" frozen dinner is a healthier choice for them.

WHITE MEATS

SIX

HEART-HEALTH TIPS AT A GLANCE

► Lean white meats eaten in moderation can be a good source of protein, B vitamins, and minerals.

► Always choose the leanest cuts of meats possible—unfortunately, these are usually the most expensive. Chicken tenders and breasts, lean ground chicken and ground turkey, turkey breast, pork tenderloin, pork chops, and veal cutlets are all good lean choices. Trim any visible fat before cooking.

► Keep your sauces simple and as low in fat as possible. Salsas are a good option, and fresh herbs, dried spices, and lemon are easy flavor boosters (see Adding Flavor without Adding Salt, page 183).

► Mix and match the sauces and salsas in this chapter with other main courses. For instance, the White Bean, Artichoke Heart, Olive, and Sun-Dried Tomato Salsa (page 200) paired here with pork tenderloin is also excellent with chicken, red meat, or fish. The Shiitake Mushroom, Green Bean, Corn, and Red Bell Pepper Salsa (page 202) served with pork chops is perfect with chicken, fish, red meats, or tofu.

► Stir-fries are a great way to combine protein and vegetables. Have all of your ingredients ready, including the rice or rice noodles, and cooking dinner will take just minutes.

► Try chicken or turkey burgers instead of hamburgers made with beef. Because ground chicken and turkey contain less fat than beef, you will need to add some moisture to the meat—plain nonfat yogurt, fat-free ricotta cheese, or reduced-fat feta works well. The chicken burgers on page 191 will get you started—then feel free to experiment with your favorite flavors.

▶ Keep your sodium intake to a minimum. Oversalting food is a habit—using less salt can also become a good habit. Always taste your food before salting it. See High-Sodium Culprits, page 187, and Salt Limits and Lingo, page 182, for the recommended uppermost limits of daily salt intake. Carefully follow any sodium restrictions outlined by your doctor or health-care provider. You may also want to consider the DASH-Sodium Diet; see High Calcium Intake from Dairy Products—or Following the DASH Diet—May Lower Blood Pressure, page 65, and Sources, page 267, for information on how to obtain a copy of the DASH Eating Plan.

▶ Avoid deep-fried foods, such as fried chicken, chicken nuggets, and deep-fried turkey. If you own a deep fryer, get rid of it.

▶ Make smart choices when dining out. Look for the heart-health ❤ symbol on menus, and ask the kitchen to prepare dishes according to your specific needs. It is always a good idea to ask for sauces and salad dressings on the side.

Chicken, Arugula, Sun-Dried Tomato, Olive, and Feta Cheese Pasta Salad

Heart-Health Benefits: Protein, vitamin C, and B vitamins

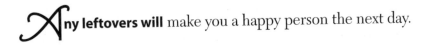ny leftovers will make you a happy person the next day.

■ *Serves 4* ■

2 cups bow-tie or other small pasta, preferably whole wheat

2 tablespoons olive oil

8 ounces boneless, skinless chicken breasts or tenders, any visible fat removed, cut into 1/4-inch dice

1/3 cup sun-dried tomatoes in oil, drained and cut into small dice

1/2 cup coarsely chopped pitted black olives, preferably Kalamata

1/4 cup crumbled reduced-fat feta cheese, cut into small dice

4 cups lightly packed baby arugula, washed and stems trimmed (if using large arugula leaves, cut them in half)

2 tablespoons toasted pine nuts (optional)

2 tablespoons balsamic vinegar, or to taste

1. Cook the pasta according to the package directions. Drain, then transfer to a large serving bowl. Add 1 tablespoon of the olive oil (to prevent the pasta from sticking together), mix, and set aside.
2. Add the remaining 1 tablespoon olive oil to a large nonstick skillet and heat over medium-high heat. Add the chicken and sauté, stirring occasionally, for 5 minutes, or until completely cooked.
3. Transfer the chicken to the bowl containing the pasta, then add the remaining ingredients and mix until well combined. Adjust the seasoning and serve at room temperature.

▶ **Substitutions:** The chicken can be replaced by an equal amount of extra-firm tofu. Drain the tofu, pat dry with paper towels, and cut into ½-inch cubes. Sautée according to the directions in Step 2, and proceed as above.

Approximate Nutritional Information: Serving size: one-quarter sautéed chicken with arugula, sun-dried tomatoes, olives, and feta cheese (pine nuts not included); Calories: 221 cals, 11%; Protein: 18 g, 36%; Total fat: 8 g, 12%; Saturated fat: 1.6 g, 8%; Cholesterol: 35 mg, 12%; Carbohydrates: 19 g, 6%; Fiber: 2 g, 7%; Sodium: 341 mg, 14%; Vitamin C: 13 mg, 22%; Niacin: 8 mg, 41%; Vitamin K: 24 mcg, 30%; Diabetic Exchange Values: 1 Starch, 2 Medium-Fat Meat, 1 Vegetable

Percentage of calories from fat: 33%

Rigatoni with Chicken, Vegetables, and Tomato Sauce

Heart-Health Benefits: Protein, calcium, vitamins A and C, B vitamins, folic acid, and magnesium

---

An **easy chicken** and vegetable dinner everyone will enjoy. Use your favorite vegetables in place of the ones called for, and substitute tofu for the chicken, if desired (see Substitutions below). A fresh green salad is the perfect side dish.

■ *Serves 6* ■

2 cups (uncooked) rigatoni, preferably whole wheat

2 tablespoons canola oil or olive oil

3 cups broccoli florets

1 medium zucchini, washed, halved lengthwise, and sliced

1 small red bell pepper, washed, cored, seeded, and cut into small dice

1 pound boneless, skinless chicken breasts or

tenders, any visible fat removed cut into $^1/_2$-inch dice

3 cups high-quality all-purpose tomato sauce (such as Rao's Homemade All Natural Premium Quality Marinara Sauce)

$^1/_2$ cup thinly sliced fresh basil leaves

2 cups shredded part-skim low-moisture mozzarella cheese

1. Have ready a 9-inch oval or square baking dish. Cook the rigatoni according to the package directions. Drain, then transfer the pasta to a large bowl. Cover with foil to keep warm; set aside.
2. Heat 1 tablespoon of the canola oil in a large nonstick skillet over medium-high heat. Add the broccoli, zucchini, and red bell pepper and sauté, stirring occasionally, for 5 minutes, or until crisp-tender; 2 minutes into the cooking time, add 3 tablespoons water to the skillet to prevent the vegetables from sticking to the pan. Do not overcook the vegetables. Transfer the vegetables to the bowl containing the pasta, re-cover, and set aside. (Do not rinse the skillet.)
3. Add the remaining 1 tablespoon canola oil to the skillet and heat over medium-high heat. Add the chicken and sauté for 5 minutes, stirring occasionally, or until the chicken is completely cooked. Add the tomato sauce to the skillet and stir until it is thoroughly heated. Transfer the chicken and sauce to the bowl containing the pasta, add the basil, and mix until well combined.
4. Preheat the broiler. Transfer the pasta mixture to the baking dish. Sprinkle the top with the mozzarella cheese, then place the baking dish under the broiler until the cheese is melted and bubbly. Watch carefully to prevent burning. Serve immediately.

▶ **Substitutions:** The chicken can be replaced by one 15-ounce package of extra-firm tofu. Drain the tofu, pat dry with paper towels, and cut into ½-inch cubes. Sauté according to the directions in Step 3, then proceed as above.

Approximate Nutritional Information: Serving size: one-sixth rigatoni with chicken, vegetables, and tomato sauce; Calories: 389 cals, 19%; Protein: 34 g, 67%; Total fat: 13.9 g, 21%; Saturated fat: 5.4 g, 27%; Cholesterol: 64 mg, 21%; Carbohydrates: 33 g, 11%; Fiber: 3 g, 13%; Sodium: 904 mg, 38%; Calcium: 331 mg, 33%; Vitamin A: 2,703 IU, 54%; Vitamin C: 94 mg, 156%; Thiamin: 0.4 mg, 28%; Riboflavin: 0.5 mg, 28%; Niacin: 12 mg, 61%; Vitamin B$_6$: 0.7 mg, 38%; Folic acid: 124 mcg, 31%; Magnesium: 80 mg, 20%; Vitamin K: 99 mcg, 124%; Diabetic Exchange Values: 2 Starch, 4 Lean Meat, 1 Vegetable

Percentage of calories from fat: 32%

SALT SUBSTITUTES AND SALT-FREE SEASONINGS

CONFUSED ABOUT THE difference between salt substitutes and salt-free seasonings? Both use potassium chloride instead of sodium chloride, but salt substitutes contain only potassium chloride and no other seasonings. Salt-free seasonings get their flavor from a blend of seasonings combined with trace amounts of potassium chloride. For comparison, ¼ teaspoon of Mrs. Dash Original salt-free seasoning contains only 10 milligrams of potassium chloride, whereas the same amount of Morton Salt Substitute contains 610 milligrams.

Salt Limits and Lingo

THERE IS NO Recommended Dietary Allowance (RDA) for sodium. The numbers you see on food labels are Daily Reference Values (DRV) set by the U.S. Food and Drug Administration, with the percentage of each nutrient's Daily Value listed next to it. The DRVs for some nutrients represent the uppermost limit that is considered desirable, and for sodium this value is set at 2,400 milligrams per day. This is not a recommended intake, but rather a reference point to the upper limit.

To add confusion, the Food and Nutrition Board of the Institute of Medicine (1997–2001), came up with another nutrition standard called Dietary Reference Intakes (DRI), which replaced the 1989 Recommended Dietary Allowances. DRIs are developed from a set of four reference values: Estimated Average Requirements (EAR), Recommended Dietary Allowances (RDA), Adequate Intakes (AI), and Tolerable Upper Intake Levels (UL). The Adequate Intake (AI) of sodium for most males and females fourteen years and older is 1,200 to 1,500 milligrams of sodium, and the Tolerable Upper Intake Level (UL) is 2,200 to 2,300 milligrams.

The American Heart Association recommends no more than 2,400 mg of sodium per day for healthy Americans. The National Institute of Heart, Lung, and Blood Disorders also recommends no more than 2,400 milligrams, but it goes a step further and states that for those with high blood pressure, a diet with no more than 1,500 milligrams of sodium per day had blood-pressure–lowering benefits.

Understanding the Salt Lingo on Labels

- ▶ Low Sodium: less than 140 milligrams of sodium
- ▶ Very Low Sodium: less than 35 milligrams of sodium
- ▶ Sodium Free or Salt Free: less than 5 milligrams of sodium
- ▶ Reduced, Less, or Fewer Sodium: a product must contain 25 percent or less sodium than the regular reference product
- ▶ Light or Lite: sodium content is reduced by 50 percent
- ▶ Unsalted, No Salt Added, or Without Added Salt: The product is made without added salt, but it still contains the sodium that is a natural part of the food itself

Adding Flavor without Adding Salt

▶ Fresh or dried leafy herbs and dried spices add flavor to everything from salad dressings and bean dips to seafood and casseroles.

▶ Curry powder livens up sauces, marinades, and salad dressings.

▶ Mustard works wonders in vinaigrettes, marinades, and other dressings, and as a condiment for meat or poultry.

▶ Freshly squeezed lemon or lime juice enhances vegetables such as broccoli and asparagus, and seafood, chicken, veal, or lamb. Grated lemon or lime zest is wonderful sprinkled over such dishes as well.

▶ Garlic is a great flavor booster for meats, poultry, fish, sauces, marinades, and salad dressings. To get the maximum health benefits of garlic, chop it about 15 minutes before cooking or using it.

▶ Chopped fresh ginger is a delicious addition to stir-fries, curries, and marinades.

▶ Lemongrass adds an Asian touch to curries, soups, and marinades.

▶ Nuts add crunch and flavor to pasta, salads, rice and other grains, vegetables, fish, chicken, and desserts.

▶ Freshly ground pepper, Tabasco, and other sauces add heat to many dishes.

Cashew Chicken with Broccoli and Red Bell Peppers

Nutrition Highlight: Protein, vitamins A and C, B vitamins, and magnesium

*H*ere is a fresh and light approach to the ever-popular cashew chicken. Serve over brown basmati rice or rice noodles.

■ *Serves 4* ■

Sauce

2 tablespoons lite soy sauce

3 tablespoons water

2 tablespoons hoisin sauce

1 tablespoon seasoned rice vinegar

1 teaspoon cornstarch

1 tablespoon canola oil

1 teaspoon toasted sesame oil

1 large garlic clove, minced

2 tablespoons minced fresh ginger

3 cups broccoli florets

1¹⁄₂ cups sliced red bell peppers

1¹⁄₄ pounds boneless, skinless chicken breasts or tenders, any visible fat removed and cut into ¹⁄₂-inch dice

¹⁄₂ cup sliced scallions

¹⁄₃ cup chopped cashew nuts, or to taste

3 tablespoons chopped fresh cilantro, for garnish (optional)

1. To make the sauce, combine all of the ingredients in a medium bowl and mix; set aside.
2. Heat 1½ teaspoons of the canola oil and the sesame oil in a large nonstick skillet over medium-high heat. Add the garlic and ginger and sauté for 30 seconds. Add the broccoli and red bell peppers and sauté, stirring occasionally, for 5 minutes, or until crisp-tender; 2 minutes into the cooking time, add 3 tablespoons water to the skillet to prevent the vegetables from sticking. Do not overcook the vegetables. Transfer the vegetables to a serving bowl and cover with foil to keep warm. (Do not rinse the skillet.)
3. Add the remaining 1½ teaspoons canola oil to the skillet and heat over medium-high heat. Add the chicken and sauté, stirring occasionally, for 5 minutes. Add the scallions, the sauce, and cashew nuts and cook, stirring, for 1 minute more, or until the sauce thickens slightly.
4. Transfer the contents of the skillet to the bowl containing the vegetables and gently mix. Adjust the seasoning, garnish with the cilantro, if using, and serve immediately.

▶ **Substitutions:** The chicken can be replaced by one 15-ounce package of extra-firm tofu. Drain the tofu, pat dry with paper towels, and cut into ½-inch cubes. Sauté according to the directions in Step 3, and proceed as above.

Approximate Nutritional Information: Serving size: one-quarter cashew chicken with broccoli and red bell peppers; Calories: 320 cals, 16%; Protein: 38 g, 76%; Total fat: 11.1 g, 17%; Saturated fat: 1.8 g, 9%; Cholesterol: 82 mg, 27%; Carbohydrates: 18 g, 6%; Fiber: 4 g, 15%; Sodium: 608 mg, 25%; Vitamin A: 2,608 IU, 52%; Vitamin C: 171 mg, 284%; Niacin: 17 mg, 86%; Vitamin B_6: 1 mg, 56%; Magnesium: 96 mg, 24%; Vitamin K: 80 mcg, 100%; Diabetic Exchange Values: 1 Starch, 5 Very-Lean meat, 2 Fat

Percentage of calories from fat: 31%

THE HIDDEN DANGERS OF CHICKEN NUGGETS

IF YOU OR your children tend to eat a lot of chicken nuggets, you may want to cut back or even cut them out. Chicken Nuggets from fast-food restaurants and frozen boxes (with a few exceptions, such as Bell & Evans All Natural Chicken Nuggets) are made from finely ground dark and light meat and skin, breading, fillers, and added fats, including trans fats from partially hydrogenated oil. A 12-nugget serving from McDonald's has 510 calories and 30 grams of total fat, meaning that nearly 60 percent of the calories come from fat. Healthier alternatives to chicken nuggets are grilled or broiled chicken sandwiches or chicken Caesar salads (go easy on the dressing, though).

Attention Parents: If chicken nuggets are a major part of your children's diets, be sure to look for those brands that are baked, not fried, and those that are made from white meat with no fillers. Or offer a grilled or broiled chicken sandwich instead of nuggets.

Chicken and Vegetable Curry Stir-Fry

Heart-Health Benefits: Protein, vitamins A and C, B vitamins, and magnesium

$\mathcal{S}$erve this flavor-packed chicken and vegetable curry over brown basmati rice or rice noodles. A salad made with Asian greens rounds off the meal perfectly.

■ *Serves 4* ■

1¼ pounds boneless, skinless chicken breasts or
   tenders, any visible fat removed, and cut into
   ½-inch slices

1 medium sweet onion, such as Vidalia, halved
   and thinly sliced

1 tablespoon mild curry powder

1 tablespoon sugar

2 tablespoons fish sauce

2 tablespoons canola oil

1½ cups broccoli florets

¾ cup sliced red bell peppers

¾ cup baby peeled carrots sliced diagonally into
   ¼-inch slices

3 scallions, trimmed and sliced into large pieces

¼ cup chopped fresh cilantro

Freshly squeezed lime juice, to taste

1. Combine the chicken, onion, curry powder, sugar, fish sauce, and 1 tablespoon of the canola oil in a bowl. Mix until well combined, then allow the chicken to marinate, covered and refrigerated, for at least 30 minutes, or overnight.
2. Heat 1½ teaspoons of the canola oil in a large nonstick skillet over medium-high heat. Add the broccoli, red bell peppers, and carrots and sauté for 5 minutes, stirring occasionally; 2 minutes into the cooking time, add 2 tablespoons water to the skillet to prevent the vegetables from sticking to the pan. Do not overcook the vegetables. Transfer the vegetables to a large serving bowl and cover with foil to keep warm. (Do not rinse the skillet.)
3. Add the remaining 1½ teaspoons of canola oil to the skillet and heat over medium-high heat. Add the marinated chicken-onion mixture and the scallions and sauté, stirring occasionally, for 3 minutes. Add ¼ cup water and continue to cook for 3 minutes, or until the chicken is fully cooked. (Note: If your skillet is on the small side, you may need to sauté the chicken in two batches. Use a splatter screen to reduce cleanup.)
4. Transfer the chicken to the serving bowl containing the vegetables and gently mix. Adjust the seasoning and garnish with the cilantro and a squeeze of lime juice. Serve immediately.

Approximate Nutritional Information: Serving size: one-quarter chicken and vegetable curry stir-fry; Calories: 280 cals, 14%; Protein: 35 g, 71%; Total fat: 9 g, 14%; Saturated fat: 1 g, 5%; Cholesterol: 82 mg, 27%; Carbohydrates: 14 g, 5%; Fiber: 3 g, 13%; Sodium: 833 mg, 35%; Vitamin A: 6,715 IU, 134%; Vitamin C: 93 mg, 154%; Niacin: 17 mg, 85%; Vitamin B$_6$: 1 mg, 53%; Magnesium: 79 mg, 20%; Vitamin K: 52 mcg, 65%; Diabetic Exchange Values: 4 Very-Lean Meat, 2 Fat, 3 Vegetable

Percentage of calories from fat: 29%

High-Sodium Culprits

AS A GENERAL rule, always choose products with as little sodium as possible in them, and preferably no added sodium. Rinse canned vegetables, beans, tuna, and other high-sodium products before cooking or serving them. If you are on a sodium-restricted diet, carefully follow your doctor's advice.

Meats and Fish: Bacon; sausages; bologna; salami; ham; corned beef; hot dogs; canned meats; sardines; canned tuna and salmon; smoked meat, chicken, or fish; frozen prepared dinners

Snack Foods: Salted chips, pretzels, tortilla chips, pork rinds, and corn chips; salted popcorn; nuts and seeds; salted crackers; rolls or breads with salt toppings; French fries; pickles; olives; fast food

Seasonings: Salt, sea salt, and "lite" salt (contains 50 percent salt); seasoned salts (such as onion, celery, and garlic salt); meat tenderizers; MSG (monosodium glutamate); bouillon cubes and powders; soy sauce; teriyaki sauce; steak sauce; salad dressings; barbecue sauce; ketchup, relish, and mustard; sauerkraut; packaged sauces and gravies; regular Worcestershire sauce

Other: Canned or packaged soups, broths, and bouillons; instant soups; processed and prepared foods; boxed meals and side dishes (such as flavored rice mixes, macaroni and cheese, etc.); canned vegetables; cheese; cottage cheese; cheese spreads; buttermilk; soft drinks; tomato juice and V-8 juice; pickles

Chicken Fajitas
with Homemade Guacamole

Heart-Health Benefits: Protein, vitamins A, C,
and K, B vitamins, folic acid, magnesium, and fiber

---

*F*ajitas are always a winner. In this recipe the chicken is sliced, marinated, and then sautéed. It can also be cooked on an indoor grill. If you use an outdoor grill, slice the chicken into large enough pieces so they don't fall through the grill. Read the labels of tortilla packages to make sure that the ones you buy don't contain partially hydrogenated oil—you'd be surprised at how many of them do. Some topping ideas include grated low-fat cheese, diced vine-ripened tomatoes or tomato salsa, guacamole or avocado slices, shredded lettuce, jarred or canned jalapeño peppers, chopped fresh cilantro, fat-free sour cream, and lime wedges. For vegetarians, the chicken can be substituted with extra-firm tofu or large portobello mushrooms.

■ *Serves 4* ■

Marinade

2 tablespoons freshly squeezed lime juice

1 tablespoon reduced-sodium Worcestershire
   sauce

1 large garlic clove, minced

$^1/_2$ teaspoon ground cumin

$^1/_2$ teaspoon dried oregano

2 teaspoons chili powder

1 teaspoon red pepper flakes (optional)

$1^1/_4$ pounds boneless, skinless chicken breasts or
tenders, any visible fat removed and cut into
long strips on the diagonal

1 tablespoon canola oil

1 large red bell pepper, washed, cored, seeded,
   and cut into strips

1 sweet onion, such as Vidalia, thinly sliced

Canola oil cooking spray, if using an indoor grill

Ten 7-inch corn or flour tortillas

Homemade Guacamole (see recipe on page 190)

1. For the marinade, combine all of the ingredients in a small bowl and mix well. Or, if you plan to marinate the chicken in a bowl rather than a zip-top bag, use a large bowl to make the marinade. Using a fork, pierce the chicken all over to allow the marinade to seep in, then place the chicken in a zip-lock bag, add the marinade, and seal. Or add the chicken to the bowl and cover with plastic wrap. Refrigerate for at least 30 minutes, or overnight.
2. Heat 1½ teaspoons of the canola oil in a large nonstick skillet over medium-

high heat. Add the red bell peppers and onion and sauté for 10 minutes. Transfer to a serving bowl, cover, and set aside. If you are sautéing the chicken, do not rinse the skillet.

3. Add the remaining 1½ teaspoons canola oil to the skillet and heat over medium-high heat until hot. Add the marinated chicken and sauté for 10 to 12 minutes, stirring occasionally, or until the chicken is completely cooked, or preheat an indoor grill to high. Spray the grill with cooking spray, add the chicken pieces, spreading them out in a single layer, and grill for 4 to 5 minutes, or until the chicken is fully cooked. Transfer the chicken to a serving dish and cover to keep warm.

4. While the chicken is cooking, heat the tortillas according to the package directions. Wrap the tortillas in a dish cloth or foil to keep them warm.

5. Serve the chicken with the tortillas, the peppers and onions, guacamole, and any other toppings.

Homemade Guacamole

Heart-Health Benefits: Vitamin K and fiber

*Y*ou can make this guacamole as simple or as doctored-up as you wish. It is best eaten the same day it is made.

■ *Makes 1 cup* ■

2 large ripe avocados, preferably Hass

2 tablespoons finely chopped red onion

1 tablespoon freshly squeezed lime juice, or to taste

2 tablespoons chopped fresh cilantro

1 small garlic clove, crushed

Salt, to taste

Dash of Tabasco sauce, or to taste

1. Cut the avocados in half and remove the pits. Cut the halves into quarters, then peel them and place in a small bowl. Using the back of a fork or a potato masher, mash the avocados to a chunky consistency. (Do not use a food processor or blender.)
2. Add the remaining ingredients and mix until well combined. Adjust the seasoning if necessary. Cover with plastic wrap pressed flush against the surface of the guacamole, and refrigerate for a couple of hours to allow the flavors to blend before serving.

▶ **Storage Tip:** This guacamole keeps refrigerated for 1 day. Some discoloration will occur, but the taste will not be affected.

Approximate Nutritional Information: Serving size: one-quarter fajitas (without guacamole); Calories: 336 cals, 17%; Protein: 37 g, 74%; Total fat: 5.2 g, 8%; Saturated fat: 0.8 g, 4%; Cholesterol: 82 mg, 27%; Carbohydrates: 35 g, 12%; Fiber: 5 g, 19%; Sodium: 198 mg, 8%; Vitamin A: 1,196 IU, 24%; Vitamin C: 74 mg, 124%; Niacin: 17 mg, 86%; Vitamin B$_6$: 1 mg, 53%; Folic acid: 83 mcg, 21%; Magnesium: 89 mg, 22%; Vitamin K: 5 mcg, 6%; Diabetic Exchange Values: 1 Starch, 4 Very Lean Meat, 1 Fat, 1 Vegetable

Percentage of calories from fat: 14%

Approximate Nutritional Information: Serving size: one-quarter marinade; Calories: 13 cals, 1%; Protein: 0.3 g, 1%; Total fat: 0.3 g, 0%; Saturated fat: 0 g, 0%; Cholesterol: 0 mg, 0%; Carbohydrates: 3 g, 1%; Fiber: 0.6 g, 3%; Sodium: 29 mg, 1; Vitamin K: 3 mcg, 3%; Diabetic Exchange Values: FREE

Percentage of calories from fat: 19% The fat value of this marinade is not important, since it will be discarded before cooking.

Approximate Nutritional Information: Serving size: one-quarter homemade guacamole (about ¼ cup); Calories: 146 cals, 7%; Protein: 2 g, 4%; Total fat: 13 g, 20%; Saturated fat: 1.8 g, 9%; Cholesterol: 0 mg, 0%; Carbohydrates: 9 g, 3%; Fiber: 6 g, 24%; Sodium: 154 mg, 6%; Vitamin K: 18 mcg, 22%; Diabetic Exchange Values: 3 Fat, 1 Vegetable

Percentage of calories from fat: 74%. **Note:** Avocadoes are a good source of heart-healthy monounsaturated fat.

Two Chicken Burgers

Feta and Fresh Basil Chicken Burgers

Heart-Health Benefits: Protein and B vitamins

A delicious burger with or without a bun. A whole-grain salad, such as the Mediterranean-Style Couscous Salad, page 99, or the Black and White Gazpacho Salad, page 105, is a perfect side dish. If you want a sauce, the Sun-Dried Tomato Sauce, page 152, is a great choice.

■ *Serves 4* ■

1 pound ground chicken, the leanest you can find

¼ cup crumbled reduced-fat feta cheese

1 tablespoon reduced-sodium Worcestershire sauce

2 tablespoons thinly sliced fresh basil leaves

1 tablespoon freshly squeezed lemon juice

1 small garlic clove, crushed

2 tablespoons thinly sliced scallion greens

¼ teaspoon salt

About 3 tablespoons all-purpose flour

Canola oil cooking spray or canola oil

1. Combine all of the ingredients except the flour and cooking spray in a large bowl and mix until well blended. Divide the mixture into 4 equal parts, then form each portion into a patty.
2. Spread the flour on a large plate. Lightly coat both sides of each patty with flour, pat off the excess, and set aside.
3. Preheat an indoor grill to high or heat a large nonstick skillet over medium-high heat. Spray the grill or skillet with cooking spray or lightly grease with canola oil. Add the burgers and cook on the indoor grill for a total of 5 to 6 minutes or in the skillet for 2 to 3 minutes on each side. Check for doneness by cutting into a burger; the middle should be fully cooked and the juices should be clear. Serve immediately.

Approximate Nutritional Information: Serving size: one-quarter feta and fresh basil chicken burgers; Calories: 147 cals, 7%; Protein: 28 g, 56%; Total fat: 2.4 g, 4%; Saturated fat: 1 g, 5%; Cholesterol: 68 mg, 23%; Carbohydrates: 2 g, 1%; Fiber: 0.1 g, 1%; Sodium: 337 mg, 14%; Niacin: 13 mg, 64%; Vitamin B_6: 0.6 mg, 32%; Vitamin K: 6 mcg, 8%; Diabetic Exchange Values: 4 Very-Lean Meat

Percentage of calories from fat: 16%

Shiitake Mushroom and Ginger Chicken Burgers

Heart-Health Benefits: Protein and B vitamins

The Sesame Ginger Noodle Salad, page 98, or the Baby Spinach Salad with Asian Dressing, page 87, go well with these ginger-flavored burgers. A little soy sauce mixed with some wasabi makes a tasty, spicy sauce.

■ *Serves 4* ■

Canola oil cooking spray or canola oil

4 ounces shiitake mushrooms, stems discarded, washed, and thinly sliced

1 small garlic clove, crushed

Salt and freshly ground pepper

1 pound ground chicken, the leanest you can find

1 tablespoon reduced-sodium teriyaki sauce or lite soy sauce

¼ cup chopped fresh cilantro

2 tablespoons thinly sliced scallion greens

1 teaspoon fresh ginger, crushed with a garlic press (use the juices and the crushed ginger)

¼ teaspoon salt

About 3 tablespoons all-purpose flour

1. Heat a large nonstick skillet over medium-high heat. Spray with cooking spray or lightly grease with canola oil, then add the shiitake mushrooms and garlic, season with salt and pepper, and sauté for 5 minutes. Transfer the mushrooms to a large bowl and cool completely.

2. Add the remaining ingredients except the flour to the mushrooms and mix until well combined. Divide the mixture into 4 equal parts, then form each portion into a patty.

3. Spread the flour on a large plate. Lightly coat both sides of each patty with flour, pat off the excess, and set aside.

4. Preheat an indoor grill to high or heat a large nonstick skillet over medium-high heat. Spray the grill or skillet with cooking spray or lightly grease with canola oil. Add the burgers and cook on the grill for a total of 5 to 6 minutes or in the skillet for 2 to 3 minutes on each side. Check for doneness by cutting into a burger; the middle should be fully cooked and the juices should be clear. Serve immediately.

Approximate Nutritional Information: Serving size: one-quarter shiitake mushroom and ginger chicken burgers; Calories: 147 cals, 7%; Protein: 27 g, 54%; Total fat: 1.5 g, 2%; Saturated fat: 0.4 g, 2%; Cholesterol: 66 mg, 22%; Carbohydrates: 5 g, 2%; Fiber: 0.7 g, 3%; Sodium: 396 mg, 16%; Niacin: 13 mg, 66%; Vitamin B$_6$: 0.7 mg, 34%; Vitamin K: 0.5 mcg, 1%; Diabetic Exchange Values: 4 Very-Lean Meat, 1 Vegetable

Percentage of calories from fat: 9%

Tips for Choosing Healthy Margarines

▶ Choose soft margarines. The more solid the margarine, the more trans fats it contains because the oils are hydrogenated to make margarine solid. Soft margarines in a tub or squeeze bottle are preferable to hard stick margarines.

▶ Choose margarine with no trans fats or trace amounts of trans fats. If the label says "fat-free" or "trans-fat–free," that means it can contain up to less than half a gram per serving, which is minimal.

▶ Choose cholesterol-lowering margarines, such as Benecol and Take Control. These contain compounds derived from pine trees and soybeans, which have been proven to reduce the absorption of dietary cholesterol in the body. Eaten in the amounts specified, they can reduce total blood cholesterol by about 10 percent on average, and LDL (bad) cholesterol even more. These margarines contain trace amounts of hydrogenated oil and trans fats.[1]

▶ Choose margarines made from heart-healthy oils. Some margarines contain olive or canola oil, both of which lower LDL (bad) cholesterol and maintain HDL (good) cholesterol levels. There's even a margarine made partly from flaxseed oil, which supplies some heart-healthy alpha-linolenic acid, similar to the omega-3 fatty acids in fish oil.

▶ Choose "light" or "diet" margarines. Like butter, margarine has about 10 grams of fat and 100 calories per tablespoon. Unlike butter, all margarines are cholesterol free. "Light" or "diet" margarines contain more water and less than half the fat and calories of regular brands. But they are not suitable for baking because of their high water content.

Really Good Turkey Loaf

Heart-Health Benefits: Protein and B vitamins

𝒜 **delicious combination** of ingredients comes together in this moist turkey loaf. Serve with baked potatoes topped with fat-free sour cream or plain nonfat yogurt and a green salad. Use the leanest ground turkey you can find.

■ *Serves 6* ■

Glaze

¼ **cup hoisin sauce**

2 **teaspoons seasoned rice vinegar**

1½ **tablespoons canola oil**

8 **ounces shiitake mushrooms, stems discarded, washed, and thinly sliced**

1 **garlic clove, minced**

2 **pounds ground turkey, the leanest you can find**

3 **slices sandwich bread, crusts removed, soaked in water and then squeezed to remove most of the water**

½ **cup chopped fresh cilantro**

1 **tablespoon Dijon mustard**

2 **tablespoons lite soy sauce**

2 **large egg whites**

½ **cup plain nonfat yogurt**

Freshly ground pepper, to taste

1½ **teaspoons salt**

1. Preheat the oven to 350 degrees F. Line a large baking pan with foil.
2. To make the glaze, mix the ingredients in a measuring cup or a small bowl; set aside.
3. Heat the canola oil in a large nonstick skillet over medium-high heat. Add the shiitake mushrooms and garlic and sauté for 5 minutes. Transfer the mushrooms to a large bowl and cool completely.
4. Add all of the remaining ingredients to the mushrooms and mix with a fork or your hands until well blended. (See Cooking Tip on page 195 to check the seasoning.) Form the mixture into a large ball and transfer it to the prepared baking pan. Using your hands, form the ball into an oval-shaped loaf approximately 10 inches long and 2½ inches high. Using the back of a spoon, coat the turkey loaf evenly with the glaze.
5. Bake for 1 hour and 15 minutes, or until completely cooked: An instant-read thermometer should read 180 degrees F and the juices should be clear when the center of the loaf is pierced with a knife or skewer. Remove the loaf from the oven, cover it loosely with foil, and allow it to rest for 10 minutes before slicing.

▶ **Cooking Tip:** To check the seasoning of the turkey loaf mixture before baking, spray a small nonstick skillet with canola oil cooking spray and cook about 1 tablespoon of the mixture until well-done. Taste the cooked meat, and adjust the seasoning in the remaining turkey mixture if necessary.

▶ **Advance Preparation:** The glaze can be made up to 2 days in advance and refrigerated. The turkey loaf can be mixed, or mixed and shaped, up to 6 hours before baking; keep refrigerated.

Approximate Nutritional Information: Serving size: one-sixth really good turkey loaf; Calories: 313 cals, 16%; Protein: 38 g, 76%; Total fat: 8.6 g, 13%; Saturated fat: 1.8 g, 9%; Cholesterol: 99 mg, 33%; Carbohydrates: 19 g, 6%; Fiber: 2 g, 6%; Sodium: 1,236 mg, 51%; Riboflavin: 0.5 mg, 29%; Niacin: 8 mg, 41%; Vitamin B$_6$: 0.8 mg, 41%; Vitamin K: 9 mcg, 11%; Diabetic Exchange Values: 1 Starch, 5 Very Lean Meat, 2 Fat

Percentage of calories from fat: 25%

A Comparison of Fat and Cholesterol in Four-Ounce Servings of White Meats

FOOD	TOTAL FAT	SATURATED FAT	CHOLESTEROL
Boneless, Skinless Chicken Breast, Raw	1.4 grams (2% Daily Value)	0.3 grams (2%)	66 mg (22%)
Boneless, Skinless Fryer/ Roaster Turkey Breast, Raw	0.7 grams (1%)	0.2 grams (1%)	70 mg (23%)
Pork Loin or Tenderloin, Raw	3.8 grams (6%)	1.3 grams (7%)	74 mg (25%)
Veal, Lean, Raw	3.2 grams (5%)	0.9 grams (5%)	94 mg (31%)

Selecting, Storing, and Cooking Poultry

Selecting

▶ Select the leanest cuts. The leanest poultry is the white meat from the breast of the chicken or turkey, without the skin. Although skinless dark meat is also lean, it has nearly twice the calories from fat as white meat.

▶ Choose low-fat ground chicken or turkey. Because regular ground poultry includes dark meat and skin, it can have as much fat as ground beef.

▶ Avoid poultry that does not feel cold to the touch. Fresh poultry needs to be kept well chilled to avoid bacterial contamination.

▶ Choose poultry that looks moist and supple. Avoid any that has signs of drying, discoloration, blemishes, or bruising. Fresh poultry has a mild scent and is free of strong odors.

Storing

▶ Use fresh poultry within 2 days. Store it in the back of your refrigerator, which tends to be the coldest place.

▶ Freeze poultry in the store packaging, adding a second layer of airtight plastic wrap to it. Use frozen poultry sections within nine months, whole poultry within a year.

▶ Thaw frozen poultry in the refrigerator. Bacteria can grow rapidly on poultry that is thawed at room temperature. Thawing in the refrigerator can take up to two days (depending on the size and cut), so plan in advance. Defrosting poultry in the microwave is another option, but you must either cook the poultry immediately after defrosting it or put it back in the refrigerator if you are marinating the meat before cooking. Defrost on the "defrost" or 50 percent power setting to avoid cooking the edges and leaving the rest of the meat frozen.

Cooking

▶ To lower the fat content, cut off the visible fat and, in most cases, the skin before cooking poultry. If roasting a whole bird, remove the skin after cooking, before you carve the meat.

▶ Avoid contaminating other foods with raw poultry juices. Use different cutting boards and knives for preparing raw poultry, meat, or fish. Wash your hands and all of the utensils and surfaces that have come in contact with raw poultry or its juices.

▶ Cook all poultry thoroughly. A food thermometer should read 180 degrees F for ground poultry, 170 degrees F for breast and thigh portions, and 180 degrees F for whole birds. Any juices should run clear and there should be no signs of uncooked or pink flesh.[2]

Veal Chops with Fresh Marjoram Sauce and Brown Rice

Heart-Health Benefits: Protein, B vitamins, and magnesium

These moist and tender chops are graced with the delicate flavor of fresh marjoram in a refreshingly light sauce. Dried marjoram does not work here.

■ *Serves 4* ■

1½ pounds bone-in veal chops (½ inch thick), any visible fat removed

Salt and freshly ground pepper, to taste

⅓ cup all-purpose flour

1½ tablespoons canola oil

1 cup lightly packed fresh marjoram sprigs, plus ¼ cup chopped marjoram leaves

3 cups boiling water, or enough to cover the veal chops in the saucepan

1 to 2 teaspoons freshly squeezed lemon juice, to taste

4 cups cooked brown rice

1. Season both sides of the veal chops with salt and pepper. Spread the flour in a large rimmed plate or in a pie dish. Lightly coat only one side of each chop with the flour; set the chops aside, floured side up.
2. Choose a saucepan large enough to hold the chops—they can be tightly packed. Add the canola oil to the saucepan and heat over medium-high heat until hot. Add the veal chops floured side down, and brown on one side for 2 minutes. Turn the chops, add the marjoram sprigs, and brown the second side for 2 minutes.
3. Remove the saucepan from the heat and slowly add the boiling water. (Note: The water will splatter when it comes in contact with the hot saucepan, so be careful not to burn yourself.) Return the saucepan to the medium-high heat and bring to a boil. Reduce the heat slightly and cook at a strong simmer, covered, for 30 minutes; turn the chops twice.
4. Uncover the saucepan and continue to simmer for 10 minutes, or until the sauce has reduced to about 1 cup.
5. Transfer the veal chops to a serving dish, then strain the sauce into a small bowl, pressing out as much liquid as possible. Add the chopped marjoram and the lemon juice, and adjust the seasoning. Serve the sauce on top of the veal chops or on the side.

Approximate Nutritional Information: Serving size: one-quarter veal chops with fresh marjoram sauce and 1 cup brown rice; Calories: 450 cals, 23%; Protein: 39 g, 79%; Total fat: 11.2 g, 17%; Saturated fat: 2 g, 10%; Cholesterol: 134 mg, 45%; Carbohydrates: 45 g, 15%; Fiber: 4 g, 15%; Sodium: 437 mg, 18%; Thiamin: 0.3 mg, 22%; Riboflavin: 0.5 mg, 34%; Niacin: 18 mg, 91%; Vitamin B_6: 1 mg, 59%; Vitamin B_{12}: 2 mcg, 38%; Magnesium: 129 mg, 32%; Vitamin K: 9 mcg, 12%; Diabetic Exchange Values: 3 Starch, 4 Lean Meat

Percentage of calories from fat: 23%

Lupita's Mexican-Style Lemon Chicken

Heart-Health Benefits: Protein and B vitamins

Serve this spicy lemon chicken with brown rice and a green salad. Chicken thighs are used in this recipe because they stay moist during cooking.

■ *Serves 6* ■

2½ pounds skinless bone-in chicken thighs, any visible fat removed

2 small onions, peeled

4½ to 5 cups water

½ cup freshly squeezed lemon juice, or to taste

½ teaspoon salt

2 dried chile peppers, such as ancho, guajillo, or chilaca (stemmed and deveined), or 2 canned or jarred hot red chile peppers, or to taste

1 garlic clove, peeled

1 bay leaf

2 whole cloves

¼ cup lite soy sauce

1 tablespoon olive oil

Cooked brown rice

1. In a large saucepan, combine the chicken thighs, 1 of the (whole) onions, 3½ cups of the water, ¼ cup of the lemon juice, and the salt and bring to a boil. Reduce the heat and simmer for 10 minutes. If the chicken pieces are not covered by the water, turn them after 5 minutes of cooking.

2. While the chicken is cooking, if using dried chile peppers, place them in a small saucepan with 1½ cups water and bring to a boil. Cook for 5 minutes, then remove the saucepan from the heat and set aside.

3. In the bowl of a food processor or blender, combine the remaining onion (cut in half), the garlic clove, bay leaf, whole cloves, soy sauce, and the remaining ¼ cup lemon juice. Add the chile peppers and their cooking liquid (or the canned or jarred chile peppers and 1 cup water) and process until smooth; set aside.

4. After the chicken has cooked for 10 minutes, remove the saucepan from the heat. Transfer the chicken thighs to a large plate lined with paper towels (drying off the thighs will reduce some of the splattering during sautéing). Strain the poaching liquid into a heatproof bowl and set aside. Rinse the saucepan and wipe it dry.

5. Add the olive oil to the saucepan and heat over medium-high heat until hot. Add the chicken thighs and lightly brown them for 3 minutes, turning once. (Note: Do not worry if the chicken sticks to the pan. The sauce will remove any stuck bits.) Add the pureed onion mixture and the strained poaching liquid, stir, and bring to a boil. Reduce the heat and cook at a strong simmer for

30 to 40 minutes, or to the desired consistency. (Note: The sauce should be fairly thin because it will be served with rice.)

Approximate Nutritional Information: Serving size: one-sixth Mexican-style lemon chicken; Calories: 201 cals, 10%; Protein: 27 g, 54%; Total fat: 7.4 g, 11%; Saturated fat: 1.4 g, 7%; Cholesterol: 110 mg, 37%; Carbohydrates: 5 g, 2%; Fiber: 0.5 g, 2%; Sodium: 692 mg, 29%; Niacin: 8 mg, 42%; Vitamin B$_6$: 0.5 mg, 25%; Vitamin K: 7 mcg, 8%; Diabetic Exchange Values: 3 Lean Meat, 1 Vegetable

Percentage of calories from fat: 34%

Well-Done Temperature Guide for Meat and Poultry

MEAT	DEGREES F AT WELL-DONE STAGE[3]
Beef	170
Pork	170
Lamb	170
Veal	170
Chicken and Turkey	
Whole	180
Breasts	170
Thigh	170
Ground	180
Ostrich[4]	
Ground	160
Fillets	145
Duck and Goose	180
Ground Beef, Veal, Lamb, and Pork	160

Pork Tenderloin with White Bean, Artichoke, Olive, and Sun-Dried Tomato Salsa

---

Heart-Health Benefits: Protein, iron, vitamin C, B vitamins, and fiber

---

$\mathcal{P}$ork tenderloin is a lean and tasty cut of meat. This recipe calls for searing the tenderloin and then briefly roasting it. The white bean salsa can be served with other dishes, such as roasted or grilled chicken, or with a meaty fish, such as swordfish or tuna.

■ *Serves 4* ■

1 to 1¼ pounds pork tenderloin (about 1½ inches thick), any visible fat removed.

1 tablespoon herbes de Provence

Salt and freshly ground pepper, to taste

White Bean Salsa (makes about 2½ cups)

1½ cups canned great northern beans, rinsed and drained

½ cup sun-dried tomatoes in oil, drained and cut into a small dice

⅓ cup sliced pitted green olives

4 canned artichoke hearts (in brine), drained and cut into small dice

1 tablespoon freshly squeezed lemon juice, or to taste

1 to 2 tablespoons olive oil, to desired consistency

½ teaspoon cayenne pepper or Tabasco sauce, to taste

2 teaspoons herbes de Provence, 1 tablespoon very finely chopped fresh rosemary, or 2 tablespoons thinly sliced fresh basil leaves

Salt, to taste

2 tablespoons canola oil

1. Preheat the oven to 400°F. Line a baking sheet with sides with foil.
2. Pat the pork tenderloin with dry paper towels, then evenly coat it with the herbes de Provence and season with salt and pepper. Cover with plastic wrap and refrigerate until ready to use. (The tenderloin can be seasoned up to 24 hours in advance.)
3. To make the white bean salsa, combine all of the ingredients in a large bowl and gently mix. Adjust the seasoning. Set aside at room temperature until ready to serve.
4. To cook the pork tenderloin, heat the canola oil in a large nonstick skillet over medium-high heat until hot. Add the tenderloin and brown on all sides, about 5 to 6 minutes, turning frequently with tongs. Transfer the tenderloin to the prepared baking sheet, and roast for 15 minutes. Or, if you prefer a slightly pink center, reduce the roasting time to about 12 minutes.

5. Remove the tenderloin from the oven, cover it loosely with foil, and allow it to rest for 10 minutes before slicing it.
6. Using a sharp knife, cut the tenderloin into ½-inch slices. Serve immediately, with the salsa.

Approximate Nutritional Information: Serving size: one-quarter pork tenderloin (without salsa); Calories: 136 cals, 7%; Protein: 24 g, 48%; Total fat: 3.8 g, 6%; Saturated fat: 1.3 g, 7%; Cholesterol: 74 mg, 25%; Carbohydrates: 0 g, 0%; Fiber: 0 g, 0%; Sodium: 57 mg, 2%; Thiamin: 1 mg, 74%; Niacin: 5 mg, 25%; Vitamin B$_6$: 0.6 mg, 29%; Diabetic Exchange Values: 4 Very-Lean Meat

Percentage of calories from fat: 27%

Approximate Nutritional Information: Serving size: one-quarter white bean, artichoke, olive, and sun-dried tomato salsa (made with 1 tablespoon olive oil); Calories: 199 cals, 10%; Protein: 9 g, 19%; Total fat: 6.8 g, 11%; Saturated fat: 0.9 g, 5%; Cholesterol: 0 mg, 0%; Carbohydrates: 27 g, 9%; Fiber: 7 g, 26%; Sodium: 597 mg, 25%; Iron: 5 mg, 25%; Vitamin C: 20 mg, 33%; Vitamin K: 5 mcg, 6%; Diabetic Exchange Values: 1 Starch, 1 Fat, 3 Vegetable

Percentage of calories from fat: 30%

THE DOWNSIDE OF BOXED MEALS

BOXED MEALS SUCH as macaroni and cheese or potatoes may be convenient, but they are not always healthy. Many brands contain partially hydrogenated oil and offer little nutrition. The words "all natural" on the label are usually a good indication that the product is free of partially hydrogenated oil and artificial products. Try to make as many dishes as possible from scratch. Or start with a box, but use only half the spice package or flavoring; these are usually loaded with salt.

Grilled Boneless Pork Chops with Shiitake Mushroom, Green Bean, Corn, and Red Bell Pepper Salsa

Heart-Health Benefits: Protein, vitamins A and C, and B vitamins

This recipe calls for Old Bay Seasoning, but feel free to use your favorite dried herbs or spices instead. Choose the leanest chops you can find.

■ *Serves 4* ■

1 pound boneless pork chops (about ½ inch thick), any visible fat removed

Old Bay Seasoning, to taste

Shiitake Mushroom Salsa (makes about 3 cups)

4 ounces fresh haricot verts or thin green beans

1 tablespoon canola oil

8 ounces shiitake mushrooms, stems discarded, washed, cut in half if large, and very thinly sliced

1 garlic clove, minced

1 cup fresh corn (from 2 ears of corn) or frozen corn

¾ cup very finely chopped red bell peppers

2 tablespoons chopped fresh marjoram or 2 teaspoons dried marjoram

1 tablespoon balsamic vinegar, or to taste

Salt and freshly ground pepper, to taste

Canola oil cooking spray

1. Pat the pork chops dry with paper towels, then sprinkle them evenly with Old Bay Seasoning. For spicier chops, use more seasoning. Cover with plastic wrap and refrigerate until ready to use. (The chops can be seasoned up to 24 hours in advance.)
2. To make the shiitake mushroom salsa, cook the haricots verts in boiling water for 3 minutes. They should be crisp; do not overcook. Drain, rinse them with cold water, and drain again. Cut them into very small pieces; set aside.
3. Heat the canola oil in a large nonstick skillet over medium-high heat until hot. Add the shiitake mushrooms and sauté for 4 minutes, or until soft and slightly browned. Add the garlic, corn, red bell peppers, and haricots verts and sauté for 1 minute, or just until heated though; do not overcook. Transfer the salsa to a serving dish and stir in the marjoram and balsamic vinegar. Adjust the seasoning and set aside at room temperature until ready to serve.
4. To grill the pork chops, preheat an indoor grill. Spray with cooking spray and grill the pork chops for 1½ to 2 minutes, depending on the thickness of the chops; do not overcook. Or to cook them on an outdoor grill, preheat the grill. Spray the grill with cooking spray and cook the chops, turning once, for a total of 4 to 5 minutes. Serve immediately with the shiitake mushroom salsa.

▶ **Cooking Tip:** If you don't have a grill, you can panfry the pork chops. Heat 1 tablespoon canola oil in a large nonstick skillet over medium-high heat. Add the pork chops and cook on each side for 1½ to 2 minutes, or until cooked through.

Approximate Nutritional Information: Serving size: one-quarter boneless grilled pork chops (without salsa); Calories: 164 cals, 8%; Protein: 23 g, 47%; Total fat: 7.1 g, 11%; Saturated fat: 2.4 g, 12%; Cholesterol: 73 mg, 24%; Carbohydrates: 0 g, 0%; Fiber: 0 g, 0%; Sodium: 57 mg, 2%; Thiamin: 1 mg, 80%; Riboflavin: 0.3 mg, 19%; Niacin: 5 mg, 25%; Vitamin B_6: 0.7 mg, 35%; Diabetic Exchange Values: 3 Lean Meat

Percentage of calories from fat: 41%. **Note:** It is more important to focus on the total fat of this low-calorie recipe which is 7 grams, or 11% Daily Value per serving, than on the percentage of calories from fat.

Approximate Nutritional Information: Serving size: one-quarter shiitake mushroom, green bean, corn, and red bell pepper salsa; Calories: 126 cals, 6%; Protein: 3 g, 6%; Total fat: 4.1 g, 6%; Saturated fat: 0.4 g, 2%; Cholesterol: 0 mg, 0%; Carbohydrates: 23 g, 8%; Fiber: 4 g, 16%; Sodium: 157 mg, 7%; Vitamin A: 1,202 IU, 24%; Vitamin C: 61 mg, 101%; Vitamin K: 12 mcg, 15%; Diabetic Exchange Values: 1 Fat, 1 Vegetable, 1 Fruit

Percentage of calories from fat: 27%

Tips for Dining Out

DINING OUT CAN be stressful when you are trying to eat healthfully. You might feel pressure to order what everyone else is ordering, to eat as much as other guests, or to drink alcohol. You might feel embarrassed to order a salad as your main course, guilty about leaving a lot of food on your plate, or cheated when everyone else is eating dessert and you're not. Here are some tips to make dining out a healthy and fun experience.

- Before you leave the house, eat some cut-up raw vegetables, nuts or seeds, whole-grain crackers with low-fat cheese, or fresh fruit so you are not starving by the time you get to the restaurant.
- Order water or a beverage with no added sugar, such as unsweetened iced tea. Avoid high-sugar soft drinks.
- Stay clear of the bread basket, especially if you are trying to lose weight. If you do eat bread, choose a whole-grain variety. Try to avoid butter.
- Choose dishes with a heart-healthy ❤ symbol on the menu.
- Choose a small portion of food, ask for a half portion, or plan to share a dish. One main course, salad, or dessert can usually feed two, so don't be embarrassed to share.
- Don't hesitate to ask for meals to be prepared according to your needs—less salt, a healthier sauce, or no sauce.
- Start with a salad to fill you up before the main course. You may eat less this way.
- Always ask for sauces and salad dressings on the side. Choose vinegar-and-oil-based salad dressings over creamy ones, or make your own salad dressing with a splash of olive oil and vinegar.
- Don't add salt without tasting first—most restaurant prepared and processed foods are over-salted.
- Choose lean cuts of meat that have the least amount of saturated fat (see The Leanest Cuts of Beef, page 207, and A Comparison of Fat and Cholesterol in White Meats, page 195).
- Choose fish or shellfish that is broiled, baked, grilled, steamed, or sautéed, not fried.
- Avoid deep-fried foods.
- Trim any visible fat from your meat or poultry.
- Remember: You do not have to clean your plate (even though you paid for it). The amount of time and energy it will take you to burn off extra calories and fat is not worth the money.
- Choose fruit or fruit-based desserts.
- If you are diabetic, keep in mind your meal plan. If you are on a new meal plan, carry a copy of it with you so you can choose wisely from the menu.

SEVEN

RED MEATS

HEART-HEALTH TIPS AT A GLANCE

▶ Try to reduce your consumption of red meats. As you can see from the nutritional information for the recipes and the information throughout the book, red meats contain higher amounts of cholesterol, total fat, and saturated fat than any other source of protein. For this reason, this chapter has the fewest recipes.

▶ Choose the leanest cuts of red meat (see The Leanest Cuts of Beef, page 207), trim all visible fat before cooking; and drain off fat that appears during cooking. Do not overcook lean cuts of meat—due to their low fat content, they tend to become tough and dry faster than fattier cuts. This is especially true for ostrich meat, buffalo meat, and Piedmontese beef (see page 210). Some cheap lean cuts, such as round roasts for pot roast, thrive with "slow and low" cooking.

▶ Branch out and try ostrich meat, buffalo meat, and Piedmontese beef. These red meats have less cholesterol and saturated fat than conventional beef. Also, try to buy grass-fed beef whenever possible—it's leaner and healthier. (Text boxes in this chapter give information on ostrich, buffalo, Piedmontese beef, and grass-fed beef, and the Sources section has mail-order information for these meats.) Some of these meats are more expensive than conventional beef, but spending more on healthier cuts of red meat can be a wise investment.

▶ If you think there is no life without beef burgers, the following burger alternatives might change your mind: Buffalo Burgers with Onion-Ketchup Sauce, page 214, Two Chicken Burgers, page 191, and Old Bay Tofu Cakes with Cocktail Sauce, page 137.

▶ Substitute white meats or tofu in your favorite red meat recipes. For instance, instead of meat loaf made with ground beef, try Really Good Turkey Loaf, page 194; instead of beef fajitas, try Chicken Fajitas with Homemade Guacamole, page 188; and instead of a beef stir-fry, try Tofu Vegetable Stir-Fry, page 144.

- ▶ Invest in an indoor grill, such as a Foreman Grill, which presses out the fat during cooking (see The Foreman Grill: A Healthy Way to Cook, page 209).

- ▶ Eat a side salad or the vegetables on your plate before you eat the meat. If you fill up on these healthy greens and vegetables, you may be inclined to eat less meat.

- ▶ Enjoy a glass of red wine instead of white with your dinner. Red wine contains the antioxidant resveratrol, which is believed to help reduce the risk of coronary heart disease (see Red Wine and Resveratrol, page 217).

- ▶ Avoid the French fries, onion rings, hush puppies, Tater Tots, and other deep-fried starches often served with red meats. Breaded items in particular are loaded with calories and fats that are soaked up during frying. Instead, try a baked potato with plain nonfat yogurt or fat-free sour cream, oven-roasted potatoes sprayed with olive oil and dusted with herbs or spices, boiled potatoes with olive oil and chopped fresh parsley, brown rice, quinoa, or any other heart-healthy whole grain.

- ▶ Reduce or eliminate fast food from your diet and your family's. If you need convincing of just how bad fast food is for you and your children, see Calories, Fat, and Cholesterol in Fast Food, page 220, and Frightening Facts about Fast Food for Kids, page 221. Almost all fast food is cooked in partially hydrogenated oil. Buns, tortillas, breading, cookies, and other foods contain partially hydrogenated oil. Also, high-fructose corn syrup and corn syrup solids are used liberally in fast food.

The Leanest Cuts of Beef

ALWAYS CHOOSE THE leanest and healthiest cuts of beef you can find. Generally the words "round" or "loin" indicate leanness, and "select" cuts are lower in fat than "choice" or "prime" cuts. Trim as much fat as possible from the meat before you cook it. Keep in mind that many of your favorite recipes that call for red meat taste just as good when replaced by a white meat, a meaty fish (such as tuna or swordfish), or even tofu. Avoid organ meats, such as liver, kidneys, heart, and tongue, which are extremely high in cholesterol.

Eye of Round (sandwich steak), lean, $^1/_4$ inch thick
Uses: Sandwiches and salads
Cooking Tips: A dry rub or dry seasoning is better than a marinade. Cook over high heat for about 1 minute. Panfrying with canola oil cooking spray works best. This meat cooks very quickly; overcooking or cooking over low heat tend to render tough meat.

Eye Round (braising steak), lean, $^3/_4$ inch thick
Uses: Steaks and kebabs
Cooking Tips: Cook over high heat for 5 minutes or so, depending on thickness. Panfrying with canola oil cooking spray works best. This meat cooks very quickly; overcooking or cooking over low heat tends to render tough meat.

Eye Round (oven roast), lean, average weight about 2.5 pounds
Best Roasts: Top round roast (also known as top round first cut or top round steak roast), bottom round rump roast (also known as round roast, bottom round pot roast, bottom oven roast), and eye round roast (also known as eye round pot roast)
Uses: Braised meat or pot roast
Cooking Tips: Roast or braise (covered) at low to moderate heat (about 300 to 350 degrees F) for about 30 to 40 minutes per pound.

New York Boneless Sirloin Steak, lean
Uses: Steaks and stir-fries
Cooking Tips: Marinate or use a dry rub. Cook over high heat for 5 to 7 minutes, depending on thickness.

Beef Tenderloin, $1^1/_2$ to 3-inch thick fillet steaks or loin
Uses: Steaks, beef Stroganoff, stir-fries, or any dishes that require very tender meat
Cooking Tips: Marinate or use a dry rub. Cook over high heat, preferably on the grill or under the broiler, or panfry using canola oil cooking spray. Cooking times will depend on the thickness.

Pot Roast with Shiitake Mushrooms and Rosemary

Heart-Health Benefits: Protein, iron, and B vitamins

$\mathcal{E}$**veryday fare never** tasted so good. Serve with noodles, roasted or boiled potatoes, or brown rice.

■ *Serves 8* ■

One 3¹⁄₄ pound pot roast (beef eye of round, choice cut), rinsed and patted dry

Salt and freshly ground pepper, to taste

2 tablespoons Dijon mustard

2 tablespoons canola oil

8 ounces shiitake mushrooms, stems discarded, washed, and quartered

1 onion, peeled and cut in half

3 garlic cloves, peeled

3 cups boiling fat-free reduced-sodium stock

3 fresh parsley sprigs

1 fresh rosemary sprig

1. Season the pot roast with salt and pepper. Using your hands or the back of a spoon, smear the entire roast with a thin coating of Dijon mustard; set aside.
2. Preheat the oven to 375 degrees F. Have ready a Dutch oven that is suitable for browning the meat, or a braising pan.
3. Heat the canola oil in a Dutch oven or a large nonstick skillet (if using a braising pan) over medium-high heat until hot. Add the pot roast and brown it on all sides, for a total of about 4 minutes, turning frequently (don't worry about the mustard or the meat sticking to the pot). Transfer the roast to the braising pan, if using, or to a large plate. In the Dutch oven or skillet, brown the shiitake mushrooms, onion, and garlic for 2 minutes. Add the stock to the pot (be careful of splattering) and scrape the bottom of the pot, then add the parsley and rosemary. Return the meat to the Dutch oven or transfer the vegetables and liquid to the braising pan. Cover and cook in the oven for 2 hours, or until the meat is fork-tender. Transfer the roast to a serving dish and cover with foil to keep warm.
4. Remove the wilted parsley sprigs and rosemary stem from the sauce, and skim off any fat from the surface. The sauce can be served as is, or, if you prefer a smoother sauce, transfer the sauce and vegetables to a blender or food processor (or use a hand-held blender) and process until smooth. Add more water to thin the sauce if necessary. For an even smoother consistency, strain the pureed sauce through a fine-mesh sieve. Slice the roast and serve immediately.

▶ **Cooking Tip:** If you do not have a Dutch oven or braising pan, you can use a Pyrex baking dish and cover the pot roast with foil during cooking.

Approximate Nutritional Information: Serving size: one-eighth pot roast with shiitake mushrooms and rosemary; Calories: 367 cals, 18%; Protein: 55 g, 110%; Total fat: 12.4 g, 19%; Saturated fat: 3.4 g, 17%; Cholesterol: 99 mg, 33%; Carbohydrates: 6 g, 2%; Fiber: 0.7 g, 3%; Sodium: 368 mg, 15%; Iron: 5 mg, 27%; Riboflavin: 0.3 mg, 20%; Niacin: 10 mg, 52%; Vitamin B_6: 0.7 mg, 39%; Vitamin B_{12}: 3 mcg, 54%; Vitamin K: 22 mcg, 28%; Diabetic Exchange Values: 1 Vegetable, 8 Very Lean Meat, 2 Fat

Percentage of calories from fat: 31%

THE FOREMAN GRILL: A HEALTHY WAY TO COOK

NAMED FOR THE heavyweight boxing champion, the George Foreman Lean Mean Fat-Reducing Grilling Machine is an indoor electric grill that can be used to cook hamburgers and steaks, fish and chicken, vegetables, and everything in between. The nonstick plates reduce the need for oil or grease, the pressure of the grill plates squeezes out fats, and the high heat source from both top and bottom cooks food in minutes. This grill is excellent for people in apartments or for those who do not want a large, expensive outdoor grill.

If you are not looking for a grill to reduce fat by "pressure cooking" and high heat, other grill brands might be a better match for your cooking style and taste. For instance, the Hamilton Beach grill has more clearance between the grill plates, and it also has a choice of heat levels. Most indoor grills come in a couple of sizes: small for one or two people, large for a family.

Cardiac-Friendly Beef: Piedmontese!

EVERY ONCE IN a while, a new product enters the market that commands notice. Piedmontese beef is one of them. Piedmontese beef has about half the calories and cholesterol and one-tenth the fat of conventional beef. What's more, despite its unbelievably low fat content, the meat is juicy, tender, and extremely flavorful. Keep in mind that it cooks faster than conventional beef, so reduce the cooking time by about one-third. Piedmontese beef is not yet widely available in grocery stores, but it can be purchased from mail-order companies; see Sources, page 269. Also see Sources, same page, for more information on Piedmontese beef.

How do the nutritional values for Piedmontese beef compare to those for conventional beef? Piedmontese beef is lower in fat, cholesterol, and calories.[1]

	PIEDMONTESE BEEF (3.5 OUNCES)	CONVENTIONAL BEEF (3.5 OUNCES)[2]
calories	104	287
protein	22 g	18 g
total fat	1.9 g	24 g
saturated fat	0.6 g	10 g
cholesterol	32 mg	70 mg

What physical traits distinguish the Piedmontese breed from conventional cattle? Piedmontese cattle can be distinguished by their double muscling. A double muscle is characterized by a hump of fleshy tissue over the withers (the neck area) that can sometimes weigh as much as forty to fifty pounds. The cattle also have a large dewlap (or lower chest area close to the front legs), big drooping ears, and a voice that sounds more like a grunt than a low. And they have outstanding resistance to certain diseases and parasites.

Another unique feature of Piedmontese cattle is the myostatin gene, which is responsible for double muscling and tender meat. Naturally occurring in all mammals, this gene restricts muscle growth. It became naturally mutated or inactivated in the Piedmontese breed, causing increased muscle growth instead of restricting it. The myostatin gene is also responsible for the natural tenderness of Piedmontese beef because it reduces the amount of connective tissue in the muscle. The less connective tissue, the softer the meat.

Where is Piedmontese beef from, and how did it get to the United States? The origin of Piedmontese cattle can be traced to the mountainous Piedmont region of northwest Italy. An indigenous ancient European breed of cattle known as Aurochs [*Bos primigenius*] populated this area. About 25,000 years ago, Zebu [*Bos indicus*], another breed of cattle common to India and Africa, began a massive migration from Pakistan that ended in northern Italy. There, the Zebus met the Aurochs. After thousands of years of mating, the Aurochs and the Zebus evolved into one breed, the Piedmontese.

The first Piedmontese animals exported to North America arrived in Saskatchewan, Canada, in 1979. These animals included one bull, Brindisi, and four females, Banana, Biba, Bisca, and Binda.

The following year, five more bulls, Captain, Champ, Corallo, Camino, and Domingo, arrived in Canada. In the early 1980s, five Piedmontese cattle were imported from Italy to the United Sates. The three bulls were Istinto, Imbuto, and Iose, and the two cows were India and Gazza. These fifteen cattle formed the genetic base for the Piedmontese breed in North America.[3]

Grass-Fed versus Grain-Fed Beef

FOLLOWING IS A list of reasons to think about switching to grass-fed beef, especially if you tend to consume large amounts of beef. It is true that grass-fed beef is considerably more expensive than grain-fed beef, but the nutritional benefits may be worth the extra dollars. Grass-fed beef is becoming increasingly available in grocery stores; if you can't find it, see Sources, page 269–70. And for further information on grass-fed beef, see Sources, page 270.

Think less saturated fat. Grass-fed beef has less saturated fat than grain-fed beef. A 4-ounce serving of grass-fed beef has about 7 to 10 grams of total fat, compared with 14 to 16 grams in the same cut of grain-fed beef. Bear in mind that both grass-fed and grain-fed beef have about the same amount of cholesterol. [4]

Think more nutritional benefits. Grass-fed beef contains heart-healthy omega-3 fatty acids (similar to those in fish) and conjugated linoleic acid (CLA); (see CLA: A Natural Trans Fatty Acid, page 63), both of which are either lacking or found only in trace amounts in grain-fed beef.[5]

Think fewer risks from food-borne illness. The incidence of *E. coli (Escherichia coli)* levels is much lower in grass-fed cattle. Meat from corn-fed cattle is more likely to be contaminated with the dangerous *E. coli* bacteria for two reasons: First, the corn interferes with a cow's normal ruminant digestion, and second, the animals are crowded together in filthy feedlot conditions.[6]

Think grass is good. Cows are herbivores. Their physiological structure is designed for a grass-based diet. Cattle are ruminants, meaning that they possess a rumen, or fermentation sac, in which resident bacteria convert cellulose from grass, plants, and shrubs into proteins and fats. Their digestive systems are designed for grass, not for starchy, low-fiber grain and other "by-product feedstuff," such as municipal garbage, stale cookies, poultry manure, chicken feathers, bubble gum, and restaurant waste.[7] Feeding cattle corn fattens them up unnaturally fast. It takes four to five years to get a grass-fed cow to a slaughterable weight, versus fourteen to sixteen months for a cow fattened in a feedlot. And, because a cow's constitution is not designed to digest corn, feedlot cows are more susceptible to a host of illnesses and infections [8]

Think fewer hormones and antibiotics. Grass-fed cattle are given fewer hormones and antibiotics. Hormones are usually administered to artificially speed up the weight gain of cattle. Overuse of antibiotics, which are sometimes administered as a prophylactic, can cause drug-resistant strains of bacteria.[9]

Filets Mignons with Sautéed Mushrooms and Balsamic Vinegar

Heart-Health Benefits: Protein, iron, and B vitamins

---

*F*ilets mignon is the ultimate red meat splurge when the occasion calls for it! Good balsamic vinegars vary in quality and price, much like fine wines. The best balsamic vinegar is aged vinegar from Modena, Italy, such as Traditional Balsamic Vinegar Gold Seal, which carries a hefty price tag of about $180 (you will understand why after you taste it). If you buy this liquid-gold vinegar, *never* cook it; just use a drop or two of it to flavor anything from poultry or fish to fresh strawberries or vine-ripened tomatoes. Since most people do not have Gold Seal vinegar hanging around their kitchens, this recipe calls for cheaper balsamic vinegar (any brand will work), which is reduced quickly to thicken it. Because this sauce is so tasty, a little bit goes a long way. Serve the filets mignons and sautéed mushrooms with boiled potatoes or brown rice and a green vegetable or salad.

■ *Serves 2* ■

2 tablespoons canola oil

2 tablespoon minced shallots

8 ounces assorted mushrooms, such as shiitake, baby bella, oyster, or chanterelles, stems trimmed (discarded if using shiitakes), washed, and thinly sliced

1 garlic clove, minced

Salt and freshly ground pepper, to taste

Balsamic Vinegar Sauce

1 tablespoon minced shallots

1 tablespoon brown sugar

$^1/_2$ cup balsamic vinegar

Two 4- to 5-ounce center-cut filets mignons (beef tenderloin steaks), about 1$^1/_4$ inches thick, dried thoroughly with paper towels

1. To sauté the mushrooms, heat 1 tablespoon of the canola oil in a large non-stick skillet over medium-high heat. Add the shallots and sauté for 30 seconds. Add the mushrooms and garlic, season with salt and pepper, and sauté, stirring occasionally, for 5 minutes, or until the mushrooms are wilted and lightly browned. Transfer the mushrooms to a bowl, cover with foil, and set aside. (Do not rinse the skillet.)

2. To make the balsamic vinegar sauce, reheat the skillet over medium-high heat. Add the shallots and sauté for 30 seconds. Sprinkle the brown sugar in the skillet, and as soon as it melts, add the balsamic vinegar (be careful, as the sauce may spatter). Simmer for a couple of minutes, until the sauce is slightly thickened and reduced to about ¼ cup; set aside.

3. To cook the meat, preheat the oven to 450 degrees F. Line a small baking pan with foil.
4. Heat the remaining 1 tablespoon canola oil in a large nonstick skillet over medium-high heat. Season the filets mignons with salt and pepper, then place them in the hot skillet. Cook the steaks, turning only once, for 2 minutes on each side, or until they are nicely browned and a crust has formed. Using tongs or a spatula, transfer the steaks to the prepared baking pan.
5. Place in the oven and roast to the desired degree of doneness: 4 minutes for very rare, 5 to 7 minutes for medium-rare, 9 minutes for medium, 12 minutes for well-done. Meanwhile, reheat the sauce over low heat. (Note: See Cooking Tip for using an indoor grill to cook the steaks.)
6. Place a steak on each plate. Drizzle the sauce over the steaks, top with the sautéed mushrooms, and serve immediately.

▶ **Cooking Tip:** To cook the steaks on an indoor grill, preheat the grill on high. Spray the grill with canola oil cooking spray, add the steaks, and cook for 3 minutes. Check doneness frequently to prevent overcooking. Filets mignons cooked on an indoor grill with grill plates that press the steaks tend to be a little less juicy than panfried and roasted steaks or steaks cooked on an outdoor grill.

Approximate Nutritional Information: Serving size: one-half filets mignons with sautéed wild mushrooms and balsamic vinegar; Calories: 403 cals, 20%; Protein: 34 g, 67%; Total fat: 17.7 g, 27%; Saturated fat: 4.5 g, 23%; Cholesterol: 95 mg, 32%; Carbohydrates: 26 g, 9%; Fiber: 2 g, 6%; Sodium: 78 mg, 3%; Iron: 5 mg, 26%; Riboflavin: 0.4 mg, 28%; Niacin: 6 mg, 28%; Vitamin B_6: 0.6 mg, 34%; Vitamin B_{12}: 3 mcg, 49%; Vitamin K: 10 mcg, 13%; Diabetic Exchange Values:1 Starch, 2 Vegetable, 4 Medium-Fat Meat

Percentage of calories from fat: 40%. **Note:** The fat content of this recipe is high, so filets mignons should be an occasional splurge.

Buffalo Burgers
with Onion-Ketchup Sauce

Heart-Health Benefits: Protein, vitamin C, and B vitamins

Bun or no bun, these buffalo (also known as bison) burgers rock—tell that to your kids! This onion-ketchup sauce is tasty enough for grown-ups and ketchupy enough for kids (but don't use the whole peppercorns or bay leaves if serving to kids). Serve with roasted or boiled potatoes on the side and a green vegetable or salad.

■ *Serves 4* ■

1 pound ground buffalo

2 tablespoons ketchup

1 tablespoon reduced-sodium Worcestershire
  sauce

1 teaspoon Dijon mustard

1/4 teaspoon salt

Canola oil cooking spray or canola oil

Onion-Ketchup Sauce

  1 1/2 tablespoons canola oil

  2 medium onions, halved and thinly sliced
    (about 3 cups sliced onions)

  5 bay leaves

  1/2 teaspoon whole black peppercorns

  1/2 cup ketchup

  2/3 cup water

1. To make the buffalo burgers, combine all of the ingredients in a bowl and mix until well incorporated. Divide the meat into 4 equal portions, and form each portion into a patty.
2. Spray a large nonstick skillet cooking spray or add a tiny amount of canola oil to the skillet and heat over medium-high heat until hot. Add the buffalo burgers and cook on each side for 4 minutes. Cover the skillet with foil and set aside. Alternatively preheat an indoor grill, spray with cooking spray, and grill the burgers for a total of about 3 minutes, or until cooked through. Then transfer to a plate and cover with foil.
3. To make the onion-ketchup sauce, heat the canola oil in a large nonstick skillet over medium-high heat until hot. Add the onions, bay leaves, and peppercorns and sauté for 10 minutes, or until the onions are golden brown.
4. Stir in the ketchup and water, add the cooked burgers, and simmer for 5 minutes, or until the burgers are heated through. Add more water to thin the sauce if necessary. Remove the bay leaves and serve immediately.

Approximate Nutritional Information: Serving size: one-quarter buffalo burgers (without onion-ketchup sauce); Calories: 124 cals, 6%; Protein: 23 g, 47%; Total fat: 1.5 g, 2%; Saturated fat: 0.5 g, 3%; Cholesterol: 52 mg, 17%; Carbohydrates: 3 g, 1%; Fiber: 0 g, 0%; Sodium: 189 mg, 8%; Niacin: 7 mg, 34%; Vitamin B$_6$: 0.6 mg, 31%; Vitamin B$_{12}$: 2 mcg, 31%; Diabetic Exchange Values: 3 Very-Lean Meat, 1 Vegetable

Percentage of calories from fat: 12%

Approximate Nutritional Information: Serving size: one-quarter onion-ketchup sauce; Calories: 103 cals, 5%; Protein: 2 g, 4%; Total fat: 3.7 g, 6%; Saturated fat: 0.3 g, 2%; Cholesterol: 0 mg, 0%; Carbohydrates: 17g, 6%; Fiber: 2 g, 10%; Sodium: 337 mg, 14%; Vitamin C: 12 mg, 20%; Vitamin K: 7 mcg, 9%; Diabetic Exchange Values: 1 Starch, 1 Fat

Percentage of calories from fat: 31%

Buffalo:
An Alternative to Beef

THE WORD IS spreading—ground buffalo meat is an excellent alternative to ground beef. It has fewer calories and less fat and cholesterol than conventional beef, and many people claim that it is tastier, too! Some stores sell preformed buffalo patties, which are convenient and easy to grill. Others sell ground buffalo, which you can use as a substitute for ground beef in burgers, spaghetti sauce, taco filling, meatballs, or meat loaf. If you cannot find buffalo in the meat or frozen section of your grocery store, see Sources, page 269, for mail-order companies.

	BUFFALO BURGER (4 OUNCES)	EXTRA LEAN (93%) GROUND BEEF BURGER (4 OUNCES)
calories	190	265
protein	20 g	21 g
total fat	11 g	19 g
saturated fat	4 g	8 g
cholesterol	50 mg	78 mg

Lamb Chops
with Cilantro-Mint Salsa

Heart-Health Benefits: Protein and B vitamins

Brown rice, quinoa, couscous, or tabbouleh would be perfect accompaniments to these lamb chops. The cilantro-mint salsa is also great with fish or shellfish, white meats, and other red meats.

■ *Serves 4* ■

Cilantro-Mint Salsa (makes ²/₃ cup)

1¹/₂ cups packed fresh cilantro leaves

1 cup packed fresh mint leaves

1 tablespoon capers

1 garlic clove

1 tablespoon freshly squeezed lemon juice, or
   to taste

5 tablespoons olive oil

Pinch of sugar

1¹/₂ pounds lamb chops (about 1 inch thick), any
   visible fat removed

Salt and freshly ground pepper, to taste

Canola oil cooking spray or canola oil

Squeeze of fresh lemon juice

1. To make the cilantro-mint salsa, combine all of the ingredients in the bowl of a food processor or blender and process until smooth. Transfer to a small serving bowl and cover with plastic wrap pressed flush against the surface of the sauce. Set aside at room temperature if using within 2 hours; otherwise, refrigerate.

2. To cook the lamb chops, season on both sides with salt and pepper. Spray a large nonstick skillet with canola oil cooking spray or add a tiny amount of canola oil to the skillet and heat over medium-high heat until hot. Add the lamb chops and cook on each side for 2 to 3 minutes. The inside of the chops should be light pink. Preheat an indoor grill, alternatively, spray with cooking spray, and grill the chops for a total of about 1½ minutes, or until cooked through. Or, if using an outdoor grill, preheat the grill to high and cook the chops for about 2 minutes on each side. Arrange the lamb chops on a serving platter and top with a squeeze of fresh lemon juice. Serve immediately with the cilantro-mint salsa on the side.

Approximate Nutritional Information: Serving size: one-quarter lamb chops (without salsa); Calories: 237 cals, 12%; Protein: 21 g, 42%; Total fat: 16.3 g, 25%; Saturated fat: 7.8 g, 39%; Cholesterol: 75 mg, 25%; Carbohydrates: 0.3 g, 0%; Fiber: 0 g, 0%; Sodium: 358 mg, 15%; Niacin: 6 mg, 28%; Vitamin B₆: .4 mg, 21%; Vitamin B₁₂: 3 mcg, 51%; Diabetic Exchange Values: 3 Medium-Fat Meat, 1 Vegetable

Percentage of calories from fat: 64%. **Note:** The fat content of this recipe is high, so lamb chops should be an occasional splurge.

Approximate Nutritional Information: Serving size: one-quarter cilantro-mint salsa; Calories: 65 cals, 3%; Protein: 0.3 g, 1%; Total fat: 6.8 g, 11%; Saturated fat: 0.9 g, 5%; Cholesterol: 0 mg, 0%; Carbohydrates: 0 g, 0%; Fiber: 0.5 g, 2%; Sodium: 33 mg, 1%; Vitamin K: 4 mcg, 5%; Diabetic Exchange Values: 1 Fat

Percentage of calories from fat: 91%. **Note:** It is more important to focus on the total fat value of this cilantro-mint salsa which is 7 grams, or 11% Daily Value, per serving than on the percentage of calorie's from fat.

RED WINE AND RESVERATROL

MANY STUDIES SUGGEST that consuming alcohol *in moderation* may reduce the risk of coronary heart disease. However, if you don't drink, you should not start just for the heart benefits. The effect appears to come from an increase in HDL cholesterol, but additional protective effects may come from the alcohol inhibiting the formation of blood clots. The benefits may also come from the nonalcoholic components of alcoholic beverages, such as the skins of red grapes in red wine, which contain an antioxidant called resveratrol. This antioxidant is also found in raspberries, peanuts, and mulberries.

Resveratrol and its role in preventing cardiovascular disease and cancer are still being studied. The amount of resveratrol in red wine is variable, but it is probably safe to say that drinking an occasional glass of red wine is not harmful to your health and may provide some small benefit. *However, do not take resveratrol pills or supplements, which have no proven health benefits and may be harmful if consumed incorrectly.*[1]

Curried Ostrich Fillets with Apple-Onion Jam and Cucumber Salsa

Heart-Health Benefit: Protein

This recipe is a good introduction to ostrich if you haven't already tried it. The apple-onion jam is great with other red and white meats, and the cucumber salsa is a welcome side dish to any meal.

■ *Serves 2* ■

Curry Dry Rub

 ¹/₂ teaspoon curry powder

 ¹/₂ teaspoon ground cumin

 ¹/₄ teaspoon ground ginger

Two 4- to 5-ounce ostrich fillets

Apple-Onion Jam (makes about ²/₃ cup)

 1 tablespoon canola oil

 1 onion, halved and very thinly sliced

 1 apple, peeled and grated

 2 tablespoons cider vinegar

 ¹/₄ teaspoon ground ginger

 ¹/₄ teaspoon chili powder

 2 tablespoon honey

 Salt, to taste

Cucumber Salsa

 ¹/₂ cup plain nonfat yogurt

 ¹/₂ cup shredded cucumber (with skin)

 1 tablespoon thinly sliced fresh mint leaves or 1 teaspoon dried mint, or to taste

 ¹/₄ teaspoon ground cumin, or to taste

 ¹/₄ teaspoon crushed garlic, or to taste (optional)

 Salt and freshly ground pepper, to taste

 Canola oil cooking spray or canola oil

1. To make the curry dry rub, combine all of the ingredients in a very small bowl and mix well. Coat each ostrich fillet with some of the dry rub. Cover and refrigerate for at least 10 minutes, or up to 24 hours.
2. To make the apple-onion jam, heat the canola oil in a medium nonstick skillet over medium-high heat until hot. Add the onion and sauté for about 10 minutes, or until golden brown. Add the remaining ingredients and simmer for 10 to 15 minutes, or until the jam has thickened to the desired consistency. Keep in mind that the jam will thicken as it cools. Set aside.
3. To make the cucumber salsa, combine all of the ingredients in a small bowl and mix until well blended. Refrigerate until ready to serve. (Note: This sauce is best if served within 3 hours of making it.)
4. To cook the ostrich, spray a large nonstick skillet with cooking spray or add a tiny amount of canola oil to the skillet and heat over medium-high heat until hot. Add the ostrich fillets and cook for 2 to 3 minutes on each side, or to desired doneness. (Note: Do not overcook the ostrich, as it tends to dry out quickly.)

Approximate Nutritional Information: Serving size: one-half curried ostrich patties (without apple-onion jam and cucumber salsa); Calories: 144 cals, 7%; Protein: 27 g, 55%; Total fat: 3.0 g, 5%; Saturated fat: 1.1 g, 6%; Cholesterol: 92 mg, 31%; Carbohydrates: 0 g, 0%; Fiber: 0 g, 0%; Sodium: 71 mg, 3%; Diabetic Exchange Values: 4 Very Lean Meat

Percentage of calories from fat: 20%

Approximate Nutritional Information: Serving size: 3 tablespoons apple-onion jam; Calories: 94 cals, 5%; Protein: 0.4 g, 1%; Total fat: 3.5 g, 5%; Saturated fat: 0.2 g, 1%; Cholesterol: 0 mg, 0%; Carbohydrates: 16 g, 5%; Fiber: 1 g, 6%; Sodium: 4 mg, 0%; Vitamin K: 5 mcg, 7%; Diabetic Exchange Values: 1 Fruit, 1 Fat

Percentage of calories from fat: 32%

Approximate Nutritional Information: Serving size: 1/2 cup cucumber salsa; Calories: 49 cals, 2%; Protein: 4 g, 7%; Total fat: 1 g, 2%; Saturated fat: 0.6 g, 3%; Cholesterol: 4 mg, 1%; Carbohydrates: 6 g, 2%; Fiber: 0.4 g, 2%; Sodium: 45 mg, 2%; Vitamin K: 8 mcg, 10%; Diabetic Exchange Values: 1/2 Fat-Free Milk

Percentage of calories from fat: 19%

Have You Tried Ostrich Lately?

OSTRICH IS GAINING in popularity in the United States for all the right reasons. The color, flavor, texture, and protein content of ostrich meat are similar to beef, but it has only about one-third of the total fat.

	BROILED OSTRICH TENDERLOIN (3 OUNCES)	BROILED BEEF TENDERLOIN (3 OUNCES)
calories	108	179
protein	20 g	24 g
total fat	3.1 g	8.5 g
saturated fat	1.2 g	3.1 g
cholesterol	80 mg	71 mg

Tips for Cooking Ostrich

Ostrich cuts are rated tender or medium-tender. Cuts rated tender, such as ostrich tenderloin or fan fillet, should be marinated and grilled, broiled, panfried, skewered for kebobs, or thinly sliced for a stir-fry or fajitas. To retain the most moisture, tender meats should first be seared over high heat, and the cooking finished over medium heat. Medium-tender cuts are best braised at a low temperature. Meat from the ostrich leg is usually ground or processed. Whatever the cut, ostrich meat is so lean that if it is even slightly overcooked, it will be dry.[2]

Ground ostrich and ostrich fillets are available in some whole foods stores, gourmet stores, and supermarkets in the fresh meat or frozen foods section. If you can't find ostrich meat, see Sources, page 269, for mail-order companies. And see Sources, same page, for more information about ostrich meat.

THE BEST HOT DOGS

AMERICANS AND HOT dogs are married to each other, for better or for würst! We start feeding our kids hot dogs at a tender age, and, soon enough, hot dogs become an addiction. When buying hot dogs, look for brands labeled "low fat" or "fat free." Chicken or turkey dogs are a good alternative to beef, as they contain less saturated fat. Tofu hot dogs, such as Tofu Pups, are yet another healthier option. As with hamburgers, try to serve hot dogs with whole wheat buns—if you can get away with it! Remember that hot dogs are high in fat and sodium, so go easy.

Calories, Fat, and Cholesterol in Fast Food

FAST FOOD NATION: The Dark Side of the All-American Meal by Eric Schlosser (Perennial, 2002), and *Super Size Me: A Film of Epic Portions*, a documentary by Morgan Spurlock, are essential reading and viewing if you have any misconceptions about exactly how dangerous fast food is to your health. In *Super Size Me*, Spurlock eats a month's worth of meals at McDonald's, agreeing to "super size" his meals whenever he is asked by a salesclerk. Spurlock's experiment proved to be a serious health hazard, especially for his liver. His basic message is, don't overconsume McDonald's food or any other fast food, because the health consequences are dire, even potentially fatal in the long run. *The following nutritional contents of fast foods show that a single meal can consume your entire daily allowance of calories, fats, and cholesterol, with very few nutritional benefits.*

	CALORIES	TOTAL FAT	SATURATED FAT	CHOLESTEROL
McDonald's Big Mac Hamburger	600 (30% Daily Value)	33 g (51%)	11 g (55%)	85 mg (28%)
McDonald's Large French Fries	540 (27%)	26 g (40%)	5 g (23%)	0 mg (0%)
Burger King Double Whopper Sandwich	980 (49%)	62 g (95%)	22 g (110%)	160 mg (53%)
Burger King Medium Onion Rings 320 calories (16%)	320 (16%)	16 g (25%)	4 g (20%)	0 (0%)

Frightening Facts about Fast Food for Kids

WITH THE RISE in the rates of obesity, diabetes, and blood pressure in children, it is vital for parents to eliminate, or at least *strictly limit*, the amount of fast food their children consume. An average fast-food meal, including a regular-size hamburger, small French fries, and ice cream dessert, is about 1,130 calories, (which is about 70 percent of a child's daily calorie needs), 44 grams of total fat (20 grams of saturated fat), and 110 milligrams of cholesterol. *The predisposition for heart disease starts in childhood, so a healthy diet early in life is the best prevention.*

	CALORIES	TOTAL FAT	SATURATED FAT	CHOLESTEROL
Burger King Whopper Jr. with Cheese Sandwich	440 (22% Daily Value)	26 g (40%)	9 g (45%)	55 mg (18%)
McDonald's Chicken McNuggets (4 pieces)	170 (9%)	10 g (15%)	2 g (10%)	25 mg (8%)
McDonald's Small French Fries	210 (11%)	10 g (15%)	1.5 g (8%)	0 (0%)
McDonald's M&M McFlurry	630 (32%)	23 g (35%)	15 g (75%)	75 mg (25%)
Wendy's Cheeseburger Kid's Meal	310 (16%)	12 g (18%)	5 g (25%)	45 mg (15%)
Wendy's Small Frosty Dairy Dessert	330 (17%)	8 g (12%)	5 g (25%)	35 mg (12%)

Attention Parents: Make the healthiest fast-food choices for your children. As fast-food chains come out with healthier options, take advantage of them. Remember that you are the boss, and that you have the power to nix unhealthy items, even if it results in a temper tantrum.

EIGHT

DESSERTS AND SNACKS

HEART-HEALTH TIPS AT A GLANCE

Desserts

▶ You can enjoy desserts on a heart-healthy diet. Make smart choices, and desserts can be a nutritious part of your meal plan.

▶ Moderation and portion control are essential. Ideally, dessert portions should never exceed 250 calories.

▶ Always opt for low-calorie, low-fat, and cholesterol-free desserts that have some nutritional benefits, such as vitamins and calcium. Some suggestions include fresh fruit salad topped with nonfat frozen yogurt or sorbet; natural fruit pops; canned fruit, such as Mandarin orange segments or pears, served with nonfat frozen yogurt; fresh berries with sweetened light whipped cream in a spray can; biscotti with a glass of Italian sweet wine, such as vin santo, for dipping; meringue with berries (see Berry Meringue Confection, page 245); fruit compotes or poached fruits (see Pears Poached in Red Wine with Orange and Cinnamon, page 227); and angel food cake (see Raspberry Angel Food Cake with Lemon Glaze, page 242).

▶ Share a dessert, particularly in a restaurant, where dessert menus showcase dangerously decadent fare. If you indulge, think quality, not quantity. Limit yourself to one bite, and you will never feel guilty.

▶ Try soy desserts, such as soy yogurt or non-dairy frozen desserts. Some of them are surprisingly good and healthy, too (see Non-Dairy Cholesterol-Free Frozen Desserts, page 235).

▶ Make your own desserts so you know exactly what goes into them. With a few adjustments, you can turn your favorite off-limits classic desserts into healthy treats. Two examples are the Vanilla Flan with Fresh Berries, page 252, and the Creamy Ricotta Kahlúa Cheesecake, page 249.

▶ Use heart-healthy oils whenever possible (see Understanding Heart-Healthy Oils, page 116), or substitute fruit purees for fat (see Cutting Some of the Fat out of Baking, page 247).

▶ Use whole-grain flours whenever possible. Start by substituting half of the all-purpose flour called for in a recipe with whole wheat flour, then try experimenting with other flours (see Whole-Grain Flours, page 250).

▶ Bake with liquid egg substitutes and/or egg whites. See Baking with Egg Substitutes, page 239, to get started, then play around with your favorite recipes. As a general rule, $1/4$ cup liquid egg substitute equals 1 egg.

▶ Choose dark chocolate over other types of chocolate. See Can't Live without Chocolate?, page 254.

▶ Be aware that most store-bought piecrusts and other boxed baking mixes contain partially hydrogenated oil. Whenever possible, make baked goods from scratch.

▶ If you just have to have a certain high-calorie, high-fat, simply-no-good-for-you dessert, make it a meal. That way, you get it out of your system, and with any luck, you realize that this was not as satisfying as a nutritious and tasty meal, and you will be less inclined to do it again. (If you are inclined to do it again, don't!)

Snacks

▶ Snacking can contribute to a healthy diet and can even foster weight loss. By snacking on healthy foods, you can quell hunger the nutritious way. As with desserts, moderation and portion control are key.

▶ The ideal snack contains between 100 and 140 calories and a minimal amount of fat (see Top Ten Hunger Busters for about 100 Calories, page 231).

▶ Some of the best snacks include fruit (fresh and dried), vegetables, nuts and seeds, fat-free dairy products, low-fat cheese, low-fat granola bars, whole-grain breads, and whole-grain crackers. For more ideas see Heart-Healthy Snacks, page 226.

▶ Snacks such as doughnuts, deep-fried pies, sticky buns, candy bars, and other artery-clogging, empty-calorie items should be avoided (see Snack No-Nos, page 228).

▶ Snacking between meals is fine, as long as snacks do not become mini meals. If they do, you will need to reevaluate your eating habits.

▶ Fiber is a great way to fill up, and fiber combined with protein will keep hunger at bay longer. For example, rice crackers or whole-grain crackers topped with low-fat cheese, peanut butter, or bean dip will go further than just the crackers alone.

▶ In general, try to cut your calorie intake from sugar and foods that contain high-fructose corn syrup. Sugar substitutes in beverages and baking are a good start (see Splenda: The Sugar Substitute, page 247).

▶ Avoid all desserts and snacks that contain partially hydrogenated oil. And do not bake with solid margarine, Crisco, or other products that contain trans fats.

▶ If you are craving a certain snack or dessert, go with it in a contained portion size and be done with it. Buy a small bag of cookies and limit yourself to half the bag—give away the other half or throw it out. This is better than buying a big bag on sale and having it tempt you for days.

Orange, Blueberry, and Date Salad with Vanilla Frozen Yogurt

Heart-Health Benefits: Vitamin C and fiber; cholesterol free

$\mathcal{A}$ **simple, refreshing fruit** salad naturally sweetened with dates.

■ *Serves 3* ■

2 large navel oranges, peeled and cut into
    segments (see Cooking Tip below)
³/₄ cup fresh blueberries, washed and picked over
10 pitted dates, thinly sliced

Dash of ground cinnamon
1¹/₂ cups fat-free or low-fat frozen vanilla yogurt
    or creamy Greek-style nonfat plain yogurt

Combine all of the ingredients except the frozen yogurt in a bowl. Toss gently. Top each serving with a scoop of frozen yogurt.

▶ **Timesaving Tip:** Use canned Mandarin orange segments, drained, instead of the fresh oranges.

▶ **Cooking Tip:** To slice oranges into segments, cut a thin slice from the top and bottom of each orange to expose the flesh. Then stand each orange on a cutting board and, using a sharp knife, working from the top of the orange to the base, slice the peel and bitter white pith from the orange. (Use the first slice as your guide to know how deep to slice to remove the peel and pith.) Working over a bowl to catch the juices, hold the orange in one hand and slice the orange segments from between the membranes, getting the knife as close to the membranes as possible and allowing the segments to drop into the bowl. Once all of the segments have been removed, squeeze the membranes over the bowl to extract as much juice as possible.

Approximate Nutritional Information: Serving size: one-third orange, blueberry, and date salad with ¹/₂ cup fat-free frozen yogurt; Calories: 224 cals, 11%; Protein: 6 g, 12%; Total fat: 0.5 g, 1%; Saturated fat: 0.1 g, 1%; Cholesterol: 1.2 mg, 0%; Carbohydrates: 53 g, 18%; Fiber: 5 g, 21%; Sodium: 54 mg, 2%; Vitamin C: 57 mg, 84%; Vitamin K: 8 mcg, 10%; Diabetic Exchange Values: 2 Starches, 1¹/₂ Fruit

Percentage of calories from fat: 2%

Heart-Healthy Snacks

WHAT IS A heart-healthy snack? It is a snack that is low in calories (between 100 and 140 calories) and fat and high in nutrients (including vitamins, minerals, and/or fiber). Always keep in mind that snacking should be done in moderation. If you do not pay attention to your snacking habits, calories and fats can quickly creep up on you.

Dairy and Soy Snacks: Nonfat (preferably light) yogurt or soy yogurt, low-fat cheese (with 3 grams or fat or less per serving), string cheese, fat-free or 1% or 2% cottage cheese, homemade or store-bought smoothies made with nonfat yogurt, fat-free frozen yogurt, frozen ice milk, and fat-free frozen soy frozen desserts

Vegetable and Fruit Snacks: Fat-free dips or salsa with cut-up raw vegetables, vegetables soup, grape or cherry tomatoes, nonfat yogurt dips with fresh fruits, dried fruit (including raisins, cranberries, dates, prunes, figs, apricots, pineapple, pears, mangoes, papaya, and cherries), canned mandarin orange slices, unsweetened applesauce or other fruit sauces, all-fruit ices or calorie-free Popsicles, sugar-free Jell-O, and fresh berries topped with By Nature Sweetened Light Whipped Cream (in a spray can)

Grain, Nut, and Seed Snacks: Whole wheat crackers, rice cakes, high-fiber cereal bars, low-fat granola bars (see Granola Bars, Cereal Bars, Diet Bars, and Trail Mixes, page 244), low-fat oatmeal cookies, popcorn, reduced-salt pretzels, whole-grain pita bread, whole-grain bagels and English muffins, instant oatmeal, whole-grain dry cereals with fat-free milk, roasted soy nuts, and all kinds of nuts and seeds.

Protein Snacks: Low-fat cheese, fat-free or 1% cottage cheese, peanut butter or other nut butter (such as almond, peanut, soy, or cashew), fruit (such as sliced apples or celery) or vegetables with nut butters, hummus, and low-fat bean dips

Attention Parents: The snacks listed above are excellent choices for children. Try to avoid empty-calorie snacks marketed toward children. Healthy snacks make healthy kids.

Pears Poached in Red Wine with Orange and Cinnamon

Heart-Health Benefits: Fiber; fat free, cholesterol free, and sodium free

These pears are gorgeous served in large wine goblets or glass bowls. A small scoop of fat-free vanilla frozen yogurt and a sprig of fresh mint would add a touch of decadence. Cutting the pears into quarters instead of poaching them whole reduces the cooking time and allows the pears to absorb more of the delicious red wine syrup.

■ *Serves 4* ■

Red Wine Syrup
2 cups red wine (any kind)
³/₄ cup sugar
1 cinnamon stick
3 strips of orange rind
1 teaspoon pure vanilla extract

4 just-ripe Bosc or Bartlett pears, peeled, quartered, and cored

1. To make the red wine syrup, combine all of the ingredients except the vanilla extract in a medium saucepan, stir, and bring to a boil.
2. Add the pears and return to a boil, then reduce heat and simmer, uncovered, for about 20 minutes, or until soft.
3. Transfer the pears and red wine syrup to a heatproof bowl, stir in the vanilla extract and cool to room temperature.
4. Cover with plastic wrap pressed flush against the pears, and refrigerate. Allow the pears to marinate for at least 3 hours, and ideally overnight, before serving.

▶ **Advance Preparation:** The pears can be made up to 3 days before serving.

Approximate Nutritional Information: Serving size: 1 pear poached in red wine with orange and cinnamon (without syrup): Calories: 96 cals, 5%; Protein: 0.6 g, 1%; Total fat: 0 g, 0%; Saturated fat: 0 g, 0%; Cholesterol: 0 mg, 0%; Carbohydrates: 26 g, 9%; Fiber: 5 g, 21%; Sodium: 0 mg, 0%; Diabetic Exchange Values: 1 ½ Fruit

Percentage of calories from fat: 2%

Approximate Nutritional Information: Serving size: 2 tablespoons red wine syrup; Calories: 57 cals, 3%; Protein: 0 g, %; Total fat: 0 g, 0%; Saturated fat: 0 g, 0%; Cholesterol: 0 mg, 0%; Carbohydrates: 10 g, 3%; Fiber: 0 g, 0%; Sodium: 0 mg, 0%; Vitamin K: 7 mcg, 9%; Diabetic Exchange Values: 1 Fruit

Percentage of calories from fat: 0%

Snack No-Nos

TRY TO AVOID snacks that have zero nutritional value and are high in calories, artery-clogging trans fats, and saturated fats. Examples are doughnuts (plain and filled), cinnamon buns, fried dough, fried fruit turnovers, and other similar deep-fried items. Consider these nutritional break-downs before biting into a fat-filled snack.

	CALORIES	FAT
Dunkin' Donuts Cinnamon Bun	510	15 grams
Krispy Kreme Glazed Crème Filled Doughnut	350	20 grams
Burger King Dutch Apple Pie	340	14 grams
Krispy Kreme Chocolate Iced Cake Doughnut	270	13 grams

Two Crisps

*W*arm from the oven, topped with a squirt of light whipped cream or a scoop of fat-free vanilla frozen yogurt, these crisps are as good as they get.

Apple-Pineapple Granola Crisp

Heart-Health Benefits: Vitamin C; cholesterol free

■ *Makes one 9-inch crisp; serves 8* ■

Apple-Pineapple Filling

5 Granny Smith apples (about 2¹/₄ pounds),
  peeled, cored, and cut into ¹/₄-inch slices

3 cups canned pineapple cubes in juice,
  drained

¹/₃ cup finely diced candied ginger

¹/₃ cup lightly packed brown sugar

1 tablespoon all-purpose flour

Granola Topping

¹/₃ cup whole wheat flour

¹/₄ cup lightly packed brown sugar

¹/₄ cup Promise margarine (Not light or
  fat-free)

1¹/₂ cups granola without fruit, preferably low-
  fat and free of partially
  hydrogenated oil (such as Heartland Granola
  Cereal Original All Natural Made with
  Rolled Oats, Brown Sugar, and Molasses)

1. Preheat the oven to 375° F. Have ready a 9-inch oval or square baking dish.
2. To make the apple-pineapple filling, combine all of the ingredients in a large bowl and mix until well blended. Transfer the filling to the baking dish; set aside.
3. To make the granola topping, mix the flour and brown sugar in a bowl. Add the margarine and slice it into the flour mixture with a table knife until the mixture resembles coarse meal. Add the granola and mix with a fork or your hands until the granola is incorporated and the topping holds together in small clumps.
4. Distribute the topping evenly over the filling. Bake for about 45 minutes, or until the juices are bubbling. Remove the crisp from the oven and allow to cool slightly before serving.

Approximate Nutritional Information: Serving size: one-eighth apple-pineapple granola crisp with candied ginger; Calories: 256 cals, 13%; Protein: 3 g, 6%; Total fat: 7.1 g, 11%; Saturated fat: 1.2 g, 6%; Cholesterol: 0 mg, 0%; Carbohydrates: 49 g, 16%; Fiber: 5 g, 18%; Sodium: 53 mg, 2%; Vitamin C: 12 mg, 20%; Vitamin K: 2 mcg, 3%; Diabetic Exchange Values: 1 Starch, 2 Fruit, 1 Fat

Percentage of calories from fat: 24%

Peach-Blueberry Granola Crisp

Health-Heart Benefits: Vitamin C; cholesterol free

■ *Makes one 9-inch crisp; serves 8* ■

5 to 6 just-ripe peaches (about 1³/₄ pounds),
   peeled, pitted, and cut into ¹/₄-inch slices
   (see Cooking Tip below for peeling
   instructions), or three 15-ounce cans lite sliced
   peaches (peaches in extra light syrup), drained
   (about 4 cups drained peaches)

3¹/₂ cups fresh blueberries, washed and picked
   over, or 3 cups frozen blueberries, thawed and
   drained
¹/₃ cup lightly packed brown sugar
2 teaspoons ground cinnamon
2 tablespoons all-purpose flour or cornstarch
1 recipe Granola Topping (page 229)

Follow the directions for Apple-Pineapple Granola Crisp, substituting the peach and blueberry filling ingredients in Step 2.

▶ **Cooking Tip:** To peel fresh peaches, bring a large pot of water to a boil. Have ready a bowl of ice water. Add the peaches to the boiling water and cook for 30 to 60 seconds, or just until their skins loosen. Transfer them to the bowl of ice water to cool, then drain them. The skins should peel off easily with a paring knife.

▶ **Advance Preparation:** The granola topping (for either crisp) can be made up to 2 days in advance and refrigerated.

Approximate Nutritional Information: Serving size: one-eighth peach-blueberry granola crisp: Calories: 251 cals, 13%; Protein: 4 g, 7%; Total fat: 7.3 g, 11%; Saturated fat: 1.2 g, 6%; Cholesterol: 0 mg, 0%; Carbohydrates: 47 g, 16%; Fiber: 5 g, 19%; Sodium: 52 mg, 2%; Vitamin C: 12 mg, 20%; Vitamin K: 14 mcg, 18%; Diabetic Exchange Values: 1 Starch, 2 Fruit, 1 Fat

Percentage of calories from fat: 25%

Top Ten Hunger Busters
for about 100 Calories

1 stick mozzarella string cheese
80 calories
5 grams fat

1 medium apple
90 calories
0 fat

2 tablespoons raisins
90 calories
0 fat

5 pieces dried apricots
90 calories
0 fat

1 cup carrots with 2 tablespoons hummus
95 calories
1 gram fat

1 cup fresh or frozen grapes
100 calories
0 fat

1 medium banana
105 calories
0 fat

1 medium peach and 6 ounces light fat-free yogurt (with about 70 calories)
105 calories
0 fat

1 cup fresh strawberries with 2 tablespoons By Nature Sweetened Light Whipped Cream
105 calories
1.6 grams fat

1 tablespoon peanut butter and 2 celery stalks
115 calories
8.5 grams fat

18 dry-roasted whole almonds
120 calories
10 grams fat

10 large dry-roasted cashews
120 calories
10 grams fat

12 walnut halves
120 calories
11 grams fat

Almond Drop Biscuits
with Strawberries and Raspberries

Heart-Health Benefits: Vitamin C and fiber; cholesterol free

A **variation on the** strawberry shortcake theme—perfect for summer when fresh berries are at their peak.

■ *Serves 6* ■

Strawberry-Raspberry Filling
1 pound (about 4^1/$_2$ cups) fresh strawberries, washed and hulled; half the strawberries sliced into quarters, or eighths if they are large, the other strawberries left whole
^{1}/$_3$ cup Splenda Blend for Baking or sugar, or to taste
1^1/$_2$ cups fresh raspberries

Almond Drop Biscuits
^{1}/$_2$ cup all-purpose flour
^{1}/$_2$ cup whole wheat flour

2 teaspoons baking powder
^{1}/$_4$ cup sugar
3 tablespoons Promise margarine (Not light or fat-free)
^{1}/$_2$ cup fat-free milk
^{1}/$_3$ cup sliced almonds, toasted

Whipped light cream in a spray can, such as By Nature Sweetened Light Whipped Cream (optional)
Confectioners' sugar, for dusting (optional)

1. To make the strawberry-raspberry filling, combine the sliced strawberries (not the whole berries) and Splenda in a bowl, mix, and set aside. Place the whole strawberries in the bowl of a food processor and pulse until they are chopped into small pieces; do *not* puree. Add the chopped strawberries to the sliced strawberries, stir, cover, and refrigerate until ready to serve. (Note: The raspberries will be added just before serving.)
2. Meanwhile, to make the almond drop biscuits, preheat the oven to 450° F. Line a baking sheet with parchment paper or lightly grease with canola oil cooking spray.
3. Combine the all-purpose and whole wheat flour, baking powder, and sugar in a large bowl and mix. Add the margarine and mix it into the flour mixture with a fork until the mixture resembles coarse meal. Add the milk and almonds and stir with a fork until just combined; do not overmix.
4. Measure scant ¼-cupfuls of the dough and arrange them on the baking sheet; you should have 6 biscuits. Bake for 10 minutes, or until light golden brown. Immediately remove the biscuits from the baking sheet and cool them on a plate or cooling rack.
5. Once they are cooled, place the biscuits in an airtight container until ready to serve.

6. To serve, slice each biscuit in half. Arrange the bottoms of the biscuits on dessert plates. Cover the bottoms with the strawberry filling and juices, and then place the raspberries on top. Garnish the filling with a squirt of whipped light cream, if desired. Position the tops of the biscuits against the cream, dust with confectioners' sugar, if using, and serve.

▶ **Cooking Tip:** An equal amount of all-purpose flour can be substituted for the whole wheat flour.

▶ **Advance Preparation:** The almond drop biscuits can be frozen for up to 1 month.

Approximate Nutritional Information: Serving size: 1 almond drop biscuit with one-sixth strawberry-raspberry filling (whipped light cream not included): Calories: 238 cals, 12%; Protein: 6 g, 11%; Total fat: 10 g, 16%; Saturated fat: 1.3 g, 7%; Cholesterol: 0 mg, 0%; Carbohydrates: 35 g, 12%; Fiber: 6 g, 22%; Sodium: 13 mg, 1%; Vitamin C: 43 mg, 72%; Vitamin K: 4 mcg, 5%; Diabetic Exchange Values: 2 Starch, 2 Fat

Percentage of calories from fat: 36%. **Note:** This percentage is high because of the almonds in the biscuits.

Patricia Terry's Pumpkin Muffins or Bread with Dried Cranberries and Pecans

---

Heart-Health Benefits: Vitamin A; cholesterol free

Make the batter the night before and enjoy these pumpkin muffins with your coffee in the morning. The smaller-size loaves make great hostess or thank-you gifts, especially around the holidays. For fewer calories, omit the dried cranberries and pecans.

■ *Makes three 8¹/₂ x 4¹/₂-inch loaves, five 5³/₄ x 3-inch loaves, or about 30 regular muffins* ■
(each large loaf serves 12, each small loaf serves 5)

Cupcake liners, or canola oil cooking spray for the
   loaf pans
2 cups all-purpose flour
1¹/₂ cups whole wheat flour
2¹/₂ cups sugar
¹/₂ teaspoon baking powder
2 teaspoons baking soda
¹/₂ teaspoon salt
2 teaspoons ground cinnamon
1 teaspoon ground nutmeg (optional)
¹/₂ teaspoon ground ginger (optional)

¹/₂ cup canola oil
¹/₂ cup unsweetened applesauce
¹/₂ cup liquid egg substitute
2 large egg whites
²/₃ cup water
One 15-ounce can solid pack pumpkin (100%
   pure pumpkin, not pumpkin pie mix)
1 cup dried cranberries or dark or light raisins
   (optional)
1 cup chopped pecans or walnuts (optional)

1. Preheat the oven to 350 degrees F. Line 30 muffin cups with cupcake liners and set aside. Or spray two 8½ x 4½ x 2½-inch loaf pans or five 5¾ x 3 x 2⅛-inch loaf pans with cooking spray and set aside.
2. In a large bowl, combine the dry ingredients and mix until well blended; set aside.
3. In another large bowl, combine the canola oil, applesauce, egg substitute, egg whites, and water and whisk to mix. Add this mixture to the dry ingredients and whisk just until combined. Add the pumpkin and dried cranberries and pecans, if using, and mix until well blended.
4. Fill each muffin cup a little more than two-thirds full, or divide the batter among the prepared loaf pans. Bake muffins for 25 minutes, or bake large loaves for about 70 minutes, small loaves for about 40 minutes, or until a toothpick inserted into the center of each muffin or loaf comes out clean. Cool completely before slicing the loaves.

▶ **Substitutions:** An equal amount of all-purpose flour can be substituted for the whole wheat flour. A tablespoon of pumpkin pie spice mix can be substituted for the cinnamon, nutmeg, and ginger.

▶ **Advance Preparation:** The batter can be made a day in advance. The muffins or loaves can be frozen for up to 1 month.

Approximate Nutritional Information: Serving size: 1 pumpkin muffin; Calories: 195 cals, 10%; Protein: 3 g, 6%; Total fat: 7 g, 10%; Saturated fat: 0.5 g, 3%; Cholesterol: 0 mg, 0%; Carbohydrates: 32 g, 11%; Fiber: 2 g, 8%; Sodium: 139 mg, 6%; Vitamin A: 2,225 IU, 45%; Vitamin K: 7 mcg, 9%; Diabetic Exchange Values: 1 Starch, 1 Fruit, 1 Fat

Percentage of calories from fat: 30%

NON-DAIRY CHOLESTEROL-FREE FROZEN DESSERTS

BELOW IS A list of non-dairy cholesterol-free frozen desserts. Check labels for calories, especially if you are trying to lose weight. Avoid desserts that have cookie crusts, such as ice cream sandwiches, and ice cream in a cone (cones usually contain partially hydrogenated oil).

Rice Dream Non-Dairy Dessert
Rice Dream Vanilla Bar
Soy Delicious Non-Dairy Frozen Dessert
Soy Dream
Sweet Nothings Non-Dairy Fat-Free Desserts
Tofutti Milk Free
Whole Soy-Frozen Cultured Soy

Attention Parents: Because most kids have a weakness for all things sweet and frozen, try sneaking some frozen soy desserts into their meal plan. You'll be surprised at what you can get away with, and you might even enjoy a bite or two.

Frozen Yogurt, Sorbet, Ice Milk, and Ice Cream

FRUIT SORBET HAS about 120 calories, 0 grams of fat, and 0 grams of cholesterol per $1/2$ cup, while rich vanilla ice cream packs 270 calories, 18 grams of fat, and 120 milligrams of cholesterol. All of the following nutritional breakdowns are for half-cup servings.

Fat-Free Frozen Yogurt
78 calories (4% Daily Value)
0 mg cholesterol
0 g total fat
0 g saturated fat
4 g protein
137 mg calcium

Frozen Cultured Soy
120 calories (6%)
0 mg cholesterol
1 g total fat (2%)
0 g saturated fat
2 g protein (4%)
42 mg calcium (4%)

Fruit Sorbet
120 calories (6%)
0 mg cholesterol
0 g total fat
0 g saturated fat
0 g protein
0 mg calcium

Flavored Ice Milk
67 calories (3%)
9 mg cholesterol (3%)
2 g total fat (3%)
1 g saturated fat (5%)
2 g protein (4%)
70 mg calcium (7%)

Low-Fat No-Sugar-Added Vanilla Ice Cream
100 calories (5%)
10 mg cholesterol (3%)
2 g total fat (3%)
1 g saturated fat (5%)
3 g protein (6%)
100 mg calcium (10%)

Regular Vanilla Ice Cream
132 calories (7%)
29 mg cholesterol (10%)
7 g total fat (11%)
4 g saturated fat (22%)
2 g protein (5%)
84 mg calcium (8%)

Rich Vanilla Ice Cream
270 calories (14%)
120 mg cholesterol (40%)
18 g total fat (28%)
11 g saturated fat (55%)
5 g protein (10%)
150 mg calcium (15%)

Smart Cookies

MOST STORE-BOUGHT cookies are loaded with partially hydrogenated oil, calories, and artificial ingredients, without any redeeming health benefits. Choose from the Smart Choice Cookies below, limit your consumption, or satisfy your cookie craving with whole wheat crackers (see Wise Crackers, page 240).

Smart Choice Cookies

365 Cookies

All Natural Frookies

Barbara's Bakery

Brent & Sam's All Natural Gourmet Cookies

Country Choice

Health Valley Natural Goodness

Heaven Scent Natural Foods

Immaculate Baking Co. ChocoBilly's

Joseph's

Mi-Del

Miss Meringue

New Morning (Cinnamon Grahams)

Newman's Own

Organica Foods

Pamela's

Quadratini

Snackimals

Attention Parents: Buy cookies from whole foods stores, which tend to sell the healthier brands mentioned above, or make them yourself using heart-healthy oils and baking-friendly soft margarines instead of butter (see Tips for Choosing Healthy Margarines, page 193). The recipe for Chocolate Oatmeal Cookies with Dried Cherries and Walnuts, page 238, uses canola oil to produce a deliciously crisp cookie. Also, most prepared cookie doughs found in the refrigerated sections of grocery stores contain partially hydrogenated oil. One frozen organic brand that does not is 600 lb. Gorillas Frozen Cookie Dough (sounds like fun!).

Chocolate Oatmeal Cookies with Dried Cherries and Walnuts

Heart-Health Benefit: Cholesterol free

These outrageously delicious, crispy, cholesterol-free cookies are well worth baking. However tempting they may be, though, limit yourself to just one cookie!

■ *Makes about 4 dozen cookies* ■

1/2 cup oat flour or whole wheat flour

3/4 cup all-purpose flour

1 tablespoon unsweetened cocoa powder

1 teaspoon baking soda

3/4 cup canola oil

1 cup lightly packed brown sugar

1/2 cup Splenda Blend for Baking or sugar

2 large egg whites

1 teaspoon pure vanilla extract

2 cups quick-cooking oats (such as Quick 1-Minute Quaker Oats)

1/2 cup dried cherries or cranberries

1/2 cup chopped walnuts

1. Preheat the oven to 350 degrees F. Have ready one or two baking sheets lined with parchment paper.
2. In a small bowl, combine the oat flour, all-purpose flour, cocoa powder, and baking soda and mix until blended; set aside.
3. In a large bowl, combine the canola oil, brown sugar, and Splenda. Beat with an electric mixer on medium speed for 1 minute. Add the egg whites and vanilla extract and beat on medium speed for 1 minute. Add the flour mixture and beat on low speed just until incorporated, scraping down the sides of the bowl as needed. Stir in the oats, dried cherries, and walnuts. (Note: The batter will be quite stiff.)
4. Scoop out 1-tablespoon mounds of dough and place them on the baking sheets about 1 inch apart. Flatten them slightly with your fingers or the back of a spoon. Bake for 12 to 14 minutes, or until light golden. Transfer to a baking rack to cool.
5. Store the cookies in an airtight container or freeze them.

▶ **Substitution:** Use 1¼ cups of all-purpose flour instead of both.
▶ **Advance Preparation:** The cookie batter can be made a day in advance and refrigerated.
▶ **Storage Tip:** The cookies can be kept in an airtight container for up to 1 week. They can be frozen for up to 1 month.

Approximate Nutritional Information: Serving size: 1 chocolate oatmeal cookie with dried cherries and walnuts; Calories: 79 cals, 4%; Protein: 1 g, 2%; Total fat: 4.7 g, 7%; Saturated fat: 0.3 g, 2%; Cholesterol: 0 mg, 0%; Carbohydrates: 9 g, 3%; Fiber: 0.7 g, 3%; Sodium: 30 mg, 1%; Vitamin K: 4 mcg, 5%; Diabetic Exchange Values: 1/2 Fruit, 1 Fat

Percentage of calories from fat: 50%. **Note:** This percentage is high because of the walnuts in the cookies.

BAKING WITH EGG SUBSTITUTES

IT'S GENERALLY NOT a problem. The rule of thumb is to substitute 1/4 cup egg substitute for each egg called for in a recipe. Because many egg substitutes contain thickeners in the form of vegetable gums, though, they can weigh down baked goods. If you want a lighter or less dense muffin, cake, or bread, try reducing the amount of egg substitute and using fresh egg whites instead. Two egg whites replace 1 whole egg. Some recipes in this book, such as High-Calcium Yogurt-Vanilla Pancakes (page 42), Cholesterol-Free Popovers (page 48), and Vanilla Flan with Berries (page 252), do require the use of egg substitute for texture and color. You will need to play around with your own favorite recipes to find the right balance.

Products that contain whites only, such as Egg-cology, All Whites, and Deb El Just Whites, do not have the same rising power as fresh egg whites. If you are baking something that relies heavily on whites, such as Cholesterol-Free Popovers (page 48), Raspberry Angel Food Cake with Lemon Glaze (page 242), or Berry Meringue Confection (page 245), it is best to use only fresh egg whites.

A handful of egg substitutes, such as Ener G Egg Replacer, contain no egg at all and therefore are not suitable for baking.

Wise Crackers

LIKE STORE-BOUGHT COOKIES, most store-bought crackers contain partially hydrogenated oil. Read labels carefully, or shop in whole foods stores, where you will find a wide assortment of healthy crackers. Look for crackers that are low in fat and high in fiber. Ideally the first ingredient listed should be whole wheat flour, not wheat flour. The words "multi-grain," "stone-ground," "100% wheat," "cracked wheat," "seven grain," or "bran" do not always mean whole-grain products. The best indicator of a cracker's whole-grain status is to check its fiber content, which should be at least 2 grams per serving.

Excellent Choice Whole Wheat Crackers

365 Baked Woven Wheats
Ak-Mak 100% Whole Wheat Stone Ground Sesame Crackers
Barbara's Bakery Wheatines
Dr. Kracker High Fiber Crackers
Finn Crisp
Frookie 50% Less Fat Snack Crackers
Frookie All Natural Snack Crackers
Hain Pure Foods All Natural Baked Crackers Wheatettes
Health Valley Low-Fat Crackers, No Salt Added
Healthy Valley Oat Bran Graham Crackers
Hol Grain Crackers
Kavli Crispbread
Nabisco Triscuit Low Sodium Baked Whole Grain Wheat Crackers
Ryvita Whole Grain Crisp Bread
Wasa

Good Choice Wheat Crackers

365 Golden Stoneground Wheat Thins
365 Sourdough Crackers
Annie's Totally Natural Real Cheddar Bunnies Baked Snack Crackers
Bisca Organic Water Crackers
Blue Diamond Nut Thins
Devonsheer Organic Melba Rounds and Water Crackers
Haute Cuisine
Kashi TLC (Tasty Little Crackers)
Late July Organic Round Saltine Crackers
Lavosh
Our Family Farm Captain's Catch Baked Cheese Crackers

Our Family Farm Field Friends Baked Wheat Crackers
Partners Wisecrackers Low-Fat Crackers
Starr Ridge Hors d'Oeuvre Crackers

Attention Parents: Almost all crackers on grocery store shelves, especially those from the large food companies, contain partially hydrogenated oil, so read labels carefully. It is advisable to buy crackers from whole foods stores, which tend to sell the crackers listed above. Start your children on these healthy crackers, and they won't ever miss the less healthy ones designed to cater to kids.

Raspberry Angel Food Cake
with Lemon Glaze

Heart-Health Benefits: Fat free and cholesterol free

---

*H*omemade **raspberry angel** food cake with lemon glaze is pure pleasure. Any store-bought or boxed angel food cake mix pales miserably in comparison. The key to getting good height on the cake is to bake it on the lowest oven rack. Also, it is essential to use cake flour (despite the fact that it is overrefined); other flours are simply too heavy (see Cooking Tip 1). If you use fresh eggs, please don't feel guilty about throwing away the yolks—they contain the cholesterol! Fresh berries softened with a tiny bit of sugar or Splenda are a delicious accompaniment to the cake, plus they add vitamins and fiber.

■ *Makes one 9-inch or 10-inch tube cake; serves 8* ■

1 cup cake flour

$1^{1}/_{3}$ cups sugar

$^{1}/_{4}$ teaspoon salt

12 large egg white ($1^{1}/_{2}$ to $1^{3}/_{4}$ cups); see Cooking
    Tip 2 on page 243 for information on baking
    with store-bought all-white egg products

1 tablespoon freshly squeezed lemon juice

1 teaspoon cream of tarter

2 teaspoons pure vanilla extract

$1^{1}/_{2}$ cups dried raspberries, such as Just
    Raspberries

Lemon Glaze (recipe follows; optional)

1. Adjust an oven rack to the lowest position and preheat the oven to 350 degrees F. Have ready an ungreased 9- or 10-inch angel food cake tube pan.
2. Sift the cake flour, ⅔ cup of the sugar, and the salt into a medium bowl or onto a piece of parchment paper; set aside.
3. In a large bowl (make sure the bowl is very clean), combine the egg whites, lemon juice, cream of tartar, and vanilla extract. Beat with an electric mixer on low speed for 30 seconds, until frothy bubbles appear. Gradually add the remaining ⅔ cup sugar, they increase the speed to high and continue beating until soft, glossy peaks form, about 3 minutes.
4. With a rubber spatula, gradually fold in the flour mixture and dried raspberries, if using, about ¼ cup at a time. Work with a slicing and lifting motion to bring up the egg whites from the bottom of the bowl. All of the flour needs to be absorbed, but try not to overmix, as that will deflate the whites.
5. Gently spoon the batter into the tube pan. With a dry paper towel, wipe any batter from the sides of the pan. Bake for 40 minutes, or until the top is golden and springs back when lightly touched.

6. Remove the cake from the oven and allow it to cool for 5 minutes. If the pan sides have "feet" to keep them elevated, simply invert the pan onto the countertop. If not, set the inverted pan on three upside-down mugs or small bowls to keep it suspended. (Note: Some people like to invert the pan onto the neck of a bottle—this works too.) Cool completely.
7. Once the cake is cooled, run a long thin knife around the sides of the pan and the center tube and invert the cake onto a serving plate.
8. Slowly pour the lemon glaze over the top of the cooled cake, letting it drip down the sides. Cover any leftovers with aluminum foil and store in a cool, dry place.

▶ **Cooking Tip 1:** Cake flour is very fine chemically bleached white flour. Its high starch content supports the high proportion of sugar in this recipe, allowing the cake to rise. Unbleached all-purpose flour is more nutritious, but it produces a cake that will not rise as high. Both flours taste the same.

▶ **Cooking Tip 2:** You can use an all-white egg product (such as All Whites or Egg-cology) but the result might be a shorter cake with large air pockets and a slightly salty flavor. By comparison, angel food cake made with fresh whites is lighter and less salty, with a better texture and crumb.

Approximate Nutritional Information: Serving size: one-eighth raspberry angel food cake; Calories: 214 cals, 11%; Protein: 7 g, 14%; Total fat: 0 g, 0%; Saturated fat: 0 g, 0%; Cholesterol: 0 mg, 0%; Carbohydrates: 46 g, 15%; Fiber: 2g, 7%; Sodium: 84 mg, 3%; Vitamin K: 2 mcg, 2%; Diabetic Exchange Values: 2 Starch, 1 Fruit

Percentage of calories from fat: 2%

Lemon Glaze

Makes about ³/₄ cup

1¹/₂ cups confectioners' sugar

1 tablespoon grated lemon zest

3 ¹/₂ tablespoons freshly squeezed lemon juice

1¹/₂ teaspoons hot water

Whisk all of the ingredients in a bowl until smooth.

Approximate Nutritional Information: Serving size: one-sixteenth lemon glaze: Calories: 45 cals, 2%; Protein: 0 g, 0%; Total fat: 0 g, 0%; Saturated fat: 0 g, 0%; Cholesterol: 0 mg, 0%; Carbohydrates: 11 g, 4%; Fiber: 0 g, 0%; Sodium: 0 mg, 0%; Diabetic Exchange: 1 Fruit

Percentage of calories from fat: 0%

Granola Bars, Cereal Bars, Diet Bars, and Trail Mixes

Granola bars, cereal bars, diet bars, and trail mixes can be a good choice for fiber and other nutrients, but many major brands contain partially hydrogenated oil, so read labels carefully. Despite their crunchy nature, most bars contain only 1 gram of fiber, though some contain up to 3 grams. The average calorie per bar is about 140, so go easy. Be sure to read labels on diet bars, which may not be as healthy as they seem.

Good Choice Bars

Barbara'a Puffins Cereal and Milk Bars
Barbara's Moist and Chewy Nature's Choice Granola Bars
Cascadian Farms Organic Granola Bars
Envirokids Organic Crispy Rice Bars
Health Valley Breakfast Bars
Health Valley Fat-Free Fruit Bars
Health Valley Organic Granola Bars
Health Valley Organic Tarts
Kashi Go Lean High Protein and Fiber Bars
Nature Valley Chewy Granola
Nature's Path Organic Granola Bars
Nature's Path Organic Toaster Pastries
Power Bar Pria
Save the Forest Organic Cereal Bars and Trail Mix Bars
Slim-Fast Succeed Snack Bars
Zone Perfect All Natural Nutrition Bars

Good Choice Trail Mix

365 Trail Mix
Soy Nut Trail Mix
Whole Foods Trail Mix

Attention Parents: The healthy-choice bars and trail mixes mentioned above are excellent snacks for kids. Most products on the shelves that cater specifically to children contain partially hydrogenated oil, so give children the healthier "adult" brands.

Berry Meringue Confection

Heart-Health Benefits: Vitamin C; fat free and cholesterol free

A **showstopper of a** dessert—friends will beg you for the recipe. The red, white, and blue of the meringue crust and berry filling are ideal when the occasion demands a patriotic dessert. The meringue crust will be hard and cracked on the outside, while the middle will be a marshmallowy consistency.

■ *Serves 6* ■

Meringue Crust

4 large egg whites

1 cup sugar

$^1/_2$ teaspoon cornstarch

1 teaspoon freshly squeezed lemon juice

1 teaspoon pure vanilla extract

1 tablespoon boiling water

4 cups assorted berries, such as strawberries, raspberries, and blueberries, washed and hulled or picked over if necessary.

Whipped light cream in a spray can, such as By Nature Sweetened Light Whipped Cream (optional)

1. Preheat the oven to 350 degrees F. Line a baking sheet with foil, shiny side up.
2. To make the meringue crust, combine the egg whites, sugar, cornstarch, lemon juice, and vanilla extract in a large mixing bowl. Beat with an electric mixer on low speed for 1 minute. Add the boiling water and beat on high speed for 3 to 5 minutes, or until stiff, glossy peaks form.
3. Spoon the meringue onto the prepared baking sheet in one big mound. Using the back of a spoon or a spatula, spread the meringue into 6-inch circle (the circle will spread further as it bakes).
4. Bake the meringue for 10 minutes, then reduce the heat to 200 degrees F and continue to bake for 40 minutes. Turn off the oven and leave the meringue in the oven for 1 hour (this will make it crispy).
5. Remove the meringue from the oven and let cool, then carefully peel off the foil.
6. Place the meringue on a large serving dish. Pile the berries in the middle of the crust. Top with rosettes of whipped cream, if using, and serve immediately.

Approximate Nutritional Information: One-sixth berry meringue (a mixture of 1$^1/_2$ cups strawberries, 1$^1/_2$ cups raspberries, and 1 cup blueberries was used for this breakdown); (whipped light cream not included); Calories: 180 cals, 9%; Protein: 3g, 6%; Total fat: 0 g, 0%; Saturated fat: 0 g, 0%; Cholesterol: 0 mg, 0%; Carbohydrates: 42 g, 14%; Fiber: 3g, 13%; Sodium: 38 mg, 2%; Vitamin C: 32 mg, 53%; Vitamin K: 8 mcg, 10%; Diabetic Exchange Values: 1 Starch, 2 Fruit

Percentage of calories from fat: 2%

Fresh Strawberry-Raspberry Pie

Heart-Health Benefits: Vitamin C; cholesterol free

This pie is a perfect way to showcase fresh ripe berries when they are in season. Use graham crackers that do not contain partially hydrogenated oil, such as New Morning Cinnamon Grahams, for the crust. A squirt of whipped light cream in a spray can, such as By Nature Sweetened Light Whipped Cream, is a nice finishing touch. This pie is best served on the day it is made.

■ *Makes one 9-inch pie; serves 8* ■

Graham Cracker Almond Piecrust
- 1¼ cups finely crushed graham cracker crumbs
- ⅓ cup finely chopped sliced almonds
- 2 tablespoons brown sugar
- 3 tablespoons canola oil

Filling
- 1 pound fresh strawberries (about 4½ cups), washed and hulled, smaller berries quartered, larger ones cut into sixths or eighths
- 12 ounces fresh raspberries (about 1½ cups)
- ¾ cup sugar
- ¼ cup cornstarch
- ½ cup water
- 1 tablespoons freshly squeezed lemon juice

1. Preheat the oven to 350 degrees F.
2. Combine all of the ingredients for the graham cracker almond piecrust in a bowl and mix until well blended. Transfer the crumbs to a 9-inch pie plate and press them evenly over the bottom and up the sides of the plate. Bake the pie shell for 12 to 14 minutes, or until it is firm to the touch. Remove from the oven and let cool before filling.
3. In a large bowl, combine the strawberries and raspberries. Transfer 2 cups of the berries to a food processor or blender and puree until smooth. (Note: The pureed berries should yield about 1⅓ cups.) Set aside the remaining berries.
4. Combine the berry puree, sugar, cornstarch, water, and lemon juice in a saucepan, bring to a simmer over medium heat, stirring constantly, and simmer for 2 minutes, stirring, or until the mixture becomes thick and shiny. Remove from the heat.
5. Place half of the reserved strawberries and raspberries in the pie shell and pour half of the hot berry mixture over them. Add the remaining strawberries and raspberries and top with the remaining hot berry mixture. Using a spoon, gently move the berries until all of them are covered with sauce and the sauce touches the sides of the piecrust.

6. Cover with plastic wrap and refrigerate for at least 4 hours, or until the filling is set. Serve chilled. Refrigerate leftovers.

Approximate Nutritional Information: One-eighth fresh strawberry-raspberry pie; Calories: 225 cals, 11%; Protein: 2g, 5%; Total fat: 8 g, 13%; Saturated fat: 0.5 g, 3%; Cholesterol: 0 mg, 0%; Carbohydrates: 38 g, 13%; Fiber: 4g, 16%; Sodium: 23 mg, 1%; Vitamin C: 55 mg, 91%; Vitamin K: 10 mcg, 12%; Diabetic Exchange Values: 1 Starch, 1½ Fruit, 1 Fat

Percentage of calories from fat: 32%. **Note:** This percentage is high because of the almonds in the piecrust.

CUTTING SOME OF THE FAT OUT OF BAKING

▶ Replace whole eggs with egg substitutes or egg whites (see Baking with Egg Substitutes, page 239).

▶ Replace whole milk with fat-free milk, fat-free evaporated milk, soy milk, or rice milk.

▶ Replace cream with fat-free milk, soy milk, rice milk, fat-free half-and-half, or silken tofu.

▶ Replace butter, lard, or shortening with soft margarine (Not light or fat-free) in a tub (see Tips for Choosing Healthy Margarines, page 193), canola oil, or olive oil. Avoid solid and soft margarines that contain partially hydrogenated oil.

▶ Replace oil or margarine with applesauce or pureed fruit.

▶ Replace regular whipped cream with a light whipped cream, such as By Nature Sweetened Light Whipped Cream in a spray can. This cream is not suitable for making mousse-like desserts.

▶ Replace sour cream with fat-free or low-fat plain yogurt, fat-free buttermilk, fat-free kefir, or silken tofu.

SPLENDA:
THE SUGAR SUBSTITUTE

THINGS TO KNOW about Baking with Splenda

▶ Splenda is very sweet, so you will probably need to use less Splenda than the amount of sugar called for in a recipe.

▶ Regular Splenda does not deliver the same crispness in crusts and cookies that real sugar does. Try Splenda Sugar Blend for Baking for crusts, cakes, cookies, and other recipes where you want crispness.

▶ Regular Splenda produces less juice in fruit fillings for pies and crisps than real sugar does, so you might need to add less flour or cornstarch than a recipe calls for. Splenda Sugar Blend for Baking will yield slightly more juices, but you will probably still need less flour or cornstarch.

▶ Splenda does not work in whipped egg whites for meringues, angel food cake, or other such desserts. Whites whipped with Splenda are grainy and deflate quickly.

Movie-House Popcorn versus Air-Popped

CRUNCHING YOUR WAY through a large tub (about twenty cups) of movie-house buttered popcorn popped in coconut oil adds about 1,500 calories and 116 grams of fat to your day! A small tub (about seven cups) contains about 580 calories and 47 grams of fat. This shocking information might convince you to smuggle your own air-popped popcorn, without butter, into your next movie. Avoid microwave popcorn brands, as most contain partially hydrogenated oil.

Smart Choice Store-Bought Popcorn

365 Organic Popcorn
Beantos Lite No Salt No Oil Organic Popcorn
Boston's 40% Less Fat White Cheddar All Natural Popcorn
Boston's Lite Popcorn 50% Less Fat
Half Naked Popcorn with a Hint of Olive Oil
Robert's American Gourmet Pirate's Booty Puffed Rice and Corn
Smartfood Popcorn White Cheddar Cheese Flavored

	CALORIES	CHOLESTEROL	SATURATED FAT	TOTAL FAT	PROTEIN
Air-Popped Popcorn (4 cups)	114 (6% Daily Value)	0 mg (0%)	1.2 g (2%)	1 g (%)	4 g (7%)
Oil-Popped Popcorn (4 cups)	222 (11%)	0 mg (0%)	12 g (19%)	2 g (11%)	4 g (8%)
Buttered Oil-Popped Popcorn (4 cups)	291 (15%)	11 mg (4%)	18 g (29%)	5 g (26%)	5 g (9%)

Creamy Ricotta Kahlúa Cheesecake

Heart-Health Benefits: Protein and calcium

The Kahlúa is fabulous, but it can be omitted if you want a more traditional cheesecake or if you are serving this dessert to children. Sliced fresh strawberries, raspberries, or blueberries, or a mixture of all three, are a wonderful accompaniment. For the crust, use graham crackers that do not contain partially hydrogenated oil, such as New Morning Cinnamon Grahams.

■ *Makes one 9- to 9¹/₂-inch cheesecake; serves 9* ■

Graham Cracker Walnut Piecrust
- 1¹/₄ cups finely crushed graham cracker crumbs
- ¹/₃ cup finely chopped walnuts
- 2 tablespoons brown sugar
- 1 teaspoon ground cinnamon
- 3 tablespoons canola oil

Ricotta Kahlúa Filling
- 16 ounces fat-free cream cheese
- 1 cup fat-free ricotta cheese
- ¹/₂ cup sugar
- 2 large egg whites
- ¹/₂ cup fat-free sour cream
- 3 tablespoons Kahlúa
- 2 teaspoons pure vanilla extract

1. Preheat the oven to 350 degrees F.
2. Combine all of the ingredients for the graham cracker walnut piecrust in a bowl and mix until well blended. Transfer the crumbs to a 9-inch pie plate and press them evenly over the bottom and up the sides of the plate. Bake the pie shell for 9 minutes, or until it is slightly firm to the touch. Remove from the oven and let cool before filling.
3. To make the ricotta Kahlúa filling, place the cream cheese and ricotta cheese in a large bowl and beat with an electric mixer on medium speed until creamy. Add the sugar and continue to beat for 30 seconds. Add the egg whites, sour cream, Kahlúa, and vanilla extract and beat until well blended.
4. Pour the filling into the crust and bake for 40 minutes, or until the center of the cheesecake is almost firm (it will firm up as it cools). Remove the cheesecake from the oven and let cool to room temperature, then refrigerate for at least 4 hours before serving. Refrigerate leftovers.

▶**Advance Preparation:** This cheesecake can be made up to 1 day before serving.

Approximate Nutritional Information: One-ninth creamy ricotta Kahlúa cheesecake; Calories: 217 cals, 11%; Protein: 12g, 24%; Total fat: 8 g, 13%; Saturated fat: 1.1 g, 6%; Cholesterol: 12 mg, 4%; Carbohydrates: 23 g, 8%; Fiber: 0.5g, 2%; Sodium: 393 mg, 16%; Calcium: 224 mg, 22%; Vitamin K: 6 mcg, 7%; Diabetic Exchange Values: 1 Fat-Free Milk, 1 Starch, 1 Fat

Percentage of calories from fat: 35%. **Note:** This percentage is high because of the walnuts in the crust.

Whole-Grain Flours

Kernels, or the seed-bearing fruit of grains, are composed of three layers. The outer layer, or bran, is filled with B vitamins and is an excellent source of soluble fiber, which has been linked to a lower risk of heart disease and stroke. The seed germ, or next inner layer, provides minerals, B vitamins, protein, vitamin E, and oils. The soft innermost layer, or endosperm, consists mainly of starch, with some protein and other nutrients. When flours are refined, the grains are milled to remove the bran and germ, destroying up to 80 percent of the grain's nutrients and much of its texture and taste. Enriched flours are fortified with some, though not all, of the lost nutrients.

Bottom line: Whole-grain flours are better for you than their refined, chlorine-dioxide–bleached all-purpose cousins. Try substituting whole wheat flour for half of the all-purpose flour called for in recipes (the recipes in this book will help you get started). When you feel comfortable with that, gradually add more whole wheat flour, or move on to other more unusual flours like the ones mentioned below.

When shopping, choose organically grown whole-grain flours from a store that has a high turnover. Check expiration dates. Place the flours in moisture-tight containers and refrigerate them for up to 4 months. Bring to room temperature before using. Mail-order companies are an excellent way to buy whole-grain flours; see Sources, page 267–68.

Whole-Grain Flours and Their Uses

Amaranth: A strong, sweet, spicy, nutty-flavored flour milled from the grain amaranth. High in fat, it should be kept refrigerated at all times. Best used as an accent in waffles, pancakes, cookies, or muffins.

Barley: Milled from hulled and partially pearled barley, this flour has a delicate nutty aroma. It delivers a moist cake-like crumb when combined with other higher-gluten wheat flours. Keep refrigerated.

Buckwheat: Milled from buckwheat groats; buckwheat is a plant, not a grain, related to rhubarb. Commonly used in combination with wheat flour for pancakes, waffles, and blintzes and in pasta.

Blue Cornmeal: Ground from blue corn, this meal is higher in protein than yellow cornmeal. It has a nutty flavor and yields moist results. Used in pancakes, muffins, breads, and corn tortillas.

Yellow or White Stone-Ground Cornmeal: Contains the germ and fibrous bran of corn. The white variety is more delicate and slightly sweeter. Used for polenta, corn bread, and muffins.

Corn: Milled from either whole or hulled degerminated corn kernels, this flour has a finer texture than stone-ground cornmeal. It can be used like cornmeal.

Millet: A high-protein nutritious flour ground from millet seed. It should be used as an accent in baked goods. If used alone, the results are dry, crumbly, and slightly bitter.

Oat Bran: Contains soluble fiber that can help lower blood cholesterol levels when eaten as part of a low-cholesterol diet. Added to muffins, breads, or other baked goods or used as a coating for chicken and seafood.

Oat: A sweet, oat-perfumed flour that can be used like whole wheat flour. It is excellent in pancakes, waffles, oatmeal cookies, muffins, and other baked goods.

Rye: Dark rye flour is the least refined and therefore most nutritious of the rye flours. It produces baked goods that are moist and dense. Due to its low gluten content, it is often mixed with whole wheat flour to increase its rising ability.

Soy: There are two types of soy flour available: full-fat and defatted. Full-fat soy flour, also called natural soy flour, is made from whole raw soybeans that have been hulled, cracked, and finely ground. It is high in fat and protein, as well as vitamins and minerals. Defatted soy flour is made from the soybean pulp left over after expressing oil from the beans to make soybean oil. Because the oil in defatted flour is removed, the protein is much more concentrated; there is no vitamin E, but all the other vitamins remain. The two types of soy flour can be used interchangeably to accent baked goods; they should be combined with wheat flour to increase rising ability. Keep refrigerated.

Whole Wheat: Whole wheat flour is the king of gluten, which accounts for its rising power. Use whole wheat flour in combination with other lower-gluten flours to help in rising.

Vanilla Flan with Fresh Berries

Heart-Health Benefits: Calcium and vitamin C

If you thought your cholesterol-lowering diet meant you had to give up flan for dessert, think again! Made with egg substitute and fresh egg whites, non-fat sweetened condensed milk, and fat-free milk, this flan is practically fat and cholesterol free. Serve it with your favorite fresh berries for added vitamins and fiber. Keep in mind that the flan needs to be refrigerated for twelve hours before unmolding, so make it at least one day before serving.

■ *Serves 8* ■

One 14-ounce can nonfat sweetened condensed milk

1¹/₂ cups fat-free milk

¹/₂ cup liquid egg substitute

2 large egg whites

2 teaspoons pure vanilla extract

Caramel

³/₄ cup sugar

¹/₄ cup water

4 cups fresh raspberries, sliced strawberries, or blueberries, or a mixture

1. Preheat the oven to 325 degrees F. Bring a kettle of water to a boil. Place a 2-quart soufflé dish or a metal ring mold with a 6-cup capacity in a baking pan; set aside.
2. In a bowl, combine the sweetened condensed milk, milk, egg substitute, egg whites, and vanilla extract and whisk until well blended; set aside.
3. To make the caramel, combine the sugar and water in a small nonstick saucepan. Cook over medium-high heat, stirring with a wooden spoon, until the sugar melts and reaches a rich caramel color. Carefully pour the caramel into the bottom of the soufflé dish or mold, then swirl the soufflé dish so the caramel comes about 1 inch up the sides of the dish. (Note: The caramel will be extremely hot, so be very careful. If you are using a metal ring mold, use pot holders to hold the mold when you swirl the caramel.) Place the empty saucepan in the sink and immediately fill it with water for easier cleanup.
4. Pour the egg mixture into the caramel-coated soufflé dish. Add enough boiling water to the baking pan to reach 1½ inches up the sides of the soufflé dish. Bake for 1½ hours. The middle will still be jiggly, but it will firm as it cools. Remove the soufflé dish from the baking pan and let cool to room temperature, then refrigerate for at least 12 hours, or overnight.
5. To serve, fill the baking pan you used to bake the flan with boiling water. Place the soufflé dish in it for at least 5 minutes, but no more than 7 to allow the caramel to melt and create a sauce. Loosen the sides of the flan by running a

sharp knife around the inside of the soufflé dish. Carefully invert the flan onto a large serving platter with sides to catch the caramel sauce. Serve with the fresh berries. Refrigerate leftovers.

▶ **Advance Preparation:** The flan can be made up to 2 days before serving.

Approximate Nutritional Information: Serving size: one-eighth vanilla flan with $1/2$ cup raspberries; Calories: 208 cals, 10%; Protein: 9 g, 18%; Total fat: 0.9 g, 1%; Saturated fat: 0.1 g, 1%; Cholesterol: 3.6 mg, 1%; Carbohydrates: 40 g, 13%; Fiber: 4 g, 16%; Sodium: 113 mg, 5%; Vitamin C: 16 mg, 27%; Calcium: 193 mg, 20%; Vitamin K: 5 mcg, 6%; Diabetic Exchange Values: 1 Fat-Free Milk, 2 Fruit

Percentage of calories from fat: 4%

Approximate Nutritional Information: Serving size: one-sixteenth caramel syrup; 35 cals, 2%; Protein: 0 g, 0%; Total fat: 0 g, 0%; Saturated fat: 0 g, 0%; Cholesterol: 0 mg, 0%; Carbohydrates: 9 g, 3%; Fiber: 0 g, 0%; Sodium: 0 mg, 0%; Diabetic Exchange Values: $1/2$ Fruit

Percentage of calories from fat: 0%

Can't Live without Chocolate?

IF YOU ARE a chocoholic, fear not, you can have your chocolate and eat it too . . . but only once in a while. Choose dark chocolate, which contains flavonoids (specifically the antioxidant epicat-echin) that have been shown to reduce the harmful effects of LDL, or bad cholesterol. Dark choco-late has about the same amount of flavonoids as half a cup of brewed black tea. But don't trick yourself into thinking that chocolate is necessary to prevent heart disease. If you eat too much chocolate, you are likely to gain weight, which is bad for your heart. Keep in mind that one ounce of plain chocolate contains 140 to 150 calories, 8 to 10 grams of fat, and 0 to 7 milligrams of cho-lesterol. Bittersweet chocolate has no cholesterol and milk chocolate has the most.

Serving Size: 1 ounce

	CALORIES	TOTAL FAT	SATURATED FAT	CHOLESTEROL
Bittersweet Chocolate	138	9.8 g (15% daily value)	5.9 g (30%)	0 mg
Semisweet Chocolate	139	10 g (15%)	5.6 (28%)	2.2 mg (1%)
Dark Chocolate	152	8.9 g (14%)	5.5 g (28%)	1.7 mg (1%)
Milk Chocolate	150	8.6 g (13%)	5.1 g (26%)	6.8 mg (2%)

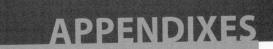

APPENDIXES

RISK CATEGORIES, LDL CHOLESTEROL GOALS, AND THERAPY

RISK CATEGORY	LDL CHOLESTEROL GOAL (MG/DL)*	INITIATE DIET, PHYSICAL ACTIVITY, WEIGHT MANAGEMENT	CONSIDER THERAPY
High risk: CHD† or CHD risk‡§ (10 year risk >20%)§§	<100 (optional goal <70)	≥100	≥100 (consider drug option with <100)
Moderately high risk: 2+ risk factors (10 year risk 10%–20%)	<130	≥130	≥130 (consider drug option with ≥160)
Moderate risk: 2+ risk factors (10 year risk <10%)	<130	≥130	≥160
Lower risk: 0–1 risk factor	<160 <160	≥160 ≥160	≥190 (160–189 LDL-lowering drug option)

*LDL is measured in milligrams per deciliter (mg/dL).

†CHD includes history of heart attack; angina; coronary artery procedures, such as angioplasty or bypass surgery; or heart ischemia.

‡CHD risk includes peripheral arterial disease, abdominal aortic aneurysm, and carotid artery disease; diabetes; and 2+ risk factors with 10-year risk for CHD >20%.

§Risk factors include cigarette smoking, hypertension (BP ≥140/90 mm Hg or on high blood pressure medication), low HDL cholesterol (<40 mg/dL), family history of early heart disease (in male first-degree relative <55 yrs; in female first-degree relative <65 yrs), and age (men ≥45 years; women ≥55 years).

§§10-year risk can be calculated at www.nhlbi.nih.gov/guidelines/cholesterol, which takes into account age, gender, total cholesterol level, HDL cholesterol level, smoking history, and blood pressure. It provides you with a risk score or your chance of having a heart attack in the next ten years.

Source: *Circulation,* "Implications of Recent Clinical Trials for the National Cholesterol Eduction Program Adult Treatment Panel III Guidelines," S. M. Grundy, J. I. Cleeman, C. N. Bairey Merz, B. Brewer, L. T. Clark, D. B. Hunninghake, R. C. Pasternak, S. C. Smith, and N. J. Stone, 2004, Volume 110, pages 227–39.

FOOD GROUPS AND SAMPLE SERVING SIZES

FOOD GROUPS	RECOMMENDED SERVINGS	SAMPLE SERVING SIZE
Fruits	1–2½ cups, or 2–5 servings	*1 serving is:* 1 medium fruit ½ cup fresh, frozen, or canned fruit ½ cup fruit juice ¼ cup dried fruit
Vegetables	1–4 cups, or 2–8 servings	*1 serving is:* 1 cup raw leafy vegetables ½ cup cut-up raw or cooked vegetables ½ cup vegetable juice
Whole Grains and Legumes	3–10 servings	*1 serving is:* 1 slice bread 1 cup dry cereal ½ cup cooked rice, pasta, or cereal ½ cup cooked dried beans
Low-Fat Dairy	3 cups, or 3 servings	*1 serving is:* 1 cup low-fat/fat-free milk or yogurt 1 cup soy milk or soy yogurt 1½ ounces of low-fat or fat-free cheese ½ cup fat-free or low-fat cottage cheese
Lean Meats and Seafood	2–7 ounces	*1 serving is:* 1 ounce cooked lean meat, poultry, or fish ¼ cup cooked tofu 1 egg or ¼ cup egg substitute
Mono- and Polyunsaturated Fats	4–13 servings	*1 serving is:* 1 teaspoon vegetable oil 1 teaspoon soft margarine 1 tablespoon regular salad dressing or 2 tablespoons reduced-fat salad dressing 1 tablespoon low-fat mayonnaise 2 tablespoons or 1 ounce avocado 8 large black or 10 large green olives 1 tablespoon peanut butter ½ ounce nuts or seeds

Three Stay Balanced Sample Menus

1,600-CALORIE STAY BALANCED MENU

Meal	Menu	Food Groups and Servings
Breakfast	½ cup oatmeal ¼ cup raisins 1 cup soy yogurt	1 whole grain 1 fruit 1 low-fat dairy
Morning Snack	1 apple 1 tablespoon peanut butter	1 fruit 1 mono/poly fat
Lunch	2 cups mixed lettuce with 2 vegetables 2 ounces chicken strips ½ whole wheat pita bread 2 tablespoons Caesar Salad Dressing with Silken Tofu (page 75) 1 cup fat-free milk	2 lean meat 1 whole grain 1 mono/poly fat 1 low-fat dairy
Afternoon Snack	1 pear	

Dinner	1 serving Lamb Chops with
	  Cilantro-Mint Salsa (page 216)
	2 tablespoons Cilantro-Mint Salsa
	  (page 216)
	1 cup cooked brown rice
	1 serving Green Bean, Tomato,
	  and Feta Salad (page 96)
		3 lean meat
		
		2 whole grain
		3 vegetable
		
		1½ mono/poly fat

Evening Snack	2 plain graham crackers 1 cup skim milk	1 whole grain 1 low-fat dairy

1,800-CALORIE STAY BALANCED MENU

Meal	Menu	Food Groups and Servings
Breakfast	1 Bran Muffin with Pineapple and Dried Cranberries (page 51)	2 whole grain
	1 cup low-fat vanilla yogurt	1 mono/poly fat 1 low-fat dairy
	1 banana	1 fruit
Morning Snack	1 cup low-sodium tomato juice	2 vegetable
	1½ ounces part-skim mozzarella cheese	1 low-fat dairy
	3 whole-grain wheat crackers	1 whole grain
Lunch	½ cup Simple Tuna Salad (page 76)	5 lean meat
	2 slices whole wheat bread	4 whole grain
	1 tablespoon low-fat mayonnaise	1 mon/poly fat
	1⅓ cups Easy Black Bean Soup with Fresh Cilantro (page 59)	
	1 apple	1 fruit
Afternoon Snack	½ cup 1% cottage cheese	1 low-fat dairy
	1 peach or ½ cup canned peaches	1 fruit
Dinner	3 ounces soy burger	3 lean meat
	1 whole wheat roll	2 whole grain
	1 serving Hearts of Palm, Tomato, and Asparagus Salad (page 94)	3 vegetable
	½ cup fresh corn or 1 ear of corn	1 mono/poly fat
Evening Snack	1 tablespoon almond butter or soy butter	1 mono/poly fat
	1 celery stalk	1 vegetable

2,000-CALORIE STAY BALANCED MENU

Meal	Menu	Food Groups and Servings
Breakfast	½ cup grape juice Cheese omelet made with ½ cup egg substitute and 2 oz low-fat cheese 2 slices rye toast 1 tablespoon soft tub margarine	1 fruit 2 lean meat 2 low-fat dairy 2 whole grain 1 mono/poly fat
Morning Snack	1 orange 1 brown rice cracker	1 fruit
Lunch	1 serving Greek Salad with Whole Wheat Flat Bread (page 86) 1 cup low-fat yogurt ½ cup blueberries 1 ounce soy nuts	3 vegetable 2 whole grain 1 low-fat dairy 1 fruit 3 mono/poly fat
Afternoon Snack	¼ cup Traditional Hummus (page 90) 3 whole-grain wheat crackers 7 baby carrots	2 whole grain 1 mono/poly fat 1 vegetable
Dinner	4 oz wild salmon, grilled or broiled 2 tablespoons Sun-Dried Tomato Sauce (page 152) ½ cup whole wheat couscous 1 cup broccoli	4 lean meat 2 mono/poly fat 1 whole grain 2 vegetable
Evening Snack	½ cup no-sugar-added low-fat vanilla frozen yogurt ½ cup strawberries	1 low-fat dairy 1 fruit

Determine Your Body Mass Index

BODY MASS INDEX CATEGORIES

Underweight = less than 18.5
Normal weight = 18.5 to 24.9
Overweight = 25 to 29.9
Obesity = 30 or greater
Extreme Obesity = 40 or greater

BODY MASS INDEX CHART

Height	Minimal Risk BMI under 25	Moderate Risk BMI 25–29.9 Overweight	High Risk BMI 30 and above Obese
4'10"	118 pounds or less	119–142 pounds	143 pounds or more
4'11"	123 or less	124–147	148 or more
5'0"	127 or less	128–152	153 or more
5'1	131 or less	132–157	158 or more
5'2"	135 or less	136–163	164 or more
5'3"	140 or less	141–168	169 or more
5'4"	144 or less	145–173	174 or more
5'5"	149 or less	150–179	180 or more
5'6"	154 or less	155–185	186 or more
5'7"	158 or less	159–190	191 or more
5'8"	163 or less	164–196	197 or more
5'9"	168 or less	169–202	203 or more
5'10"	173 or less	174–208	209 or more
5'11"	178 or less	179–214	215 or more
6'0"	183 or less	184–220	221 or more
6'1"	188 or less	189–226	227 or more
6'2"	193 or less	194–232	233 or more
6'3"	199 or less	200–239	240 or more
6'4"	204 or less	205–245	246 or more

To calculate your exact BMI value, multiply your weight in pounds by 703, divide by your height in inches, then divide again by your height in inches. Or, use your weight in kilograms divided by height in meters squared (kg/m^2).

Source: Adapted from Obesity Education Initiative: Clinical Guidelines on the Identification, Evaluation, and Treatment of Overweight and Obesity in Adults, National Institutes of Health, National Heart, Lung, and Blood Institute, *Obesity Research* 1998, 6 Edition Supplement 2:51S–209S.[1]

Body Mass Index for Children and Teens

IN CHILDREN AND teens, body mass index (BMI) is used to assess underweight, overweight, and risk for overweight. Children's body fatness changes over the years as they grow. Also, girls and boys differ in body fatness as they mature. This is why BMI for children, also referred to as BMI-for-age, is gender and age specific.[2] BMI-for-age is plotted on gender-specific growth charts. These charts are used for children and teens from two to twenty years (see below).

To measure BMI, multiply weight in pounds by 703, divide by height in inches, then divide again by height in inches. Or, use your weight in kilograms divided by height in meters squared (kg/m^2).

Health-care professionals use the following established percentile cutoff points to identify underweight and overweight children.

BMI-FOR-AGE AND PERCENTILES

Underweight   BMI-for-age less than or equal to 5th percentile
At risk of overweight   BMI-for-age 85th percentile to less than 95th percentile
Overweight   BMI-for-age greater than or equal to 95th percentile

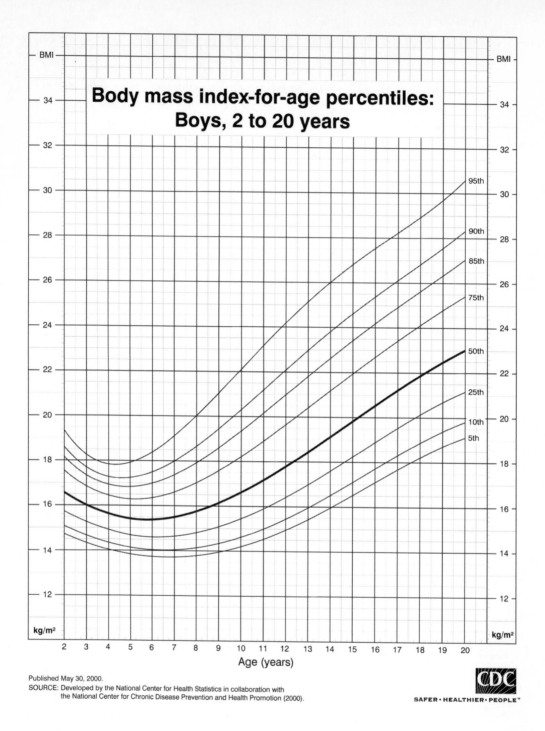

Body mass index-for-age percentiles: Boys, 2 to 20 years

BMI

95th
90th
85th
75th
50th
25th
10th
5th

kg/m²

Age (years)

Published May 30, 2000.
SOURCE: Developed by the National Center for Health Statistics in collaboration with the National Center for Chronic Disease Prevention and Health Promotion (2000).

CDC
SAFER · HEALTHIER · PEOPLE™

Source: CDC Growth Charts: United States. Developed by the National Center for Health Statistics in collaboration with the National Center for Chronic Disease and Prevention and Health Promotion (2002).

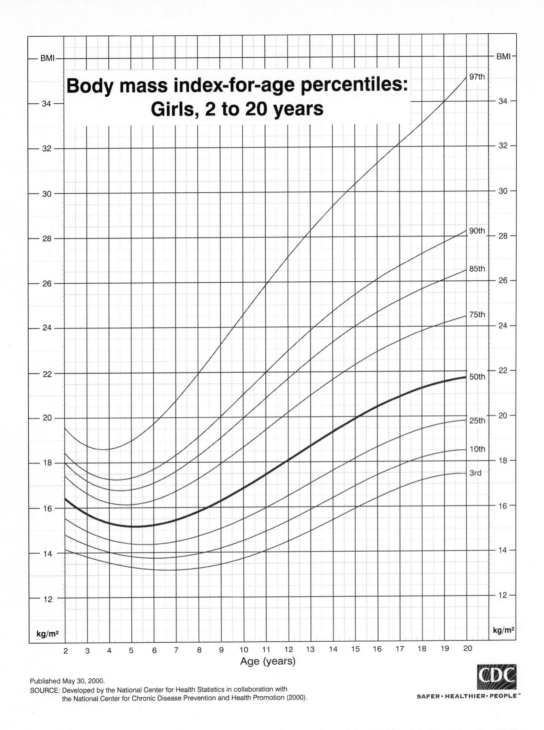

Body mass index-for-age percentiles:
Girls, 2 to 20 years

Published May 30, 2000.
SOURCE: Developed by the National Center for Health Statistics in collaboration with
the National Center for Chronic Disease Prevention and Health Promotion (2000).

Source: CDC Growth Charts: United States. Developed by the National Center for Health Statistics in collaboration with the National Center for Chronic Disease and Prevention and Health Promotion (2002).

Dietary Reference Intakes:
Selected Vitamins and Elements

Life Stage	Folate	Niacin	Pantothenic Acid	Riboflavin	Thiamin	Vit A	Vit B6	Vit B12
	µg/d	mg/d	mg/d	mg/d	mg/d	µg/d	mg/d	µg/d
Infants (mos)								
0-6	65*	2*	1.7*	0.3*	0.2*	400*	0.1*	0.4*
7-12	80*	4*	1.8*	0.4*	0.3*	500*	0.3*	0.5*
Child (y)								
1-3	150•	6•	2*	0.5•	0.5•	300•	0.5•	0.9•
4-8	200•	8•	3*	0.6•	0.6•	400•	0.6•	1.2•
Males (y)								
9-13	300•	12•	4*	0.9•	0.9•	600•	1.0•	1.8•
14-18	400•	16•	5*	1.3•	1.2•	900•	1.3•	2.4•
19-30	400•	16•	5*	1.3•	1.2•	900•	1.3•	2.4•
31-50	400•	16•	5*	1.3•	1.2•	900•	1.3•	2.4•
50-70	400•	16•	5*	1.3•	1.2•	900•	1.7•	2.4•
>70	400•	16•	5*	1.3•	1.2•	900•	1.7•	2.4•
Females (y)								
9-13	300•	12•	4*	0.9•	0.9•	600•	1.0•	1.8•
14-18	400•	14•	5*	1.0•	1.0•	700•	1.2•	2.4•
19-30	400•	14•	5*	1.1•	1.1•	700•	1.3•	2.4•
31-50	400•	14•	5*	1.1•	1.1•	700•	1.3•	2.4•
50-70	400•	14•	5*	1.1•	1.1•	700•	1.5•	2.4•
>70	400•	14•	5*	1.1•	1.1•	700•	1.5•	2.4•
Pregnancy (y)								
≤18	600•	18•	6*	1.4•	1.4•	750•	1.9•	2.6•
19-30	600•	18•	6*	1.4•	1.4•	770•	1.9•	2.6•
31-50	600•	18•	6*	1.4•	1.4•	770•	1.9•	2.6•
Lactation (y)								
≤18	500•	17•	7*	1.6•	1.4•	1,200•	2.0•	2.8•
19-30	500•	17•	7*	1.6•	1.4•	1,300•	2.0•	2.8•
31-50	500•	17•	7*	1.6•	1.4•	1,300•	2.0•	2.8•

Vit=Vitamin; Ca=Calcium; Mg=Magnesium; Mn=Manganese; Phos=Phosphorus; Se=Selenium; mos=months; y=years

The * represents Recommended Dietary Allowances (RDAs). The • represents Adequate Intakes (AIs).

Sources: *Dietary Reference Intakes for Calcium, Phosphorous, Magnesium, Vitamin D, and Fluoride* (1997); *Dietary Reference Intakes for Thiamin, Riboflavin, Niacin, Vitamin B6, Folate, Vitamin B12, Pantothenic Acid, Biotin, and Choline* (1998); *Dietary Reference Intakes for Vitamin C, Vitamin E, Selenium, and Carotenoids* (2000); and *Dietary Reference Intakes for Vitamin A, Vitamin K, Arsenic, Boron, Chromium, Copper, Iodine, Iron, Manganese, Molybdenum, Nickel, Silicon, Vanadium, and Zinc* (2001). These reports may be accessed via www.nap.edu.

The table is adapted from the DRI reports.

Vit C	Vit D	Vit E	Vit K	Ca	Iron	Mg	Mn	Phos	Se	Zinc
mg/d	µg/d	mg/d	µg/d	mg/d	mg/d	mg/d	mg/d	mg/d	µg/d	mg/d
40*	5*	4*	2.0*	210*	0.27*	30*	0.003*	100*	15*	2*
50*	5*	5*	2.5*	270*	11*	75*	0.6*	275*	20*	3
15*	5*	6*	30*	500*	7*	80*	1.2*	460*	20*	3*
25*	5*	7*	55*	800*	10*	130*	1.5*	500*	30*	5*
45*	5*	11*	60*	1,300*	8*	240*	1.9*	1,250*	40*	8*
75*	5*	15*	75*	1,300*	11*	410*	2.2*	1,250*	55*	11*
90*	5*	15*	120*	1,000*	8*	400*	2.3*	700*	55*	11*
90*	5*	15*	120*	1,000*	8*	420*	2.3*	700*	55*	11*
90*	10*	15*	120*	1,200*	8*	420*	2.3*	700*	55*	11*
90*	15*	15*	120*	1,200*	8*	420*	2.3*	700*	55*	11*
45*	5*	11*	60*	1,300*	8*	240*	1.6*	1,250*	40*	8*
65*	5*	15*	75*	1,300*	15*	360*	1.6*	1,250*	55*	9*
75*	5*	15*	90*	1,000*	18*	310*	1.8*	700*	55*	8*
75*	5*	15*	90*	1,000*	18*	320*	1.8*	700*	55*	8*
75*	10*	15*	90*	1,200*	8*	320*	1.8*	700*	55*	8*
75*	15*	15*	90*	1,200*	8*	320*	1.8*	700*	55*	8*
80*	5*	15*	75*	1,300*	27*	400*	2.0*	1,250*	60*	12*
85*	5*	15*	90*	1,000*	27*	350*	2.0*	700*	60*	11*
85*	5*	15*	90*	1,000*	27*	360*	2.0*	700*	60*	11*
115*	5*	19*	75*	1,300*	10*	360*	2.6*	1,250*	70*	13*
120*	5*	19*	90*	1,000*	9*	310*	2.6*	700*	70*	12*
120*	5*	19*	90*	1,000*	9*	320*	2.6*	700*	70*	12*

Definitions:
- Estimated Average Requirement (EAR): a nutrient intake value that is estimated to meet the requirement of half the healthy individuals in a group.
- Recommended Dietary Allowance (RDA): the average daily dietary intake level that is sufficient to meet the nutrient requirement of nearly all healthy individuals in a group. The process for setting the RDA depends on being able to set an EAR. The RDA is derived from the nutrient requirement so if an EAR cannot be set, no RDA will be set.
- Adequate Intake (AI): a value based on observed or experimentally determined approximations of nutrient intake by a group (or groups) of healthy people-used when an RDA cannot be determined. The main intended use of the AI is as a goal for the nutrient intake of individuals.

SOURCES

INTRODUCTION

Information on Cholesterol

American Heart Association
(adults and children)
National Center
7272 Greenville Avenue
Dallas, TX 75231
800-242-8721
www.amheart.org
Information for children:
www.americanheart.org/
presenter.jhtml?identifier=4499

Nemours Foundation
Kids Health
www.kidshealth.org

Mayo Clinic
www.mayohealth.org
www.mayoclinic.com

National Cholesterol Education Program
National Heart, Lung, and Blood Institute
National Institutes of Health (NIH)
8600 Rockville Pike
Bethesda, MD 20894
For web site information:
NHLBI Health Information Center: Attention
Web Site
P.O. Box 30105
Bethesda, MD 20824-0105
301-592-8573

www.nhlbi.nih.gov/guidelines/cholesterol
/index.htm
www.nlm.nih.gov/medlineplus/cholesterol.html

WebMDHealth
http://mywebmd.com

Institute of Medicine of the National Academies
500 Fifth Street, N.W.
Washington, D.C. 20001
202-334-2352
www.iom.edu

Information on Exercise

AARP (The American Association for Retired
Persons)
601 E Street, N.W.
Washington, D.C. 20049
888-687-2277
www.aarp.org

American Alliance for Health, Physical Education, Recreation, and Dance
1900 Association Drive
Reston, VA 20191
800-213-7193
info@aahperd.org
www.aahperd.org

American College of Sports Medicine
P.O. Box 1440
Indianapolis, IN 46206-1440
317-637-9200
www.acsm.org

American Council on Exercise
4851 Paramount Drive
San Diego, CA 92123
800-825-3636
www.acefitness.org

American Heart Association
National Center
7272 Greenville Avenue
Dallas, TX 75231
800-242-8721
www.amheart.org
Information for children:
www.americanheart.org/presenter.jhtml?identi-
    fier=4596
www.americanheart.org/presenter.jhtml?identi-
    fier=3007589

American Physical Therapy Association
1111 North Fairfax Street
Alexandria, VA 22314-1488
800-999-2782
www.apta.org

Centers for Disease Control and Prevention
Physical Activity for Everyone
1600 Clifton Road
Atlanta, GA 30333
800-639-3534; 404-639-3311
www.cdc.gov/nccdphp/dnpa/physical

Fifty Plus Lifelong Fitness
2483 East Bayshore Road
Suite 202
Palo Alto, CA 94303
650-843-1750
www.50plus.org

Nemours Foundation
Kids Health
www.kidshealth.org

The President's Council on Physical Fitness
Department W
200 Independence Avenue, S.W.
Room 738-H
Washington, D.C. 20201-0004
202-690-9000
www.fitness.gov

U.S. Department of Agriculture
My Pyramid
USDA Center for Nutrition Policy and Promotion
3101 Park Center Drive
Room 1034
Alexandria, VA 22302-1594
www.mypyramid.gov

Information on Weight Loss

Aim for a Healthy Weight
National Institutes of Health (NIH)
National Heart, Lung, and Blood Institute
8600 Rockville Pike
Bethesda, MD 20894
www.nhlbi.nih.gov/health/public/heart/obesity/
    lose_wt

American Heart Association
National Center
7272 Greenville Avenue
Dallas, TX 75231
1-800-242-8721
www.amheart.org
Information for children:
www.americanheart.org/presenter.jhtml?identi-
    fier=4670
www.americanheart.org/presenter.jhtml?identi-
    fier=3007590

American Obesity Association
1250 24th Street, N.W.
Suite 300
Washington, D.C. 20037
202-776-7711
www.obesity.org

National Center for Chronic Disease Prevention
    and Health Promotion
Nutrition and Physical Activity
Centers for Disease Control and Prevention
    (CDC)
4770 Buford Highway, NE, MS/K-24
Atlanta, GA 30341-3717
770-488-5820
www.cdc.gov/nccdphp/dnpa

Nemours Foundation
Kids Health
www.kidshealth.org

Nutrisystem
200 Welsh Road
Horsham, PA 19044
800-585-5483; 215-706-5300
www.nutrisystem.com

Overeaters Anonymous
World Service Office
P.O. Box 44020
Rio Rancho, NM 87174-4020
505-891-2664
www.oa.org

Smallsteps.gov
U.S. Department of Health and Human Services
200 Independence Avenue, S.W.
Washington, D.C. 20201
877-696-6775; 202-619-0257
www.smallstep.gov

WIN Weight Control Information Network
National Institute of Diabetes and Digestive
    and Kidney Diseases (NIDDK)
U.S. Department of Health and Human Services
National Institutes of Health (NIH)
1 WIN Way
Bethesda, MD 20892-3665
877-946-4627; 202-828-1025
www.win.niddk.nih.gov

Information to Help You Quit Smoking

American Cancer Society
1599 Clifton Road, N.E.
Atlanta, GA 30329
404-320-3333
www.cancer.org

American Heart Association
National Center
7272 Greenville Avenue
Dallas, TX 75231
800-242-8721
www.amheart.org

American Lung Association
1740 Broadway
14th Floor
New York, NY 10019
800-586-4872
www.lungusa.org

National Cancer Institute
800-422-6237
www.cancer.gov

Centers for Disease Control and Prevention
Office on Smoking and Health
www.cdc.gov/tobacco

Nicotine Anonymous
877-879-6422
www.nicotine-anonymous.org

Smokefree.gov
www.smokefree.gov

You Can Quit Smoking
www.surgeongeneral.gov/tobacco/conquits.htm

Information on Stress Management

American Heart Association
National Center
7272 Greenville Avenue
Dallas, TX 75231
800-242-8721
www.amheart.org/presenter.jhtml?identi-
    fier=360

Mayo Clinic
www.mayoclinic.com/invoke.cfm?id=SR00001

CHAPTER ONE: GREAT BEGINNINGS

Mail-order source for Froth au Lait
Froth au Lait, Inc.
2421 West 205th Street D106
Torrance, CA 90501
Phone: 310-212-5345
Fax: 310-212-5643
e-mail: sales@frothaulait.com
www.frothaulait.com

CHAPTER TWO: SOUPS

Source for the DASH Eating Plan
NHLB Health Information Center
P.O. Box 30105
Bethesda, MD 20824-0105
Phone: 310-592-8573
TTY: 301-629-3255
Fax: 301-592-8563
www.nhlbi.nih.gov/hbp/prevent/h_eating.htm

CHAPTER THREE:
SALADS, GRAINS, AND LEGUMES

Mail-order sources for whole grains and whole-
    grain flours
Arrowhead Mills, Inc.
The Hain Celestial Group
4600 Sleepytime Drive
Boulder, CO 80301
800-434-4246
www.arrowheadmills.com

Bob's Red Mill Natural Foods
5209 SE International Way
Milwaukie, OR 97222
800-349-2173
www.bobsredmill.com

Eden Foods, Inc.
701 Tecumseh Road
Clinton, MI 49236
888-441-3336
www.edenfoods.com

Hodgson Mill, Inc.
1203 W. Niccum Avenue
Effingham, IL 62401
800-347-0105
www.hodgsonmill.com

King Arthur Flour
135 Route 5 South
P.O. Box 1010
Norwich, VT 05055
802-649-3881
www.kingarthurflour.com

Lundberg Family Farms
5370 Church Street
Richvale, CA 95974
530-882-4551
www.lundberg.com

Westbrae Natural Foods
The Hain Celestial Group
4600 Sleepytime Drive
Boulder, CO 80301
800-434-4246
www.westbrae.com

Mail-order sources for nuts and seeds
Jaffee Bros. Natural Foods
28560 Lilac Road
Valley Center, CA 92082
760-749-1133
www.organicfruitsandnuts.com

Sun Ridge Farms
1055 17th Avenue
Santa Cruz, CA 95062-3033
831-462-1280
www.sunridgefarms.com

CHAPTER FOUR: VEGETABLE AND SOY DISHES

Sources for more information on soy
The American Soybean Association
12125 Woodcrest Executive Drive Suite 100
St. Louis, MS 63141
800-688-7692
www.amsoy.org
www.soygrowers.com

Soyfoods Association of North America (SANA)
1001 Connecticut Avenue, N.W., Suite 1120
Washington, D.C. 20036
202-659-3520
www.soyfoods.org

Soyatech
1369 State Highway 102
Bar Harbor, ME 04609
800-424-7692
www.soyatech.com

United Soybean Board
424 Second Avenue West
Seattle, WA 98119
800-825-5769
www.talksoy.com
www.soyfoods.com

Books and cookbooks on soy
Amazing Soy: A Complete Guide to Buying and Cooking This Nutritional Powerhouse, with 240 Recipes, Dana Jacobi, Morrow, New York 2001.

This Can't Be Tofu!: 75 Recipes to Cook Something You Never Thought You Would—and Love Every Bite, Deborah Madison, Broadway, New York, 2000.

The New Soy Cookbook: Tempting Recipes for Soybeans, Soy Milk, Tofu, Tempeh, Miso, and Soy Sauce, Lorna Sass, Chronicle, San Francisco, 1998.

The Whole Soy Cookbook, 175 Delicious, Nutritious, Easy-to-Prepare Recipes Featuring Tofu, Tempeh, and Various Forms of Nature's Healthiest Bean, Patricia Greenburg, Three Rivers Press, New York, 1998.

CHAPTER FIVE: FISH AND SHELLFISH

Mail-order sources for wild salmon
Ed's Kasilof Seafoods
P.O. Box 18
Kasilof, AK 99610
800-982-2377
www.kasilofseafoods.com

SalmonGram.Com
2773 Murphy Place
Bellingham, WA 98226
800-996-9980
www.salmongram.com

SeaBear Smokehouse
605 30th Street
P.O. Box 591
Anacortes, WA 98221
800-645-3474
www.seabear.com

Vital Choice Seafood
605 30th Street
Anacortes, WA 98221
800-608-4825
www.vitalchoice.com

Sources for information on wild salmon
www.wildsalmoncenter.org/faq.php
    (The Wild Salmon Center)
www.goldseal.ca/wildsalmon
    (Wild Salmon Spotlight)
www.asf.ca/overall/atlsalm.html
    (The Atlantic Salmon)
www.wdf.wa.gov (Washington Department of
    Fish and Wildlife)
www.sciencenews.org/articles/20010602/fob5.asp
    (Science News Online, "Salmon Hatcheries
    Can Deplete Wild Stocks")
www.sierraclub.org/e-files/wild_salmon.asp
    (Sierra Club, "When It Comes to Salmon, Buy
    Wild")
www.newsinfo.iu.edu/news/page/nor-
    mal/1225.html (Indiana University, Media
    Relations, "Farmed Salmon More Toxic than
    Wild Salmon, Study Finds; Eating Salmon
    May Pose Health Risks")

CHAPTER SEVEN: RED MEATS

Mail-order sources for buffalo meat
Broadleaf
5600 South Alameda Street
Suite 100
Vernon, CA 90058
800-336-3844
www.broadleafgame.com
(all cuts, including smoked buffalo)

Blackwing Meats
17618 Edwards Road
Antioch, IL 60002
800-326-7874
www.blackwing.com
(buffalo fillet, ground buffalo, and ground buf-
    falo patties)

Mail-order sources for ostrich
Blackwing Ostrich Meats, Inc.
17618 Edwards Road
Antioch, IL 60002
800-326-7874
www.blackwing.com

Broadleaf
5600 South Alameda Street
Suite 100
Vernon, CA 90058
800-336-3844
www.broadleafgame.com

Source for information on ostrich meat
American Ostrich Association
P.O. Box 163
Ranger, TX 76470
254-647-1645
www.ostriches.org

Mail-order sources for Piedmontese beef
Half Circle Ranch Organic Piedmontese Beef
15980 Rocky Mountain Road
Belgrade, MT 59714
406-388-0563
www.organicpiedmontesebeef.com

Montana Range All Natural Piedmontese Beef
P.O. Box 3094
Billings, MT 59103
888-251-1847
www.montanarange.com

Sources for information on Piedmontese beef
Piedmontese Association of the United States
343 Barrett Road
Elsberry, MO 63343-4137
Phone: 573-384-5685
Fax: 573-384-5567
www.pauscattle.org

North American Piedmontese Association Ser-
    vices
306-329-8600
www.piedmontese-napa.com

Mail-order sources for grass-fed beef
Note: Products are shipped frozen; grass-fed
    beef is not necessarily organic, so if you
    want an organic product, make sure you
    inquire before buying

American Grass Fed Beef
HC4 Box 253
Doniphan, MS 63935
866-255-5002
www.americangrassfedbeef.com
(organic grass-fed beef)

Organic Valley Beef
Highway 1
Moss Landing, CA 95039
888-674-2642
www.diamondorganics.com
(organic grass-fed beef and bison)

Slanker's Grass-Fed Meats
R.R. 2, Box 175
Powderly, TX 75473
866-752-6537; 903-732-4653
www.texasgrassfedbeef.com

U.S. Wellness Meats [formerly Grassland Beef]
R.R. 1, Box 20
Monticello, MS 63457-9704
877-383-0051
www.grasslandbeef.com
(grass-fed beef, lamb, bison, and free-range
   chicken)

Sources for information on grass-fed beef
www.eatwild.com (*Eat Wild: The Clearinghouse
   for Information about Pasture-Based Farming,* "Grass-Fed Basics")
www.foodrevolution.org/grassfedbeef.htm
   (*The Food Revolution: How Your Diet Can
   Help Save Your Life and the World,* "What
   about Grass-Fed Beef?")
www.alderspring.com/health_benefits/htmll
   (Alderspring Ranch, "Nutritional Benefits")
www.chetday.com/grassfedbeefsuppliertips.htm
   ("Ten Tips for Choosing a Grass-Fed Beef
   Supplier")

Introduction

What do the Numbers Mean?

1 *Journal of the American Medical Association*, "Implications of Recent Clinical Trials for the National Cholesterol Education Program Adult Treatment Panel III Guidelines," 2001, Volume 285, pages 2486–2497.

How Often Do I Need to Have My Cholesterol and My Children's Cholesterol Checked?

2 *Pediatrics*, "American Academy of Pediatrics, National Cholesterol Education Program: Report of the Expert Panel on Blood Cholesterol Levels in Children and Adolescents," 1992, Volume 89, pages 525–584.

Is a Low-Fat Diet Safe for Children?

3 American Heart Association [Internet]. 2005 [cited May 2005]. "Cholesterol and Atherosclerosis in Children." Available from: www.americanheart.org/presenter.jhtml?identifier=4499.

4 *Circulation*, "Nutrition and Children. A Statement for Healthcare Professionals from the Nutrition Committee, American Heart Association," E. A. Fisher, L. Van Horn, and H. C. McGill, Jr., May 6, 1997, Volume 95, pages 2332–33.

Is There An Ideal Diet For Losing Weight?

5 *Journal of the American Medical Association*, "Comparison of the Atkins, Ornish, Weight Watchers, and Zone Diets for Weight Loss and Heart Disease Risk Reduction: A Randomized Trial," M. L. Dansinger, J. A. Gleason, J. L. Griffith, H. P. Selker, and E. J. Schaefer, 2005, Volume 293, pages 293:43–53.

What is the Latest on Vitamins, Minerals, Antioxidants and Heart Health?

6 *Journal of the American College of Nutrition*, "The Effects of a Multivitamin/Mineral Supplement on Micronutrient Status, Antioxidant Capacity, and Cytokine Production in Healthy Older Adults Consuming a Fortified Diet," D. L. McCay, G. Perrone, H. Rasmussen, G. Dallal, W. Hartman, C. Guohua, R. L. Prior, R. Roubenoff, and J. B. Blumberg, 2002, Volume 19, pages 613–21.

7 *Annals of Internal Medicine*, "Effect of a Multivitamin and Mineral Supplement on Infection and Quality of Life," T. A. Barringer, J. K. Kirk, A. C. Sataniello, K. Long Foley, and R. Michletutte, 2003, Volume 138, pages 365–71.

8 *American Journal of Clinical Nutrition*, "Antioxidant Vitamins and Coronary Heart Disease Risk: A Pooled Analysis of 9 Cohorts," P. Knekt, J. Ritz, M. A. Pereira, E. J. O'Reilly, K. Augustsson, G. E. Fraser, U. Goldbourt, B. L. Heitmann, G. Hallmans, S. Lui, P. Pietinen, D. Spiegelman, J. Stevens, J. Virtamo, W. C. Willett, E. B. Rimm, A. Ascherio, December 2004, Volume 6, pages 1508–20.

9 *Journal of the American Medical Association*, "Effects of Long-Term Vitamin E Supplementation on Cardiovascular Events and Cancer: A Randomized Controlled Trial," L. E. Bosch, S. Yusuf, P. Sheridan, J. Pogue, J. M. Arnold, C. Ross, A. Arnold, P. Sleight, J. Probstfield, and G. R. Dagenais, HOPE and HOPE-TOO Trial Investigators, March 16, 2005, Volume 293(11), pages 1387–90.

Chapter One: Great Beginnings

Cholesterol-Busting Oats

1 FDA, U.S. Food and Drug Administration [Internet]. *FDA Consumer Magazine*: November–December 1998 [cited May 2005]. "Staking a Claim to Good Health: FDA and Science Stand Behind Health Claims on Foods," Paula Kurtzweil. Available from: http://vm.cfsan.fda.gov/~dms/fdhclm.html.

How Much Caffeine Is Okay?

2 Caffeine values for all coffees, teas, hot cocoa, caffeinated soft drinks, and energy drinks are from the following source: "Caffeine Content of Popular Drinks" [Internet]. Information compiled from the National Soft Drink Association, U.S. Food and Drug Administration (FDA), and Bunker and McWilliams, Pepsi [cited March 2005]. Available from: http://wilstar.com/caffeine.htm.

Caffeine values for Baker's chocolate, dark chocolate, milk chocolate, and chocolate-flavored syrup are from the following source. CERHR [Internet]. *Caffeine,* "Caffeine Levels in Foods and Drinks," August 18, 2003 [last updated October 2003; cited May 2005]. Available from http://cerhr.niehs.nih.gov/gen-pub/topics/caffeine-ccae.html.

Caffeine values for caffeinated water, Anacin, Midol, Excedrin, NoDoz, and over-the-counter diet pills are from the following source: *University of California, Berkeley Wellness Letter, The Newsletter of Nutrition, Fitness, and Self-Care,* "Not Just Coffee," June 2003, Volume 19, Issue 9, page 8.

The Benefits of Green and Black Teas

3 *Journal of Nutrition Biochemistry*, "A Review of Latest Research Findings on the Health Promotion Properties of Tea," C. J Dufresne and E. R. Farnworth, 2001, Volume 12 (7), pages 404–21.

Chapter Two: Soups

What Is PHO and Why Is It Bad for You?

1 Trans fatty acids are unsaturated fatty acids that contain at least one double bond in the trans configuration. The trans double bond configuration results in a greater bond angle than the cis configuration. This results in a more extended fatty acid carbon chain more similar to that of saturated fatty acids than that of cis unsaturated double bond containing fatty acids. Partial hydrogenation of polyunsaturated oils causes an increase in the trans fatty acid content and the hardening of fat. Foods containing hydrogenated oils tend to have a higher trans fatty acid content than those that do not contain hydrogenated oils.

This definition comes from the Institute of Medicine of the National Academies, *Letter Report on Dietary Reference Intakes for Trans Fatty Acids*. It has been posted as a pdf file on The National Academies web site at www.iom.edu/fnb. It is excerpted from the full report, *Dietary Reference Intakes for Energy, Carbohydrate, Fiber, Fat, Fatty Acids, Cholesterol, Protein, and Amino Acids*, 2002, National Academies Press, Washington, D.C.

Conjugated Linoleic Acid: A Natural Trans Fatty Acid

2 Institute of Medicine of the National Academies, *Letter Report on Dietary Reference Intakes for Trans Fatty Acids*, 2002, National Academies Press, Washington, D.C.

Lipids, "Conjugated Linoleic Acids: Are They Beneficial or Detrimental to Health?" W. J. Klaus, S. D. Heys, and D. Rotondo, 2004, Volume 43, pages 553–87.

High Calcium Intake from Dairy Products May Lower Blood Pressure

3 *American Journal of Clinical Nutrition,* "Effects on Blood Lipids of a Blood Pressure-Lowering Diet: The Dietary Approaches to Stop Hypertension (DASH) Trial," DASH Research Group, E. Obarzanek, F. M. Sacks, W. M. Vollmer, G. A. Bray, E. R. Miller 3rd, P. I. Lin, N. M. Karanja, M. M. Most-Windhauser, T. J. Moore, J. F. Swain, C.W. Bales, and M. A. Proschan, July 2001, Volume 74(10), pages 80–89.

New England Journal of Medicine, "Effects on Blood Pressure of Reduced Dietary Sodium and the Dietary Approaches to Stop Hypertension (DASH) Diet," DASH-Sodium Collaborative Research Group, F. M. Sacks, L. P. Svetkey, W. M. Vollmer, L. J. Appel, G. A. Bray, D. Harsha, E. Obarzanek, P. R. Conlin, E. R. Miller, 3rd, D.G. Simons-Morton, N. M. Karanja, and P. H. Lin, January 4, 2001, Volume 344 (1), pages 3–10.

How Much Calcium Do You Need?

4 Institute of Medicine of the National Academies, *Dietary Reference Intakes for Calcium, Phosphorous, Magnesium, Vitamin D and Fluoride,* Standing Committee on the Scientific Evaluation of Dietary Reference Intakes, Food and Nutrition Board, 1997, National Academies Press, Washington, D.C.

Chapter Three: Salads, Grains, and Legumes

Heart-Health Claim for Olive Oil

1 FDA, U.S. Food and Drug Administration [Internet]. FDA News [cited May 2005]. "FDA Allows Qualified Health Claim to Decrease Risk of Coronary Heart Disease." Available from: http://cfsan.fda.gov/~dms/qhcolive.html.

Go Nuts for Nuts

2 *University of California, Berkeley, Wellness Letter, The Newsletter of Nutrition, Fitness, and Self-Care,* "Nuts Are on a Roll," May 2003, Volume 19, Issue 8, page 1.

Healthy Seeds

3 *University of California, Berkeley, Wellness Letter, The Newsletter of Nutrition, Fitness, and Self-Care,* "Good Seeds," December 2002, Volume 19, Issue 3, page 3.

Chapter Four: Vegetable and Soy Dishes

Folic Acid for a Healthy Heart

1 American Heart Association [Internet]. 2005 [cited May 2005]. "Homocysteine, Folic Acid, and Cardiovascular Disease." Available from: www.americanheart.org/presenter.jhtml?identifier=4677.

2 *Chesapeake Dietetic Lines,* "How's Your Homocysteine?" Rebecca M. Smith, 2004, Volume 64(5)4.

Soy Power

3 A meta-analysis (basically an analysis of all the studies that have been done in an area to come up with an overall consensus) of soy studies revealed that an additional average daily intake of 40 grams of soy protein lowered cholesterol by an average of 9 percent, LDL cholesterol by 13 percent, and triglycerides by 11 percent.
   New England Journal of Medicine, "Meta-Analysis of the Effects of Soy Protein Intake on Serum Lipids," J. W. Anderson, B. M. Johnstone, M. E. Cook-Newell, et al., 1995, Volume 333, pages 276–82.

4 FDA, U.S. Food and Drug Administration [Internet]. *FDA Consumer Magazine,* May–June 2000 [cited May 2005]. "Soy: Health Claims for Soy Protein, Questions About Other Components," John Henkel. Available from: www.fda.gov/fdac/features/2000/300_soy.html.

5 The protein values for fresh green soybeans and soy yogurt are from Nutritionist Pro software. The value for soy nut butter is from the nutrition facts label on the I. M. Healthy Soy Nut Butter jar. All other protein values cited are from *FDA Consumer Magazine,* "Soy: Health Claims for Soy Protein, Questions about Other Components," by John Henkel, cited above.

Welcome to the World of Soy

6 *Whole Foods Catalog: A Complete Guide to Natural Foods,* Nava Atlas, A Fawcett Columbine Book, Ballantine Books, New York, 1988.
   Amazing Soy: A Complete Guide to Buying and Cooking This Nutritional Powerhouse, with 240 Recipes, Dana Jacobi, William Morrow, New York, 2001.

Soluble Fiber Reduces LDL Cholesterol

7 *Expert Opinion Pharmacotherapy,* "Pharmacotherapy of Dyslipidemia-Current Therapies and Future Agents," H. Bays and E. A. Stein, 2003, Volume 4 (11), pages 1901–38.

8 FDA, U.S. Food and Drug Administration [Internet]. *FDA Consumer,* November–December 1998 [cited May 2005]. "Staking a Claim to Good Health: FDA and Science Stand Behind Health Claims on Foods," Paula Kurtzweil. Available from: http://vm.cfsan.fda.gov/~dms/fdhclm.html.

9 A meta-analysis (basically is an analysis of all the studies that have been done in an area to come up with an overall consensus) demonstrated that the consumption of psyllium-enriched cereal in addition to a low-fat diet modestly improved LDL cholesterol compared to a low-fat diet alone.
   Journal of Nutrition, "Psyllium-Enriched Cereals Lower Blood Total Cholesterol and LDL Cholesterol, but Not HDL Cholesterol, in Hypercholesterolemic Adults; Results of a Meta-Analysis," B. H. Olson, S. M. Anderson, M. P. Becker, et. al., 1997, Volume 127(10), pages 1973–80.

High Calcium Intake from Dairy Sources Boosts Weight Loss

10 *Nutrition Reviews,* "Dietary Calcium and Dairy Modulation of Adiposity and Obesity Risk," M. B. Zemel and S.L. Miller, 2004, Volume 62(4), pages 125–31.

11 A recent study group looked at this data and confirmed that calcium-rich diets accelerate fat loss. There were three groups of obese patients: The control group received a low-calcium diet, with 400–500 milligrams of calcium per day. A second group, the high-calcium group, received a regular diet, with 800 milligrams of calcium supplements per day. A third group, the high-dairy group, received three to four servings of low-fat dairy products per day with a total calcium intake of 1,200 to 1,300 milligrams per day. The control group lost 5.4 percent body weight. The high-calcium group lost a bit more, and the high-dairy group lost 10.9 percent body weight.

Obesity Research, "Dietary Calcium and Dairy Products Accelerate Weight and Fat Loss during Energy Restriction in Obese Adults," M. B. Zemel, W. Thompson, A. Milstead, et al., 2004.

Preventing Osteoporosis

12 FDA, U.S. Food and Drug Administration [Internet]. FDA *Consumer Magazine*, September–October 2002 [cited May 2005]. "Osteoporosis and Men," Carol Lewis. Available from: www.fda.gov/fdac/features/2002/502_men.html.

13 National Osteoporosis Foundation [Internet]. 2004 [cited May 2005]. "Osteoporosis in Men." Available from: www.nof.org/men.

Chapter Five: Fish and Shellfish

What Are Omega-3 Fatty Acids and Why Are They Good For You?

1 FDA, U.S. Food and Drug Administration [Internet]. *Center for Food Safety and Applied Nutrition/Office of Nutritional Products, Labeling, and Dietary Supplements,* September 8, 2004 [cited May 2005]. "Questions and Answers: Qualified Health Claim for Omega-3 Fatty Acids, Eicosapentaenoic Acid (EPA), and Docosahexaenoic Acid (DHA)." Available from: www.cfsan.fda.gov/~dms/labo3qa.html.

2 FDA, U.S. Food and Drug Administration [Internet]. *FDA News,* September 8, 2004 [cited May 2005]. "FDA Announces Qualified Health Claims for Omega-3 Fatty Acids." Available from: www.fda.gov/bbs/topics/news/2004/NEW01115.html.

3 American Heart Association [Internet]. 2004 [cited May 2005]. "Fish and Omega-3 Fatty Acids." Available from: www.americanheart.org/presenter.jhtml?identifier=4632.

Eat Seafood Twice a Week

4 American Heart Association [Internet]. 2004 [cited May 2005]. "Fish and Omega-3 Fatty Acids." Available from: www.americanheart.org/presenter.jhtml?identifier=4632

American Heart Association Recommendations for Omega-3 Fatty Acid intake

5 American Heart Association [Internet]. 2004 [cited November 2004]. "Fish and Omega-3 Fatty Acids." Available from: www.americanheart.org/presenter.jhtml?identifier=4632

Omega-3 Supplement Warning

6 FDA, U.S. Food and Drug Administration [Internet]. *FDA News,* September 8, 2004 [cited May 2005]. "FDA Announces Qualified Health Claims for Omega-3 Fatty Acids." Available from: www.fda.gov/bbs/topics/news/2004/NEW01115.html.

Omega-3 Sources

7 *Circulation* [Internet]. 2002 [cited May 2005]. "Fish Consumption, Fish Oil, Omega-3 Fatty Acids, and Cardiovascular Disease," Penny M. Kris-Etherton, William S. Harris, and Lawrence J. Appel, Volume 106, page 2747. Available from: www.circ.ahajournals.org/cgi/content/full/106/21\2747/TBL3.

Mercury Levels and Fish Consumption: Warnings for Women and Children

8 EPA, U.S. Environmental Protection Agency [Internet]. *Fish Advisories, Consumption Advice, Joint Federal Advisory for Mercury in Fish,* "What You Need to Know about Mercury in Fish and Shellfish," [last updated March 16, 2005; cited May 2005]. Available from: www.epa.gov/waterscience/fishadvice/advice/html.

How to Buy and Cook Fish and Shellfish

9 *Seafood Twice a Week,* Evie Hansen and Cindy Snyder, National Seafood Educators, 1997, Richmond Beach, Washington.

What about Shellfish?

10 Yale-New Haven Hospital [Internet]. *Nutrition Advisor,* "Shellfish and Cholesterol" [last updated March 10, 2005; cited May 2005]. Available from: www.ynhh.org/online/nutrition/advisor/shellfish.html.

Choose Wild Salmon over Farm-Raised

11 Sierra Club [Internet]. "When It Comes to Salmon, Buy Wild," [cited May 2005]. Available from: www.sierraclub.org/e-files/wild_salmon.asp.

12 *Science News On Line* [Internet]. "Salmon Hatcheries Can Deplete Wild Stocks," June 2, 2001 [cited November 2004]. Available from: www.sciencenews.org/articles/20010602/fob5.asp.

Chapter Six: White Meats

Tips for Choosing Healthy Margarines

1 An intake of 2 to 3 grams per day of plant phytostanols dissolved in fat products (i.e., Benecol) has been shown to significantly lower LDL cholesterol blood levels by approximately 10 percent to 15 percent, which can be achieved by consuming 1 to 1.5 tablespoons of phytostanol-enriched margarine each day.

   Current Opinion in Lipidology, "Regulation of Cholesterol Metabolism by Dietary Plant Sterols," T. A. Mieltinen and H. Gylling, 1999, Volume 10, pages 9–14.

Selecting, Storing, and Cooking Poultry

2 Mayo Clinic [Internet]. *Food and Nutrition Center,* "Poultry, Meat, and Seafood: Pros of Protein," Mayo Clinic Staff [last updated June 18, 2003; cited May 2005]. Available from: www.mayoclinic.com; type the name of the article in the search box.

Well-Done Temperature Guide for Meat and Poultry

3 Excerpt from *U.S. Department of Agriculture and Garden Bulletin,* Number 248, August 1995.

4 The source for the ostrich cooking temperature is the American Ostrich Association. "Because of its low fat content, ostrich cooks faster than other meat products. Steaks and whole muscles should be cooked medium rare to medium (140 to 160 degrees F). Cooking ostrich to well done is not recommended."

   American Ostrich Association [Internet]. "About Ostrich Meat," 2004 [cited May 2005]. Available from: www.ostriches.org/AboutOstrichMeat.html.

Chapter Seven: Red Meats

Cardiac-Friendly Beef: Piedmontese!

1 The nutritional values for Piedmontese beef are taken from a composite average of ten Piedmontese cuts compiled by Warren Analytical Laboratory, 1997. The nutritional values for conventional beef are from the U.S. Department of Agriculture (USDA) Handbook #8.

  Piedmontese Nutrition [Internet]. 1998 [cited May 2005]. "Piedmontese Compared to Other Cuts." Available from: www.beefalobeef.com/piednutrition.htm.

2 *Research Note:* To verify the nutritional values of conventional beef supplied by USDA Handbook #8, Nutritionist Pro software was used to calculate 4 cuts of beef (3.5 ounces each), including beef short loin, T-bone steak, Choice, separable lean and fat, ¼ inch fat, broiled; beef rib eye, steak, separable lean and fat, 0 trim, broiled; beef short loin, porterhouse steak, Choice, separable lean and fat, 0 fat, broiled; and beef chuck, blade steak, separable lean and fat, 0 trim, braised. The average values for these four cuts of beef were fairly similar to the USDA values. The Nutritionist Pro values were: 286 calories; total fat, 19.5 grams; saturated fat, 7.6 grams; protein: 25 grams; and cholesterol, 71 milligrams.

3 Piedmontese Association of the U.S. (PAUS) [Internet]. "Welcome to PAUS" and "Breed Origins," 2001–2004 [cited May 2005]. Available from: http://pauscattle.org/breed/history.html.

Grass-Fed versus Grain-Fed Beef

4 *University of California, Berkeley, Wellness Letter, The Newsletter of Nutrition, Fitness, and Self-Care,* "Beef—Back to the Future," February 2003, Volume 19, Issue 5.

5 *Eat Wild: The Clearinghouse for Information about Pasture-Based Farming* [Internet]. "Health Benefits of Grass-Fed Products," 2002–2004 [cited May 2005]. Available from: www.eatwild.com/nutrition.html.

  Some references used for the above article that pertain to this text box include:

  Journal of American Medical Association, "Dietary Intake and Cell Membrane Levels of Long Chain n-3 Polyunsaturated Fatty Acids and the Risk of Primary Cardiac Arrest," T. E. Raghunathan, D.S. Siscovick, et al., 1995, Volume 274 (17), pages 1363–67.

  Dairy Science, "Conjugated Linolenic Acid Content of Milk from Cows Fed Different Diets," G. R. Anand, T. R. Dhiman, et al., 1999, Volume 82 (10), pages 2146–56.

  Cancer, "Conjugated Linoleic Acid. A powerful Anti-Carcinogen from Animal Fat Sources," C. Ip, J. A. Scimeca, et al., 1994, Volume 74 (3 supplements), pages 1050–54.

6 *Eat Wild: The Clearinghouse for Information about Pasture-Based Farming* [Internet]. "Eating Grass-Fed Beef Lowers Your Risk of E. Coli Infection" [cited May 2005]. Available from: www.eatwild.com/nutrition.html.

  Reference for the above article: *Microbes Infect,* "Potential Effect of Cattle Diets on the Transmission of Escherichia Coli to Humans," F. Diez-Gonzalez, N. Jarvis, and J. B. Russell, 2000, Volume 2, Number 1, pages 45–53.

7 *Eat Wild: The Clearinghouse for Information about Pasture-Based Farming* [Internet]. "How Much Garbage Is Being Fed to Our Livestock?" [cited May 2005]. Available from: www.eatwild.com/nutrition.html.

8 *University of California, Berkeley, Wellness Letter, The Newsletter of Nutrition, Fitness, and Self-Care,* "Beef—Back to the Future," February 2003, Volume 19, Issue 5.

9 *Eat Wild: The Clearinghouse for Information about Pasture-Based Farming,* [Internet]. "Grass-Fed Basics," 2002–2004 [cited May 2005]. Available from: www.eatwild.com/nutrition.html.

Red Wine and Resveratrol

10 *Circulation,* "Alcohol and Heart Disease," Thomas A. Pearson, 1996:94, pages 3023–25.

Have You Tried Ostrich Lately?

11 from: www.ostriches.org/AboutOstrichMeat.html.

Chapter Eight: Desserts and Snacks

Whole-Grain Flours

1 *The Whole Foods Catalog: A Complete Guide to Natural Foods,* Nava Atlas, Fawcett Columbine, Ballantine Books, New York, 1988, pages 91–105.

Appendixes

Determine Your Body Mass Index

1 American Heart Association [Internet]. 2005 [cited May 2005]. "Body Composition Tests." Available from: www.americanheart.org/presenter.jhtml?identifier=4489.

Body Mass Index for Children and Teens

2 Centers for Disease Control and Prevention, Department of Health and Human Services [Internet]. 2005 [cited May 2005]. "BMI for Children and Teens, BMI Is Used Differently with Children than It Is with Adults." Available from: www.cdc.govv/nccdphp/dnpa/bmi/bmi-for-age.htm.

ACKNOWLEDGMENTS

FROM CATHERINE JONES

*M*y **deepest appreciation** goes to Elaine Trujillo for helping me give our readers the latest heart-health information in the most understandable way. Her contribution to this book makes the world a healthier place for us all. Lynn Rudolf, a friend and caterer in Bethesda, Maryland, and Christian Zagler, an Austrian friend and cook, helped me create and test the recipes. Ria Garcia and her family were my faithful critics—they tasted almost all of the dishes and offered valuable comments and suggestions. Matthew Lore and Kylie Foxx at Marlowe & Company shared my vision of this book and helped me achieve it. I am sincerely grateful to Judith Sutton for her superb copyediting, and to my agent, Lisa Ekus, for her support.

My mother's heart attack in 2004 was the primary inspiration for *Eating for Lower Cholesterol.* My other motivation was my eight-year-old daughter, who was diagnosed with high cholesterol at an annual check-up. I thank her pediatrician, Dr. Guillermo Balfour, for his unparalleled care over the years, and for convincing me that a health-and-nutrition cookbook with information on high cholesterol in kids was desperately needed.

My family—Mary, my mom, and Bob Abernethy; Elizabeth Abernethy; Brandon and Mariana Grove; Jack and Hannah Grove; Paul and Martha Grove; and Mark Grove and Troy Queen—has always been my greatest source of strength and support. My sister-in-law, Dr. Catherine Johnsen, reviewed the medical information in the introduction and offered insightful suggestions, for which I am grateful. My husband, Paul, and children, Aleksandra and Hale, are the joys of my life. If I give them back half of what they give me, I am happy.

FROM ELAINE TRUJILLO

$\mathcal{W}$**hen Catherine Jones** asked me to coauthor *Eating for Lower Cholesterol*, I had no idea what an inspirational and rewarding endeavor it would be. I am grateful to her for giving me the opportunity to share my knowledge and the experience I have gained from all of my many patients over the years at the Cardiac Rehabilitation and EECP Center, Shady Grove Adventist Hospital. Their questions about eating, shopping, and cooking, and their concerns about heart-health, provided the groundwork for the material in this book.

I am grateful to my colleagues Barbara Courtney, Debbie Truxillo, Mike Payne, Matt Desmond, Jan Shuman, Gail Driskill, Judy Kibby, Nancy Moore, Erica Crum, and Sharon Anthanio at the Cardiac Rehabilitation and EECP Center for their encouragement. I am indebted to Malcom Robinson, Danny Jacobs, Stacy Bell, Patt Queen Samour, Maureen MacBurney, Linda Cashman, Karen Stone Moreland, and John Milner for being my mentors in the field of nutritional science and for their assistance through the years. I thank Susan Percival for her feedback on the Stay Balanced Pyramid.

A special thanks to my parents, Anthony and Clare Barbella, for a lifetime of love. I am grateful to my sister and best friend, Liz Renda, and her family for always being at my side. My brothers, Frank, Don, and Brian Barbella, and their wives and children have cheered me on. My mother-in-law, Lupita, is constantly inspiring me in the kitchen, and my father-in-law, Roberto, and my brothers-in-law, Toño, José, and Gustavo Trujillo and their families are forever encouraging.

I am deeply grateful to my husband, J. Roberto, for his unwavering support and confidence in me. My children, Danny and Jacquelyn, are my pride and joy, and I thank them for filling my life with purpose.

H

Haddock with Baby Spinach, Red Bell Peppers, and Basil Pesto, 149
Hain Celestial Group, The, 268
Half Circle Range Organic Piedmontese Beef, 269
halibut, Atlantic versus Greenland, 153
Halibut Steaks, Broiled Marinated, with Sun-Dried Tomato Sauce, 152–53
hardening of the arteries, 1
Harissa Sauce, 141
HDL cholesterol (good)
desirable levels, 2–4
estrogen and, 6
fats and, 14–15, 62, 63, 193
heart-healthy oils and, 116
moderate alcohol consumption and, 217
nuts and, 93
role of, 1–2
trans fats and, 14
heart attack symptoms, 16
heart disease
BMI and dying from, 13
from plaque, 1
predisposition starts in childhood, 221
risk factors, 5
from stress, 17
vitamin supplements and, 15
warnings signs, 6
in women, 6–7
heart-healthy eating
about, 8–12
breakfast, 25–26
desserts, 222–23
fish and shellfish, 147–48
meats, 177–78, 205–6
salads, whole grains, and legumes, 72–73
snacks, 223–24
soup, 52–53
vegetable and soy, 111–12
heart-healthy pantry, 20–23. *See also* shopping for heart-healthy foods
Hearts of Palm, Tomato, and Asparagus Salad, 94
Heart Truth Campaign, 7
Hearty Mixed Grain Pancakes, 47
hereditary factors, 5
high blood pressure (hypertension)
about, 5, 7–8
calcium for, 65

DASH diet for, 65
maximum sodium intake, 182
physical activity and, 16
High-Fiber Foods list, 103
high-sodium culprits, 187
Hodson Mill, Inc., 268
Hoisin Dressing, Quinoa with Chicken and, 108
homocysteine, 121
hot breakfast menus, 28
hot dogs, 220
Hummus, 90–92
hydrogenated oils. *See* trans fatty acids
hydrogenation process, 63
hypertension. *See* high blood pressure

I

iceberg lettuce, 80
infants
nonrestrictive diet for, 4
soy milk warning, 10
insoluble fiber, 111–12
Institute of Medicine of the National Academies, 272n1(Chpt. 2)
insulin resistance, 7

K

Kale with Black-Eyed Peas, Sautéed, 123
kasha, 106
Ketchup-Onion Sauce, 214
Kim Chee Salsa, 170, 171
King Arthur Flour, 268
Krispy Kreme donuts, 228

L

lactose intolerance, 145
Lamb Chops with Cilantro-Mint Salsa, 216–17
lasagna, 142–43
LDL cholesterol (bad)
arteries clogged by, 1
chocolate and, 254
desirable levels, 2–4
estrogen and, 6
fats and, 14–15, 61, 62, 150, 193
fiber and, 39, 111–12, 141
heart-healthy oils versus, 116
risk categories and goals, 256
risk factors related to, 4–5
soy products and, 129, 141

LDL cholesterol (bad) *(continued)*
　teas and, 50
　treatment for, 5–6
legumes. *See also* chickpeas; soybeans and
　soy products
　about, 72–73
　amount per serving, 257
　Bean, Mushroom, and Tofu Chili,
　　138–39
　Bean Salad, 83
　Black and White Gazpacho Salad, 105
　Black Bean Soup with Fresh Cilantro, 59
　Lentil Salad with Tomatoes and
　　Radishes, 79
　Lentil Soup with Brown Rice, 60
　Romaine Lettuce with Chickpeas, Feta,
　　and Lemon-Shallot Vinaigrette, 88
　Sautéed Kale with Black-Eyed Peas, 123
　Stay Balanced recommendation for, 10
　Sweet Potatoes with Black Beans and
　　Chili Dressing, Baked, 128
　Tomato and Great Northern Bean Salad
　　with Fresh Basil, 81
　Turkish-Style Red Lentil Soup with
　　Mint, 64
Lemon Chicken, Mexican-Style, 198–99
Lemon Glaze, 242–43
Lemon-Olive Oil Dressing, Coleslaw with,
　78
Lemon-Oregano Marinade, 152–53
Lemon-Shallot Vinaigrette, 88
Lentil Salad with Tomatoes and Radishes, 79
Lentil Soup, Turkish-Style Red, with Mint,
　64
Lentil Soup with Brown Rice, 60
linolenic acid
　about, 159
　alpha-linolenic acid, 93, 97, 150, 155,
　　157, 193
　conjugated linolenic acid, 63, 116, 211
lipid levels, high, 7
loose leaf lettuce, 80
low-fat dairy. *See* dairy products
low-fat diets, 4
Lundberg Family Farms, 268

M
margarine, shopping for, 193
marinades
　about, 148, 161, 183, 207
　for chicken fajitas, 188, 190

Lemon-Oregano Marinade, 152–53
　for tofu, 144–45
　for vegetables, 126–27
Mayo Clinic, 265
mayonnaise, shopping for, 82
McDonald's fast food restaurants, 45, 220,
　221
meats
　about buying, 21–22
　about dry rubs, 148, 161, 207
　amount per serving, 257
　Cajun Dry Rub, 168
　Curry Dry Rub, 218
　Stay Balanced recommendation for, 10
　temperature guide for cooking, 199
meats, red. *See also* beef
　about, 205–6, 269–70
　Buffalo Burgers with Onion-Ketchup
　　Sauce, 214
　Curried Ostrich Filets with Apple-
　　Onion Jam and Cucumber Salsa,
　　218–19
　Lamb Chops with Cilantro-Mint Salsa,
　　216–17
　Piedmontese beef, 205, 210–11, 276n7
meats, white. *See also* chicken and turkey;
　pork loin and pork tenderloin
　about, 177–78
　about veal, 195, 199
　comparison of fat and cholesterol in,
　　195
　Veal Chops with Fresh Marjoram Sauce
　　and Brown Rice, 197
meats you're better off without, 25, 187
medications
　grapefruit warning, 25, 30
　for lowering cholesterol, 5–6
　omega-3 fatty acid supplements and,
　　157
Mediterranean-Style Couscous Salad, 99
menopause, 5
mental symptoms of stress, 17
menus
　breakfast, 28–29
　Stay Balanced samples, 258–60
mercury levels in fish, 159, 167
Meringue Crust, 245
metabolic syndrome, 7, 16
methylmercury, 164, 167
Mexican-Style Lemon Chicken, 198–99
milk. *See* dairy products